Paediatric Exams

A Survival Guide

*To Chagit and Eden with all my love,
and my parents for their endless support.*

For Churchill Livingstone:

Commissioning Editor: Ellen Green
Project Development Manager: Janice Urquhart
Project Manager: Frances Affleck
Design direction: Erik Bigland/Judith Wright
Illustrated by: Peter Lamb

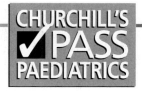

Paediatric Exams

A Survival Guide

Paul Gaon
MB BS MRCP(UK) MRCPCH
Trust Fellow in General Paediatrics, Great Ormond Street Hospital for Children, London, UK

Foreword by

Professor Anthony Milner
MD FRCP FRCPCH DCH
Professor of Neonatology, Guy's, King's and St Thomas' School of Medicine, London, UK

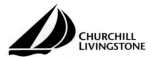

EDINBURGH LONDON NEW YORK PHILADELPHIA ST LOUIS SYDNEY TORONTO 2000

CHURCHILL LIVINGSTONE
An imprint of Harcourt Publishers Limited

© Harcourt Publishers Limited 2000

 is a registered trademark of Harcourt Publishers Limited

The right of Paul Gaon to be identified as author of this work has been asserted by him in accordance with the Copyright, Designs and Patents Act 1988.

All rights reserved. No part of this publication may be reproduced, stored in a retrieval system, or transmitted in any form by any means, electronic, mechanical, photocopying, recording or otherwise, without either the prior permission of the publishers (Harcourt Publishers Limited, Harcourt Place, 32 Jamestown Road, London NW1 7BY), or a licence permitting restricted copying in the United Kingdom issued by the Copyright Licensing Agency Ltd, 90 Tottenham Court Road, London, W1P 0LP UK.

First published 2000

ISBN 0 443 06272 2

British Library Cataloguing in Publication Data
A catalogue record for this book is available from the British Library.

Library of Congress Cataloging in Publication Data
A catalog record for this book is available from the Library of Congress.

Medical knowledge is constantly changing. As new information becomes available, changes in treatment, procedures, equipment and the use of drugs become necessary. The author and the publishers have, as far as it is possible, taken care to ensure that the information given in this text is accurate and up to date. However, readers are strongly advised to confirm that the information, especially with regard to drug usage, complies with current legislation and standards of practice.

The publisher's policy is to use **paper manufactured from sustainable forests**

Printed in China

Foreword

There is now a plethora of text books on how to pass the various parts of paediatric examinations including the MCQs, data interpretation and case histories. This begs the question as to whether there is a need for yet another book, bearing in mind the many texts on clinical paediatrics that are also available. To me, this book is special and fulfils a real need. Dr Gaon has distilled the knowledge that is required for a successful outcome in the Membership Part 2 examination in a form that is logical, readily available, and eminently readable. The majority of the chapters are system based and cover the basic physiology that is often needed for the viva, the presentation of clinical problems and their investigation and management. He also provides the clinical scenarios which are likely to be encountered. Finally, he provides excellent advice on how the clinical examination should be carried out to satisfy the Examiners. Although primarily designed for those planning to take the Part 2 Membership, this text will be of great value also for Part 1 and other paediatric examinations.

It is not surprising therefore that there is already a considerable waiting list of those who wish to borrow and read my pre-publication copy!

Professor Anthony Milner
Professor of Neonatology,
Guy's, King's and St Thomas' School of Medicine,
London, UK

Preface

Examinations pose necessary hurdles throughout your medical career. They aim to test knowledge and skills in the chosen specialty and are seen as an indicator that you are fit and ready for the next stage of clinical responsibility in professional life. This is certainly the case in paediatrics.

Paediatric examinations are demanding both because of the vast knowledge required at a relatively junior level, and secondly because they coincide with pressurised clinical responsibilities. Time now has to be rationed between demanding clinical and on call duties and examination revision. This is no easy task. It is with this in mind that the book was designed.

There are many paediatric textbooks on the market as well as an increasing number of examination orientated books. Unfortunately as is too often the case the larger general books will give an excellent basis of paediatric knowledge for clinical practice but will not prepare you adequately for examinations. You will need to determine what will be the most productive and economical use of your time. On the one hand, logic might tell you that a good wading through a large paediatric textbook would surely be enough to pass the exam. Colleagues who have taken the exams will tell you that this is a sure way to fail. On the other hand, others tell you that the only way to pass is to do lots and lots of questions. This might stand you in good stead for the written papers but you might slip up in the clinical when faced by clinicians of long standing who will easily find deficiencies in your knowledge. Clinical experience is of course essential but again time is limited. In fact there is no easy option and of course hard work will be required. Since textbooks can be vast I don't advise reading these from beginning to end. On the other hand, the increasing number of question and answer books on the market is growing rapidly and the task of reading through these *and* remembering the answers can be equally as awesome a task.

It is for these reasons that the idea of this book first came about. The wasted hours that I spent looking through books searching for information that was not to be found or found only in a fragmented fashion in several sources were innumerable. I thought that it would be a good idea to have most of the common relevant information in *one* place to save time searching through endless books for information that comes up time and again in the examinations. This book is not a complete textbook of paediatrics and was never meant to be. What it is intended is a collection of key points and methods that are essential for passing the written and clinical parts of paediatric examinations. Information that is readily available from textbooks is deliberately left out. Included is information that comes up frequently in the examinations and I have tried to pinpoint likely potential topics. I have included general rules on how to attempt the commonly asked questions, useful ways to approach complicated paediatric topics as well as tips for the clinical examination. I hope that having so many useful points in one reference guide will cut the revision time and effort significantly and reduce the frustrating wading through large textbooks and endless questions. I hope that this will as a result increase the confidence of the candidate sitting the examination.

To aid this, the book is divided up into systematic chapters which cover most topics. Each chapter includes the theory behind answering common data interpretation type questions and ways of tackling them. I have tried to emphasise the knowledge required to recognise the commonly asked clinical slides as well as being able to answer relevant questions. I have included sections on clinical scenarios which give the relevant background information needed to recognise and answer questions relating to the more greyer cases. I have also given disproportionate amounts of space to relatively rarer topics that come up commonly in the exam. I have also given more space to certain topics that are more complicated and not explained well in other texts. You will find some basic science topics included, since this area is becoming more popular as topics for discussion especially in the viva. In many chapters there are sections on radiology which I hope will be useful not only for slide questions but also in the clinical examination.

I have included easy to follow guides through the clinical examinations of the major systems, methods of interpreting the clinical findings and the all important presenting of findings to the examiners. I have attempted to present this in a clear and unambiguous way in order to give the candidate a smooth and professional examination technique. I have also included a chapter on the approach to the long case which will be useful independent of the nature of the long case with which you are confronted. A chapter is devoted to paediatric syndromes since you are expected to be familiar with many of these.

The information covered in this book will be useful for candidates taking the MRCPCH parts 1 and 2 as well as those taking the DCH. The book will be useful for paediatricians in training at all levels as well as medical students. The ideas in the book have been compiled from information from many texts, from advice from my many teachers including experienced MRCPCH examiners (to whom I am indebted) as well as ideas from numerous other sources including fellow registrars, and from my own experience of having gone through the exams myself. I hope that in writing this book I have achieved what I intended at the outset. That was to reduce the revision time and frustration for the candidate and also to provide useful knowledge and methods that will help in actually passing the examinations. Good luck!

Dr. Paul Gaon MB BS MRCP(UK) MRCPCH

Contents

1: **Genetics**	1
2: **Cardiology**	13
3: **Respiratory system**	37
4: **Nephrology**	67
5: **Neurology**	93
6: **Gastroenterology**	135
7. **Endocrinology**	169
8. **Haematology**	199
9. **Immunology**	235
10. **Metabolic diseases**	247
11. **Rheumatology**	271
12. **Dermatology**	287
13. **Vision and hearing**	305
14. **Paediatric syndromes**	317
15. **The long case**	333
Bibliography and recommended further reading	337
Index	339

Genetics

Genetics questions appear in the examination mainly as pedigrees in the data interpretation section. A broader knowledge of basic genetic issues is, however, expected and this reflects the general importance of this topic in paediatrics.

CLASSIFICATION OF CONGENITAL ABNORMALITIES

A common problem faced by paediatricians is the child with structural defects. A nomenclature has arisen to describe the genesis of such deformities.

— *Malformation:* A structural defect resulting from abnormal development.
— *Deformation:* This is where mechanical outside forces have altered the previously normal shape of body parts. Examples include oligohydramnios leading to pulmonary hypoplasia and talipes.
— *Disruption:* An extrinsic force alters a normal fetus usually by a destructive process (mechanical, vascular or infectious). Examples include amniotic bands leading to amputations and congenital rubella.
— *Sequence:* When a single error results in a chain or cascade of subsequent events resulting in a series of abnormalities. Examples include the posteriorly placed tongue in Pierre–Robin syndrome that results in micrognathia and a cleft palate.
— *Malformation syndrome:* This occurs when there are multiple structural defects present that cannot be explained by a sequence (see above). Examples of this are polydactyly and exomphalos. In a large number of cases the cause is not known. Other causes include genetic causes (single/multiple gene effect/chromosomal defects/multifactorial), teratogens such as viruses (leading to congenital infection), drugs, chemicals and irradiation.
— *Association:* This refers to cases where there are a number of malformations present that occur more often together than would be expected by chance alone, for example VATER/VACTERL and CHARGE syndromes (see chapter 14). In one-tenth of all infants with a congenital

malformation there will generally be another malformation associated with it. If you find one malformation, always look for others.

DEVELOPMENT AND TERATOGENESIS

The effect of a particular teratogen on the fetus will depend on the nature of the teratogen and the fetal age, in addition to other factors.

Weeks 1–3
Embryonic stage. At this stage teratogens act in an all or nothing fashion — either killing the fetus or not affecting it at all.

Weeks 3–10
Organogenesis. This is when organ systems are the most susceptible to damage.

Weeks 10–40
Fetal growth and maturation. At this stage unlikely to be teratogenic but may interfere with growth and physiological functioning of the normally formed fetal tissues and organ systems.

GENETIC PEDIGREES

Genetic pedigrees routinely come up in the data interpretation part of the examination and you should have a good system for dealing with these questions. A certain amount of assumed knowledge is expected here such as the theory behind the different types of inheritance (found in most paediatric textbooks).

You must know the commonly used symbols for genetic pedigrees (Fig. 1.1).

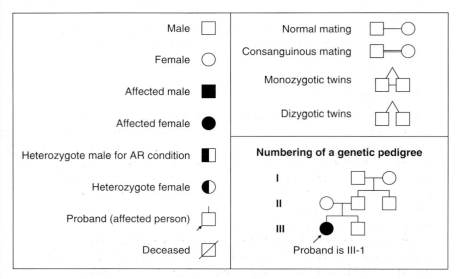

Fig. 1.1 A summary of the main symbols used in genetic pedigrees.

Essential genetic pedigree knowledge

Autosomal recessive (AR) conditions

— The affected individual has two heterozygote (carrier) parents. There is usually no antecedent history; the disease appears out of the blue.
— If both parents are heterozygotes then half the offspring will be carriers, a quarter will be affected and a quarter will be normal.
— The spontaneous mutation rate for recessive conditions is extremely rare.
— Autosomal recessive conditions and their genes are very rare but the same recessive genes are more likely to be present in the gene pool of families or smaller races that do not intermarry. Thus consanguinous relations are more likely to give rise to affected individuals. This is because heterozygotes for a particular condition are more likely to come in contact with each other producing the abnormality (homozygous individuals).
— The male:female (M:F) ratio is 1:1.

  Examples include: cystic fibrosis (carrier rate 1/25, one-quarter of children will be affected so that incidence in population is 1/2500), sickle cell disease, beta thalassaemia, most inborn errors of metabolism and spinal muscular atrophy.

Autosomal dominant (AD) inheritance

— The condition is inherited from one affected parent.
— Half of the offspring will be affected and half will be normal.
— The spontaneous mutation rate is relatively high (compared to autosomal recessive conditions).
— Male/female ratio is 1:1.
— Compared to AR disease AD disease displays a great deal of variation in expression.

  Examples include: hereditary spherocytosis, myotonic dystrophy, retinoblastoma, tuberose sclerosis, Friedreich ataxia and polycystic kidneys.

X-linked recessive conditions

— Males are affected. This is because the abnormal gene is on an X chromosome. Females have an extra X chromosome to protect them and therefore only become carriers, whereas males with only another 'empty' Y chromosome are affected. During cell division, however, a process that is called lyonisation can occur where there is a random inactivation of one of the X chromosomes in all the female cells, and thus some heterozygote females may have some of the features of the fully expressed X-linked condition. An example of this is haemophilia B where female heterozygotes may have prolonged clotting times. Another example is the raised creatine phosphokinase (CPK) levels found in heterozygote females in Duchenne muscular dystrophy.

The lyonisation process that results in an inactive X chromosome is also responsible for the Barr body seen in cells as a densely stained mass of chromatin within the nuclei (sample cells are most conveniently taken from a buccal smear). As a rule the number of Barr bodies seen will be one less than the total number of X chromosomes. Thus normal females will have one Barr body and girls with Turner syndrome will have none.

— A female carrier parent will result in half the male offspring being affected and half the female offspring being carriers.
— An affected male parent will result in all the female offspring being carriers and normal male offspring children since they inherit the normal Y chromosome from the father.

X-linked dominant conditions

These conditions are extremely rare. According to the pedigrees affected males will have affected daughters and normal sons (cf. AD inheritance). Affected females pass the condition to half of their offspring independent of their sex. Males pass the condition on to all their daughters and none of their sons. In practice a number of these conditions appear to be lethal to males (who may be stillborn) and thus only females are affected. You should know a couple of examples such as X-linked hypophosphataemic rickets and incontinentia pigmentii (lethal to males).

Useful rules in determining inheritance pattern in genetic pedigrees

1. Count the numbers of males and females affected and determine the M:F ratio.
   — If ratio is 1:1 then the condition is likely to be AR or AD. Smaller numbers of affected individuals will usually be present in a genetic pedigree of AR inheritance.
   — If females are affected more commonly than males think of X-linked dominant inheritance.
   — If no females are affected think of X-linked recessive inheritance.
2. If an affected male gives rise to an affected male think of AD inheritance (AR also possible but extremely rare). This is in contrast to X-linked dominant inheritance (affected males never give rise to an affected male). Sometimes it is difficult to distinguish between AD and X-linked dominant inheritance and therefore large pedigrees are necessary to demonstrate male to male transmission (and thus AD inheritance).
3. Remember that most individuals affected by AR conditions are usually sterile or die early.

Examples

In these examples (as is common in the examination) only affected individuals will be indicated (shaded in) and carriers will not be shown. Work through these examples (Fig. 1.2) using the rules above.

Example 1

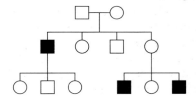

Fig. 1.2a This is an example of X-linked dominant inheritance. If asked for an example, say X-linked dominant hypophosphataemic rickets rather than incontinentia pigmentii since the latter is lethal to males.

Example 2

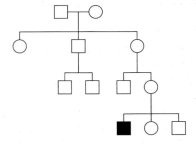

Fig. 1.2b This is an example of an X-linked recessive disorder.

Example 3

Fig. 1.2c This is an example of AR inheritance.

Example 4

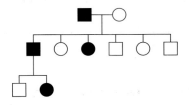

Fig. 1.2d This is an example of AD inheritance.

Another commonly asked question includes the following:

A couple come for genetic counselling about the risk that their child will have cystic fibrosis. The husband's sister has it, but the husband is not affected and there is no history in the wife's family of the disease.

Answer: Cystic fibrosis is inherited in an autosomal recessive condition. Therefore since the sister is affected, both the parents must be carriers. Since the brother is not affected there is a two-thirds chance that the brother is a carrier. We know that the carrier risk in the general population is 1/25. Thus we assume that that this is also the wife's risk of being a carrier.

Therefore the risk of their child being affected is 2/3 (father's risk of being a carrier) multiplied by 1/25 (mother's risk of being a carrier) multiplied by 1/4 (risk of child being affected with two carrier parents).

— You should know about the rare diseases that demonstrate mitochondrial inheritance. Here we see that some mitochondrial proteins are encoded for by the mitochondrial chromosome (rather than the nuclear genes). Since mitochondria are derived from the mother then these diseases demonstrate maternal inheritance. Male and female offspring are equally likely to develop the condition. Examples include MELAS and MERRF (see chapter 10).

CHROMOSOME ANALYSIS

This is another popular data interpretation question. In classic chromosomal analysis one finds that there are 23 pairs of chromosomes (22 autosomes and a pair of sex chromosomes). They are sorted by size, position of the centromere and banding pattern so that the autosomes are labelled from 1–22 and the sex chromosomes are called X and Y. In the top left hand side are the large chromosomes with median placed centromeres. As one passes from left to right the chromosomes become smaller in size and the centromere moves distally forming progressively more acrocentric chromosomes. The short arm of the chromosome is called the p arm and the long arm is called the q arm. An older nomenclature divided similar looking chromosomes into seven groups designated A–G + the sex chromosomes — Patau classification. Genetic testing is most conveniently carried out using peripheral blood lymphocytes but almost any tissue may be used. The chromosomes are arrested in metaphase and stained. In order to diagnose the problem you must label the chromosomes from 1–22 and the sex chromosomes.

Examples

Example 1

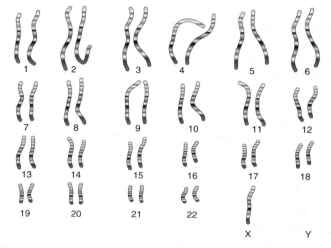

Fig. 1.3a If there is one lone X chromosome then the individual has Turner syndrome.

Example 2

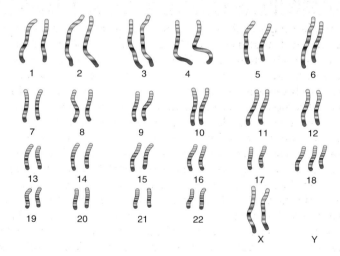

Fig. 1.3b If there is an extra chromosome at chromosome pair number 18 then the individual has Edward syndrome.

Example 3

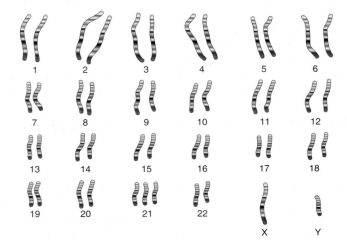

Fig. 1.3c This shows an extra chromosome at position 21. This is trisomy 21 (Down syndrome).

Example 4

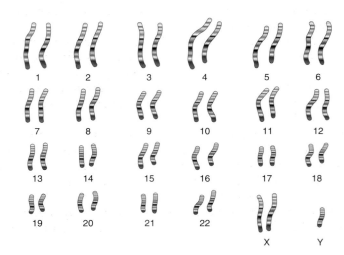

Fig. 1.3d If there is an extra X chromosome (in addition to the normal male X and Y) then the individual has Klinefelter syndrome.

CHROMOSOMAL NOMENCLATURE

You will be expected to express karyotypes in the conventional way (Paris nomenclature).

First you mention the total number of chromosomes, then you mention the sex chromosome constitution and finally the genetic abnormality.
Normal: 46 XX.
Turner syndrome: 45 XO.
Klinefelter syndrome: 47 XXY.
Cri du chat syndrome: 46 XY, del (p5).
46, XY, t(5;10)(p13;q25). This is a balanced translocation between chromosomes 5 and 10 at the break points indicated in brackets at the end.

SPECIFIC EXAMPLES OF GENETIC TOPICS

Down syndrome:

Since Down syndrome is so common you must know about its inheritance in detail. The typical phenotypic description is found in chapter 14.

The risk of Down syndrome and most chromosomal abnormalities increase with increasing maternal age (increasing the non-disjunction type of inheritance). At the maternal age of 20 the corresponding risk is 1:2000, at age 30 1:700, at age 40 1:100 and at age 45 1:50. Sixty per cent of first trimester spontaneous abortions are secondary to chromosomal abnormalities. This figure falls to about 0.5% of all live births.

Inheritance of Down syndrome

In 95–97% of cases the cause is non-disjunction during the first meiotic division. The result of this is an extra 21 chromosome in all body cells. The recurrence rate for non-disjunction is 1%.

In about 2–3% of cases a translocation is responsible for the condition. A translocation is the transfer of chromosomal material between two or more homologous chromosomes which is usually reciprocal in nature, that is an exchange of genetic material. In this case the total genetic material in the person is complete (in other words balanced, none having been lost).

A Robertsonian translocation describes the particular case when the long arms of two acrocentric chromosomes (chromosomes with centromeres close to one end: that is, chromosome numbers 13, 14, 15, 21 and 22) fuse at their centromeres. Since both chromosomes have fused the total complement of chromosomes will be 45; however since the total genetic make-up is unaltered (balanced) the person will be phenotypically normal. A balanced translocation carrier may give rise to chromosomally unbalanced offspring.

If a child has an unbalanced translocation giving rise to Down syndrome there is a 25% risk that the parent has a balanced Robertsonian translocation (most commonly between chromosomes 14 and 21) and a 75% risk that it is a de novo translocation. This is the reason why when a baby is born with Down syndrome secondary to a translocation, a karyotype of both parents is needed.

It is worthwhile working through an example of the paternal/maternal balanced Robertsonian translocation carrier. During gametogenesis five types of gametes can be formed. See Fig. 1.4.

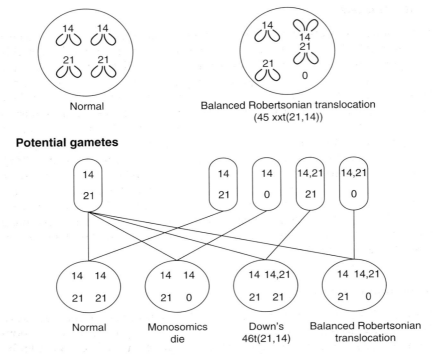

Fig. 1.4 A genetic description of how a Down syndrome translocation may occur.

You will see that the chances of a Down syndrome baby is 1:4 but the monosomy-21 fetuses abort so that the risk is actually 1:3. However a large number of Down syndrome babies abort naturally so the risk falls to 1:10 or 10% in mother carriers. The risk is 2% in carrier fathers (lower than in female carriers due to sperm immotility). It is impossible to distinguish between the non-disjunction type and translocation type solely on phenotype. The last possibility is mosaicism occurring in about 1% of cases: here some of the cells display trisomy 21 and others do not. Phenotypically these children are usually affected to a lesser degree, as compared to those derived from non-disjunction or translocation types.

Maternal serum alphafetoprotein

Know a little about maternal serum AFP. It is taken at about 16–18 weeks of pregnancy. High alpha fetoprotein levels are associated with neural tube defects (80% detection rate). It is also associated with multiple pregnancies, abdominal wall defects, Turner syndrome and intrauterine death. Low levels are associated with Down syndrome. In addition the triple test which uses two other maternal serum markers (hCG — high and unconjugated oestriol — low) has increased the detection rate to about 60% with about a 5% false positive rate (compared to 20% with serum AFP alone). The ratio gives the mother a risk (though not a certainty) of having a child with Down syndrome.

Cystic fibrosis

The genetic defect responsible for cystic fibrosis is located on chromosome 7 (q-long arm). It encodes for a membrane protein responsible for chloride transport called cystic fibrosis transmembrane regulator (CFTR). It functions via cAMP. The gene is large and many mutations (more than 200) have been described that result in the disease. The commonest mutation is a three base pair deletion (and subsequently a single amino acid deletion — phenylalanine) at position delta F508, occurring in about 70% of individuals in Europe and North America (however this prevalence varies with different racial groups for example Ashkenazi Jews — approximately 20%). Approximately two-thirds of individuals with cystic fibrosis appear to be homozygous and one-third heterozygous for the mutation. In the heterozygotes the delta F508 mutation will be paired with another mutant allele for the CFTR. Using genetic analysis via chorionic villus sampling (8–10 weeks) and amniocentesis (16–18 weeks) antenatal diagnosis is possible. See chapter 3.

Duchenne muscular dystrophy

The defective gene has been located to the X chromosome and it is very large indeed, accounting for 1% of its size. There is a very high ratio of intron (non-coding) regions to exon (coding) regions. The protein usually encoded for by this gene is called dystrophin and its deficiency results in the disease. Spontaneous mutations have been noted in about one-third of cases. DNA analysis detection techniques have enabled us to detect carriers and affected individuals thus allowing antenatal diagnosis. Males are affected, but because of lyonisation some of the muscle cells in carrier females will contain the abnormal allele and result in release of CPK resulting in levels outside the normal range in some female carriers.

Angelman syndrome and Prader–Willi syndrome

These two conditions have led to the concept of genomic imprinting (see chapter 14 for phenotypic descriptions). Genomic imprinting describes the influence of parental chromosome origin on the expression of a particular gene. Both Prader–Willi syndrome and Angelman syndrome may be the result of a deletion in the long arm of chromosome 15 (15q 11–13). If this chromosome is maternally derived then Angelman syndrome results, but if it is paternally derived then Prader–Willi results. It has been found that if both 15 chromosomes are derived from the mother then Prader–Willi phenotype will occur (and conversely if both derived from father then Angelman syndrome will occur). This is called uniparental disomy and it thus seems that the lack of a paternally derived 15 q 11–13 will result in the Prader–Willi phenotype (and the lack of a maternally derived 15 q 11–13 will result in Angelman syndrome). The description above describes about half the cases of Angelman and Prader–Willi syndromes and the remainder will have either normal karyotypes or other genetic abnormalities.

Fragile X syndrome

Fragile X is the most common inheritable type of mental retardation in males accounting for about 30% of the total number of cases. It also causes 10% of mild mental retardation in females (heterozygotes). A chromosome marker called the fragile X site can be seen at the end of the long arm of the X chromosome when the chromosomes are incubated in a folate deficient medium. The carrier frequency in females is about 1:1000. The fragile site is only a marker and not reliable in all cases and now the fragile X gene has been identified. It is an overamplified section of DNA with various lengths of CGG repeats. (See chapter 14 for phenotypic description).

Genetic anticipation

This describes the case where the severity of the inheritable disease increases with each subsequent generation. It has been noted that in a number of these conditions there is an increased frequency of trinucleotide repeats than one would normally expect. The diseases that demonstrate such anticipation include Huntington chorea, myotonic dystrophy and fragile X syndrome.

Cardiology

FETAL CARDIOVASCULAR PHYSIOLOGY

The 'basic science' nature of this topic — as well as the potential pathological implications in paediatric cardiology — make it a likely viva question.

Oxygenated blood from the placenta returns to the fetus via the umbilical vein (of which there is only one). Fifty per cent traverses the liver and the remaining 50% bypasses the liver via the ductus venosus into the inferior vena cava. In the right atrium blood arriving from the upper body from the superior vena cava (low oxygen saturation) preferentially crosses the tricuspid valve into the right ventricle and then via the ductus flows into the descending aorta and back to the placenta via the umbilical arteries (two) to reoxygenate. The relatively oxygenated blood from the inferior vena cava, however, preferentially crosses the foramen ovale into the left atrium and left ventricle to be distributed to the upper body (including the brain and coronary circulation). Because of this pattern of flow in the right atrium we have highly oxygenated blood reaching the brain and deoxygenated blood reaching the placenta. High pulmonary arteriolar pressure ensures that most blood traverses the pulmonary artery via the ductus.

Changes at birth

1. Occlusion of the umbilical cord removes the low-resistance capillary bed from the circulation.
2. Breathing results in a marked decrease in pulmonary vascular resistance.
3. In consequence, there is increased pulmonary blood flow returning to the left atrium causing the foramen ovale to close.
4. Well-oxygenated blood from the lungs and the loss of endogenous prostaglandins from the placenta results in closure of the ductus arteriosus.

CONGENITAL HEART DISEASE

You should know the approximate incidence of congenital heart disease which is approximately 8/1000 live births.

Ventricular septal defect — 30% Coarctation of the aorta — 6%
Patent ductus arteriosus — 8%   Aortic stenosis — 6%
Pulmonary stenosis — 8%   Transposition of the great vessels — 4%
Atrial septal defect — 8%   Atrioventricular septal defect — 4%
Tetralogy of Fallot — 6%

It is important to be familiar with what lesion is likely to present when, since this will be vital when answering a possible clinical scenario in the written or clinical examinations.

Cardiovascular lesion chronology

— *Within the first few hours:* pulmonary or aortic atresia/critical stenosis, hypoplastic left heart syndrome.
— *Within the first few days:* transposition of the great arteries, tetralogy of Fallot, hypoplastic left heart syndrome, patent ductus arteriosus (PDA) in small premature infants.
— *Within the first few weeks:* critical aortic stenosis, coarctation of the aorta.
— *Within the first few months:* any of the left to right (L–R) shunts (caused by falling pulmonary vascular resistance).

Presentation of congenital cardiovascular disease

A useful way at looking at congenital heart disease (CHD) and its presentation is to divide it up into three categories. These are of course simplifications but nevertheless useful.

1. **Those that are ductal dependent for pulmonary blood flow or mixing**
   Main presenting clinical feature is *cyanosis*.
   — *Decreased pulmonary blood flow:* pulmonary stenosis, pulmonary atresia –/+ventricular septal defect, Ebstein anomaly, tetralogy of Fallot, single ventricle or double outlet right ventricle with pulmonary stenosis.
   — *Increased pulmonary blood flow:* transposition without significant mixing.

2. **Those that are ductal dependent for systemic blood flow**
   Main presenting clinical features are those of *systemic hypoperfusion* (decreased peripheral perfusion, reduced urine output, metabolic acidosis). Remember that the important differential diagnosis of this type will be neonatal sepsis or a metabolic disorder.
   Examples: coarctation of the aorta, interruption of the aortic arch, critical aortic stenosis, hypoplastic left heart. There are of course non-ductal dependent cardiac causes of systemic hypoperfusion such as cardiomyopathy, myocarditis and supraventricular tachycardia (SVT).

3. **Those that are unlikely to be ductal dependent**
   The main presenting clinical feature will be *respiratory distress* and increased shadowing on the chest X-ray (CXR). Examples:
   — *Mixing lesion*: Total anomalous pulmonary venous drainage (TAPVD) with no obstruction and adequate foramen ovale, truncus arteriosus, single ventricle without pulmonary stenosis.

Table 2.1 Cardiac catheter

	Normal values	
	O₂ saturation	Pressure (mmHg)
Vena cava (VC)	75%	0–5
Right atrium (RA)	75%	m = 3
Right ventricle (RV)	75%	25/3
Pulmonary artery (PA)	75%	25/8
Left atrium (LA)	98%	m = 8
Left ventricle (LV)	98%	110/8
Aorta	98%	110/65

— *Right to left lesions*: patent ductus arteriosus, ventricular septal defect, atrioventricular canal defect.

CARDIAC CATHETER DATA

Cardiac catheter data is still a popular topic for the Part 2 examination. In order to attempt any of these questions it is of course vital to know the normal values of pressure and saturation in the various chambers of the heart and the major vessels (see Table 2.1)

— The way of attempting these types of questions is to follow the pressures and saturations around the heart (through the great vessels and chambers) systematically noting any deviations from the normal values (Table 2.1) and noting any unexpected step-ups or step-downs in saturation or pressure.

— In a left to right or right to left shunt the exact point of the step-up or step-down in oxygen saturation (in the right or left sides of the heart respectively) indicates the level of the shunt.

— A higher than expected pressure in a chamber or vessel can be explained by either a stenosis ahead of it, by a shunt such as a left to right shunt (towards the chamber or vessel) or simply by a backlog of pressure.

— A drop in pressure between a ventricle and an artery implies a stenosis in the artery.

— Equal ventricular pressures may be due to a large ventricular spetal defect (VSD), Eisenmenger syndrome, common arterial trunk and tetralogy of Fallot.

Let us now go through the lesions that are likely to come up in the examination.

1.

	O₂ saturation	Pressure
RA	88%	5
RV	87%	35/5
PA	87%	35/12
LA	97%	6
LV	97%	100/8
Aorta	97%	100/58

This is the result of an atrial septal defect. There is a rise in saturation going from the vena cava (not given!) to the right atrium. This can also be caused by TAPVD where blood from the pulmonary veins drain directly or indirectly into the right atrium. This is rarer and remember that this lesion can be cardiac, supracardiac or infracardiac, the latter type being associated with obstruction.

2.

	O_2 saturation	Pressure
SVC	75%	—
RA	75%	3
RV	75%	35/5
PA	88%	35/14
LA	95%	8
LV	95%	100/8
Aorta	95%	100/55

There is a step-up in saturation and pressure between the right ventricle and the pulmonary artery. This is an example of a patent ductus arteriosus (PDA).

3.

	O_2 saturation	Pressure
SVC	68%	—
IVC	64%	—
RA	72%	12/8
RV	84%	85/7
PA	85%	20/8
LA	98%	10/5
LV	91%	90/5
Aorta	88%	90/55

There is a step-up in oxygen saturation between the right atrium and right ventricle implying a left to right shunt at the level of the ventricles. The pressures also show a step-up at the same level. This is the pattern one would expect with a VSD. However, in addition to this we notice a step-down in pressure from the right ventricle to the pulmonary artery and this implies a stenosis. We also notice a desaturation as we pass through the left side of the heart and the low saturation in the systemic circulation (aorta). These additional features make the diagnosis tetralogy of Fallot.

4.

	O_2 saturation	Pressure
LA	98%	10/5
LV	98%	152/60
Aorta	98%	90/50

There is clearly a higher pressure than we would expect in the left ventricle for a paediatric patient and we also see a step-down in pressure between the left ventricle and the aorta implying that this is a coarctation of the aorta. The commonest site is just distal to the left subclavian artery.

5.

	O_2 saturation	Pressure
VC	30%	—
RA	32%	—

RV	32%	90/10
PA	92%	60/7
LA	93%	7
LV	94%	60/7
Aorta	35%	88/60

We can see here that the pressures and saturations in the pulmonary artery and aorta match those of the left ventricle and right ventricle respectively: that is, the reverse to what we would expect in practice. The diagnosis is transposition of the great arteries.

6.

	O_2 saturation	Pressure
RA	65%	—
RV	65%	90/10
PA	68%	100/60
LA	95%	—
LV	82%	100/12
Aorta	83%	100/55

Here we can see high pulmonary pressures which can be caused by large VSD or AV canal defects which if present for long periods result in irreversible pulmonary hypertension and reverse right to left shunting – Eisenmenger syndrome.

CYANOSIS AND THE HYPEROXIC TEST (NITROGEN WASHOUT TEST)

This is a common topic and you should be familiar with the theory. This is a useful test to help to distinguish between cardiac and respiratory disease causing cyanosis in a baby. An arterial blood gas is taken (preductal) and repeated after breathing 100% oxygen for 10–15 minutes. A PO_2 of less than 20 kPa (usually less than 10 kPa) is suggestive of a fixed right to left shunt (which implies a lesion in which there can be no increase in pulmonary blood flow or mixing of systemic and pulmonary circulations, for example tetralogy of Fallot) or severe pulmonary hypertension. A PaO_2 of more than 25–30 kPa definitely excludes it as the cause of cyanosis. In this case one would have to consider lung pathology, large left to right shunts causing pulmonary oedema and patients with mixing of their pulmonary and systemic circulations. Lung pathology is also more likely if there is a raised PCO_2 in the blood gas.

Remember the potential danger posed to the patient by the test if they are dependent on maintaining right to left mixing through a patent ductus arteriosus (PDA for example in critical pulmonary stenosis). The oxygen may stimulate the duct to close. Prostaglandin PGE1 should be available during the procedure.

Example
A baby is cyanosed. He is given 100% oxygen to breathe for 15 min. The following results are obtained.

FiO_2	PO_2	PCO_2
Air	7.8	5.2
100% O_2	17.1	5.7

This implies a right to left shunt type of congenital heart disease: the clinician would go down the cardiovascular route of investigation and treatment.

Remember that in addition to cardiac and respiratory causes of central cyanosis there may be other causes to consider: central depression including fits, polycythaemia and methaemoglobinaemia.

There are questions describing a well baby who appears cyanosed without obvious respiratory or cardiac disease and who has a normal hyperoxic test. Furthermore the blood remains a brownish colour after breathing oxygen. One must then think of methaemoglobinaemia as a cause and one would perform a methaemoglobin concentration and investigate a reason for it (see chapter 8 for details of methaemoglobinaemia).

You should know that cyanosis appears when arterial blood contains more than 5 g per cent of deoxygenated haemoglobin. In polycythaemia cyanosis is common because of the large amount of haemoglobin in the blood and rare in anaemia because it is difficult to produce sufficient amount of deoxygenated haemoglobin to produce cyanosis (even though tissue hypoxia is more likely in anaemia). Peripheral cyanosis can be the result of central cyanosis causes as well as reduced blood flow to the skin (e.g. vasoconstriction caused by the cold) because of oxygen extraction.

PAEDIATRIC ECGS

These come up frequently and you should be familiar with the general rules relating to paediatric ECGs and the common patterns. Approach this in a systematic way.

Normal axis

This will vary according to the age of the child. At birth between +60 to +180 (approx. +80 by 1 month of age), at 1 year +10 to +100 and at 10 years of age +30 to +90°.

P wave

- Remember that 1 mm on an ECG is equal to 0.04 seconds and 10 mm in amplitude equals 1 mv.
- P waves should always precede a QRS complex in sinus rhythm. Sinus arrhythmia is very common in children.
- P waves should be positive in 1,11 and aVF. P waves should be less than 2.5 mm.
- Right atrial hypertrophy/enlargement: P wave in lead 11 > 2.5 mm (P pulmonale).
- Left atrial hypertrophy/enlargement: bifid P wave (P mitrale) usually > 0.09 seconds.

PR interval

Measured from the start of the P wave until the start of the QRS complex. This is usually between three and five small squares (0.12 and 0.2 s). This will be reduced in Wolff–Parkinson–White syndrome and prolonged in first, second and third degree heart block.

QRS complex

- Look in turn at the duration, presence of Q waves, hypertrophy and QRS progression.
- Duration is normally up to three small squares (0.12 s). Abnormal Q waves are more than 4 mm deep. However Q waves can be normal in 11,111, aVF, V5 and V6. Abnormal Q waves can be seen in ischaemia and hypertrophic cardiomyopathy.
- There are criteria that you should know for the diagnosis of right and left ventricular hypertrophy:
   In right ventricular hypertrophy < 3/12: R wave in V1 > 15 mv at all ages.
   \> 3/12: R wave in V1 > 10 mv.
   In addition one would expect RAD > 180°.
- In left ventricular hypertrophy the R wave in V6 < 3/12 > 20 mv.
   \> 3/12 < 25 mv.

QRS progression

There is a gradual change from right ventricular dominance to left ventricular dominance as the child grows up; see Fig. 2.1.

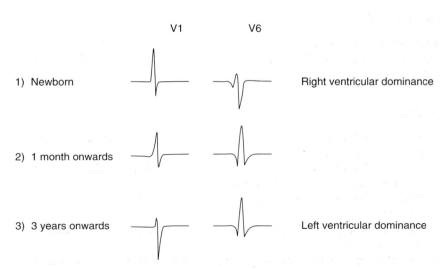

Fig. 2.1 QRS progression throughout childhood.

Any deviation from the normal patterns shown here away from that appropriate for the age towards (1) or (3) indicates either right or left ventricular hypertrophy respectively.

Bundle branch block is indicated by a prolongation of the QRS complex (> 0.12 seconds). In right BBB the rules of M pattern in V1 (RSR pattern) and W pattern in V6 (with slurred S wave) apply (**MarroW**). In LBBB there is a W pattern in V1 and M pattern in V6 (**WilliaM**).

QT interval

This is measured from the beginning of QRS complex to the end of the T wave, and is usually between 0.35–0.45 seconds. It varies with rate and you should therefore refer to QT tables in order to be accurate.

Increased in congenital long QT syndromes for example in Jervell–Lange–Nielson syndrome (associated with sensorineural deafness) and Romano–Ward syndrome is seen. These syndromes may be associated with sudden death. The QT interval may also be increased in hypocalcaemia, hypomagnesaemia, hypothermia, hypothyroidism, severe rheumatic carditis and with drugs such as amiodarone, quinidine and tricyclic antidepressants.

T waves

T waves are upright in V1 at birth. T waves in V1 then invert by the end of the first week. Then they become upright again by puberty. T waves are always upright in V6 and if they are inverted one must consider a myocarditis or possibly cardiomyopathy.

You must know the following patterns since they come up regularly: see Fig. 2.2 for some common examples.

Heart block

There is a prolonged PR interval (> 0.2 s). Called first degree if the P wave is always followed by a QRS complex and second degree if the P wave is not always followed by a QRS complex. This latter group is called Mobitz type 1 (Wenkebach) if the PR interval gradually increases in length until there is a dropped beat and Mobitz type 2 if there is a fixed PR interval where dropped beats are regular e.g. 2:1 or 3:1. This type is more likely to progress to CHB (and thus has a worse prognosis).

Third degree heart block (see CHB above) displays no relationship between P and QRS complexes and there is a ventricular rate of about 30/min. Neonatal CHB is associated with maternal SLE with anti-Ro antibodies and can also be associated with cardiac surgery. P waves are not conducted to the ventricles and there is a spontaneous escape rhythm (approximately 30/min). There may also be pacing spikes superimposed on the ECG. Clinically there may be a variable first heart sound and the presence of giant A waves (cannon waves) on the JVP (also seen in ventricular tachycardia and nodal tachycardia) as a result of atrial contraction against closed AV valves.

1. Atrial flutter with 4:1 block

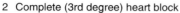

2. Complete (3rd degree) heart block

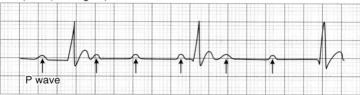

3. Dextrocardia

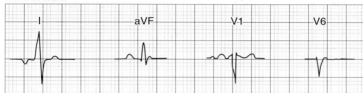

4. Wolff-Parkinson-White syndrome

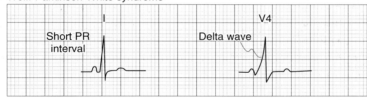

5. Atrial septal defect — ostium secundum with right axis deviation and incomplete right bundle branch block

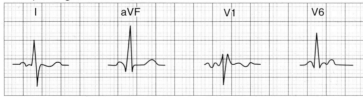

6. Miscellaneous

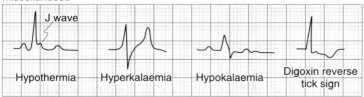

Fig. 2.2 Some common examples of paediatric ECG questions.

Right bundle branch block and left bundle branch block
Remember Marrow and William patterns. An incomplete bundle branch block occurs when the QRS complex is less than 0.12 s but features of Marrow and William (see above) are present.

Dextrocardia
Inverted P wave in lead 1, upright in aVF and loss of normal QRS progression as one goes from V1 to V6.

Wolff–Parkinson–White syndrome
Delta wave (slurred upstroke of the QRS complex) and shortened PR interval. Predisposes to paroxysmal SVT.

Atrial flutter and atrial fibrillation
In atrial flutter there is a saw tooth pattern with an atrial rate of approximately 300. There is usually a 2:1 block giving a ventricular response of 150/min. The degree of AV block can be increased with vagal manoeuvres. In atrial fibrillation there is chaotic atrial activity giving rise to an irregular ventricular response and therefore an irregular QRS interval and irregular baseline.

The commonest causes of these types of arrhythmias are post-surgical e.g. post-ASD repair, CHD e.g. Ebstein anomaly, disease resulting in dilated atria and myocarditis.

Left and right ventricular hypertrophy
Right ventricular hypertrophy is caused by L to R shunts (for example, VSD, ASD, PDA) right ventricular outflow tract obstruction (such as pulmonary atresia or stenosis) and cor pulmonale. Left ventricular hypertrophy is caused by left outflow tract obstruction (aortic stenosis or coarctation), ASD (ostium primum defect), VSD, PDA and tricuspid atresia.

Ventricular tachycardia
A wide complex regular tachycardia. A BBB with SVT is another cause of a broad complex tachycardia. They can be distinguished by: (a) the presence or absence of cannon waves (seen in VT); (b) the effect of carotid sinus massage (no effect in VT); (c) VT more likely in older patient with history of heart disease; (d) in BBB the QRS complexes look the same in SVT as when in normal rhythm whereas the old ECG in VT usually shows normal QRS complexes; (e) the rhythm in VT is very regular; (f) LAD is commoner in VT; (g) QRS >150 msec is more likely to be a result of VT; (h) evidence of AV dissociation-independent P waves, fusion or capture beats (in VT).

Left axis deviation in a neonate
This is found in (a) atrioventricular septal defect (b) tricuspid atresia and (c) pulmonary stenosis in Noonan syndrome.

ASD
— *Ostium primum*: Left axis deviation and right bundle branch block.
— *Ostium secundum*: Right axis deviation and right bundle branch block usually incomplete.

Hypothermia

Hypothermia can cause bradycardia: J waves seen as a hump on the descending limb of the QRS complex, increased QT interval and ventricular fibrillation. Beware of the shivering artefact on the ECG.

Electrolyte imbalance

— *Hypokalaemia* causes prolongation of the PR interval, ST depression, T depression/inversion, prominent U wave.
— *Hyperkalaemia* firstly produces peaking of the T waves which is followed by loss of P waves and then prolongation of the QRS complexes.
— *Hypocalcaemia* produces prolongation of the QT interval and hypercalcaemia causes shortening of the QT interval.

Increase in the PR interval

This may be caused by hypokalaemia, myocarditis, rheumatic fever, atrial septal defect (ASD) Ebstein anomaly, ischaemia, hypoxia and digoxin therapy. A decreased PR interval is seen in Wolff–Parkinson–White syndrome and the Lown–Ganong–Levine syndrome.

Digoxin

You should be familiar with the effects of digoxin on the ECG. A common change seen in children on digoxin is a prolonged PR interval and 'reversed tick' ST segment depression. Cardiac toxicity may produce any arrhythmia and ventricular bigemminy (alternating ventricular extrasystole and normal ventricular complex) is one of the commoner abnormalities. Toxicity is made more likely with hypokalaemia.

CARDIAC OPERATIONS

This is an important area for potential questions throughout the exam. Here are some of the commoner ones.

Blalock–Taussig (BT) Shunt

This is the commonest palliative shunting procedure used in conditions where there is a severe reduction in pulmonary blood flow: for example, pulmonary atresia, tetralogy of Fallot. The classic type involves connecting the subclavian artery to the ipsilateral pulmonary artery. The modified type uses a Teflon tube graft between the two arteries (usually right sided). Occasionally a child may become recyanosed some time after the procedure. Exclude a blocked shunt with a V/Q scan which will demonstrate reduced lung perfusion.

Rashkind procedure

This is the balloon atrial septostomy that can be used as an emergency measure to produce mixing in the cases of tricuspid atresia and TOGA. It is performed during cardiac catheterisation.

TOGA procedures

1. The Jatene operation involves the switch operation where there is reimplantation of the coronary arteries and swapping the pulmonary artery and aorta to their proper positions. The Senning and Mustard operations use intra-atrial baffles to redirect blood along more anatomical routes (the Senning operation uses less foreign material than the Mustard).

2. The Fontan procedure involves the connection between systemic venous vessels and chambers (IVC, SVC and right atrium) to the pulmonary arteries. This therefore bypasses the right ventricle. This can be used for tricuspid atresia, single ventricle anatomy and pulmonary atresia. It requires a normal pulmonary artery pressure as well as adequate size of the pulmonary artery. Complications include right heart failure including pericardial and pleural effusions, sick sinus syndrome and other arryhthmias.

Norwood procedure

This is used for hypoplastic left heart syndrome. It is a two-stage procedure which essentially links the right ventricle to the aorta. The pulmonary artery is divided and the proximal segment is linked to the ascending aorta and the distal segment to the descending aorta via a Blalock–Taussig shunt. An atrial septectomy produces continuity between both atria. Thus blood is pumped from the right ventricle into the aorta via the pulmonary valve with pulmonary blood flow supplied by the systemic to pulmonary shunt. Stage 2 involves the Fontan procedure. An alternative treatment involves cardiac transplantation at birth.

PAEDIATRIC CARDIOLOGY AND RADIOLOGY

— All the left to right shunts usually give rise to a large heart, large pulmonary artery and plethoric lung fields. Beware of confusing cardiomegaly with the normal thymus gland in the neonate (sail sign).

— *Aortic stenosis* may give a prominent left ventricle and post-stenotic dilatation of the aorta.

— *Coarctation of the aorta* may give rise to a prominent left ventricle and possibly rib-notching caused by erosion of the under surface of the ribs by collateral circulation (seen in children over the age of four or five).

— *Pulmonary stenosis* may give rise to post-stenotic dilatation of the pulmonary artery.

— *Tetralogy of Fallot* gives rise to the boot-shaped heart with the apex above the left diaphragm and a concave left heart border and small pulmonary artery with oligaemic lung fields.

— *Transposition of the great arteries* gives rise to the egg-on-side appearance. This is caused by a narrow base since the great vessels are superimposed rather than side by side and also a result of the absence of the main pulmonary artery segment arising from its usual location.

— *Total anomalous pulmonary venous drainage.* There is a small heart with increased pulmonary vascularity and venous congestion. In the infracardiac types that are associated with obstruction there may be extensive shadowing and even a total white out which can often be misdiagnosed as lung disease (especially confused with RDS and group B streptococcal pneumonia) caused by an increase in interstitial fluid.

— *Ebstein anomaly.* X-ray shows a very large heart and reduced pulmonary perfusion. The other main cause of a massive heart is cardiomyopathy.

— *Pulmonary hypertension.* Peripheral pulmonary markings are lost (pulmonary pruning).

CLINICAL SCENARIOS

As in clinical paediatrics pattern recognition plays a vital role and here are some examples that you should be familiar with for the data interpretation, grey cases and viva.

— After the first few weeks of life, a baby is now having difficulty completing feeds, has failure to thrive or excessive weight gain (> 25–30 g/day), sweating, tachypnoea post feeds, irritability, cyanosis or recurrent chest infections. *Heart failure* should be in your differential diagnosis.

— Do not forget *hypertensive encephalopathy* in a child who is fitting or in coma. There will usually be papilloedema and possibly retinal haemorrhages. In the clinical history there may be evidence of a cause – for example, the child having had proteinuria 3+ which was not picked up eight months ago when he attended the A&E department.

— Do not forget the heart as a possible focus of infection. The presence of pyrexia, murmurs (especially if new or changing), microscopic haematuria, splenomegaly, the presence of central lines or features of heart failure should lead you to exclude infective endocarditis. Was the heart previously normal? Look for embolic/immune phenomena of Roth spots (round retinal haemorrhages with pale/white centres), Osler nodes (painful red subcutaneous nodules at the finger tips) and Janeway lesions (blanchable red macules on the thenar and hypothenar eminences) and infected emboli, glomerulonephritis and splinter haemorrhages (IGS). Microscopic haematuria may be found. Splenomegaly is common. Clubbing is usually late. Arthritis of the large joints is common.

— Remember the three main ways that *congenital heart disease* can present in the neonatal period. Remember that ductal dependent lesions will only become symptomatic when the duct closes, which can be any time from day one until as long as the end of the first month. Remember that type 2 CHD lesions may resemble sepsis and metabolic presentations and these should always be considered in your differential diagnosis.

Remember that respiratory distress as a result of cardiac lesions is mainly caused by pulmonary congestion and oedema secondary to heart failure but also may be the result of a direct compression effect on the airways, for example double aortic arch, or secondary to metabolic acidosis with respiratory compensation.

— There are several cardiac causes that should be considered in *a child who collapses*. These include cardiac arrhythmias caused by supraventricular tachycardia, complete heart block, long QT syndrome and the vasovagal attacks. Valvular disorders such as aortic stenosis should also be considered. It is three times more common in boys. It may present with dyspnoea, chest pain or syncope, especially with exercise. In the majority of cases the aortic valve itself is narrow (valvular) and often bicuspid instead of tricuspid. Supravalvular aortic stenosis is associated with William syndrome and subvalvular aortic stenosis is associated with hypertrophic obstructive cardiomyopathy or a fibrous diaphragm. Treatment is required if there is a pressure gradient across the valve over 55–70 mmHg. As with all cardiac lesions antibiotic prophylaxis is required for dental and other types of surgery.

— Beware of the child who is described as a mouth breather, who also snores at night time and who develops cor pulmonale (right heart disease secondary to respiratory disease) with possible clinical signs such as peripheral oedema. The cause is *chronic hypoxia* leading to pulmonary hypertension, right ventricular hypertrophy and eventually right-sided heart failure. You may be shown cardiac catheter data of pulmonary hypertension or ECGs with right ventricular hypertrophy and P pulmonale. This should be treated promptly otherwise the pulmonary vascular changes become irreversible.

— You should be familiar with the numerous syndromes that have cardiac lesions as part of their repertoire (see chapter 14).

Friedreich ataxia — HOCM;
Glycogen storage disease — type 2-cardiomyopathy;
Romano–Ward syndrome — long QT interval;

Marfan syndrome — aortic dissection; aneurysm and regurgitation;
Noonan syndrome — pulmonary stenosis;
Tuberous sclerosis — rhabdomyoma.

— You should also be aware of some of the teratogens causing heart disease.

Alcohol-ASD,
Phenytoin-pulmonary stenosis
Lithium-Ebstein anomaly

Rubella-PDA, coarctation of the aorta and Fallot.

— *Peripheral pulmonary artery stenosis* may be caused by congenital rubella infection, Alagille syndrome and William syndrome.

— Remember that a baby with a stable cardiac defect such as a VSD may suddenly become decompensated and go into heart failure with an intercurrent respiratory illness such as *RSV infection*. A stable cardiac defect with the concurrent development of anaemia can produce a similar picture with cardiovascular compromise and heart failure.

— Another clinical scenario that sometimes comes up is the term baby who suddenly goes into heart failure in the first couple of weeks of life with a normal ECG, a normal or slightly enlarged cardiac shadow on the CXR and a normal echocardiogram. There may be a wide pulse pressure on examination. The answer is an *arteriovenous malformation* (AVM) which may be anywhere, but listen especially over the liver, skull and kidneys for bruits. Cyanosis may be present if a pulmonary AV malformation is present (R to L shunt). Remember however that the commonest cause of cardiovascular collapse and cyanosis in the first few hours with normal CXR and ECG is transposition of the great arteries.

— Another favourite trick question is the baby who is cyanosed centrally but in whom all cardiac investigations are normal. Think of *methaemoglobinaemia* (see chapter 8).

— *Constrictive pericarditis* can often give clinical signs that do not clearly fit a classic picture. Remember however, that it mainly gives signs of right-sided heart failure with ascites, peripheral oedema and hepatomegaly. Remember that all types of pericarditis can give rise to constrictive pericarditis (except rheumatic fever). The question may give hints as to the likely aetiology: in an Asian family, for example, think of TB.

— Onset of heart failure in the first few months of life, together with ischaemic changes on the ECG, may be caused by an *anomalous left coronary artery* (that is, arising from the pulmonary artery). It usually presents after a couple of months when the pulmonary vascular resistance falls. Deep Q waves may be seen on the ECG and the infant may develop mitral regurgitation. Treatment involves reimplantation of the left coronary artery.

— You may encounter questions where the child has underlying cardiovascular disease and then develops acutely neurological signs such as a hemiparesis. A couple of possibilities should be considered: they include either the development of a cerebral abscess from an infected embolus from a right to left cardiac lesion or from an infected embolus on a valve. The other possibility is a cerebral thrombosis secondary to polycythaemia caused by chronic hypoxia. Other causes of the co-existence of cardiovascular and neurological features include rheumatic fever, SLE, Lyme disease and syphilis.

— You should be aware of the features to look out for in a child suffering from heart transplant rejection. These include fever, prolongation of the PR interval on the ECG, reducing QRS voltages on the ECG and increasing heart size on the CXR.

— Pulsus paradoxus describes when there is an exaggeration of the normal drop in systolic blood that occurs on inspiration pressure (that is, >10 mmHg). It may be caused by tamponade, severe asthma, hypovolaemic shock and tension pneumothorax.

Paroxysmal SVT

A baby or child who is having recurring episodes of pallor and sweating: always think of paroxysmal SVT. Remember that sinus tachycardia rarely exceeds 180/min and SVT is usually over 210/min. There is an extremely regular narrow complex tachycardia on the ECG. Remember the causes of SVT which include: 50% idiopathic and the remainder caused by CHD, for example Ebstein anomaly, WPW syndrome, post-cardiac surgery and sick sinus syndrome. Treatment involves ABC resuscitation followed by vagal manoeuvres (unilateral carotid massage, valsalva manoeuvre in older children, eyeball pressure — beware the rare complication of retinal detachment, diving reflex — ice cold flannel applied to face of the baby), intravenous adenosine and if this fails call cardiologist and consider synchronous DC shock. Recurrence of SVT is very common in children. Other differential diagnoses of this presentation, together with paroxysmal pallor and sweating, include phaeochromocytoma, recurrent hypoglycaemic attacks and benign paroxysmal vertigo.

Tetralogy of Fallot

The previously pink child who is having cyanotic spells is a common examination scenario. This may be the result of pulmonary infundibular spasm associated with tetralogy of Fallot. This occurs most commonly from a few months until a couple of years of age, often precipitated by physical activity. The patient is usually distressed, anxious, cyanosed, often tachypnoeic and, if old enough, may be squatting. This latter manoeuvre raises systemic blood pressure reducing the right to left shunting. Treatment involves oxygen, knee-chest position, morphine and intravenous beta-blocker administration. Bicarbonate may be needed if there is a significant acidosis and — very rarely — emergency surgery.

Remember that the intensity of the murmur in tetralogy of Fallot is inversely proportional to the severity of the stenosis (that is, the more severe the stenosis the less the intensity of the murmur) because of the VSD present (the reverse to what one would expect if there was no VSD). There is only a single second heart sound in Fallot. The degree of cyanosis in Fallot is proportional to the severity of the pulmonary stenosis and not the size of the VSD. The pulmonary stenosis protects against pulmonary hypertension.

Rheumatic fever

Although rare nowadays rheumatic fever still comes up in the exam. There may or may not be a history of sore throat which may be followed 2–4 weeks later by the features described below. The first attack mainly occurs between 5 and 15 years. Jones' major criteria are: (a) Migratory polyarthritis (usually medium or larger joints) common; (b) Carditis (common). There is a pancarditis and there will be clinical signs related to whether myocarditis, endocarditis or pericarditis is present (there may be a tachycardia greater than expected for the fever, presence of new murmurs — most often mitral and aortic regurgitation, and Carey–Coombs murmur: a mid-diastolic rumbling murmur at the apex due to mitral valve oedema); (c) Sydenham's chorea (occuring in about 10% of rheumatic cases) may be several weeks to months following the acute infection. Sydenham's chorea rarely exists in the presence of cardiac involvement. Children are described as fidgety with sudden involuntary movements, often with altered speech (and may demonstrate the 'milking sign'); (d) Erythema marginatum — a non-pruritic maculopapular rash on the trunk and limbs with a serpiginous border and central clearing; and (e) Subcutaneous nodules — seen on the extensor surfaces of the knees, elbows, wrist or even scalp and spine (usually nodules are seen after recurrent or chronic rheumatic fever). Minor criteria include fever, arthralgia, previous rheumatic fever, raised acute phase reactants (ESR, CRP), leucocytosis, prolonged PR interval (also look for raised ST segments of pericarditis, inverted or flattened T waves of myocarditis or various degrees of heart block). The presence of two major or one major and two minor required in addition to supporting evidence of preceding streptococcal infection (increased anti-streptolysin antibodies (ASOT) titre, positive throat culture or recent scarlet fever). The following differential diagnosis should be considered: systemic lupus erythematosus, juvenile chronic arthritis, Lyme disease, leukaemia, gonococcal disease and Kawasaki disease, all of which have similarities in presentation. Treat with bed rest, high dose aspirin, steroids for carditis, and prophylaxis against recurrence (most common if there is persisting cardiac damage) with daily oral penicillin or monthly intramuscular penicillin. Chronic rheumatic fever (usually more than 10 years after the initial attack) causes valvular damage mainly affecting mitral and aortic valves.

Pericarditis

A child who presents with retrosternal chest pain that may radiate to the neck or left shoulder tip should have pericarditis excluded from the differential diagnosis. The pain is central, sharp, poorly localising and varies with respiration, posture and movement, and is often relieved by sitting forward. If diaphragmatic involvement occurs then left shoulder pain may occur because of innervation by the phrenic nerve (C3,4,5). On examination there may be a scratchy sound heard best at the left sternal edge.

An effusion may develop causing a 'silent heart' and the pericardial rub to disappear. If there is sufficient fluid build up, especially if it occurs rapidly, then tamponade may develop (the clinical condition is dictated by the rate of accumulation of fluid in the pericardium). Beck's triad: pulsus paradoxus (increase in the normal physiological fall in pulse pressure on inspiration, > 10 mmHg), increased jugular venous pressure (JVP) which increases on inspiration (Kussmaul's sign) and decreased blood pressure. ECG changes include saddle elevation (concave elevation) of the ST segments (except aVR) with possible T wave inversion. A CXR may show a large globular heart shadow if there is an effusion. An echocardiogram will demonstrate pericardial fluid. Causes include infections, more likely if accompanied by fever and associated source of infection such as pneumonia. In these cases a purulent pericarditis may occur. Viruses (about one-third of cases) for example Cocksackie, Echo. Bacteria (about one-third of cases) e.g. *Haemophilus influenzae, Staph. aureus, Strep. pneumoniae*, tuberculosis and fungal. Other causes include JCA (especially systemic onset), SLE, rheumatic fever, malignancy including leukaemic infiltration, uraemia, hypothyroidism, post-cardiotomy syndrome, trauma and irradiation. Treat first by addressing the underlying cause. Administer NSAIDs for pain. Drainage is necessary for tamponade. Antibiotics should be given for a purulent pericarditis.

A CARDIOVASCULAR CLINICAL GUIDE

Cardiovascular cases are extremely common short cases and long cases. It is essential to have the examination of the cardiovascular system rehearsed to the extent that it becomes second nature to you. This makes you look confident in front of the examiners and also enables you to concentrate on the diagnosis and creating a rapport with the patient. Here is an ordered system that will take you smoothly through the examination and will also enable you to pick up any pathology on the way.

If given the choice to present as you examine or present at the end of your examination it is much better to present after you have finished your examination. First, you will have the opportunity to impress the examiner with your smooth uninterrupted examination technique. Second, it is much easier presenting your case after having examined the whole system since you will have time to consider all your evidence in a systematic fashion. Third, any mistakes made early on in your presentation are more difficult to reverse and only provide the examiner with ammunition to attack you later. Finally it is also much more difficult to perform two tasks well at the same time. This refers to any examination system.

— Introduce yourself to the patient +/− mother.

— Ask permission and then remove the clothing from the upper part of the body (to the waist). Then place the child at an angle of 45°. (Always remember minor adjustments will have to be made for the smaller infant.)

— Observe the child from the end of the bed, particularly looking for dysmorphic features, cyanosis, respiratory distress, plethoric facies and obvious scars from previous cardiac surgery.

— Take both hands and look at both aspects of each for clubbing, splinter haemorrhages, Osler nodes and tendon xanthomata. Examine the palmar creases for pallor.

— Quickly feel both radials but then move swiftly to the brachial arteries. They can be palpated better and the character of the pulse assessed more accurately, especially in the smaller infant. Put one of your own thumbs on each of the patient's brachials (both pulses simultaneously). Assess for the presence, rate, rhythm and character, and at the same time assess the respiratory rate. Lift the right arm upwards while still feeling the pulse for the 'water hammer' pulse of aortic regurgitation.

— Look at the conjunctivae for anaemia (only one eye needed).

— Ask the patient to open his mouth and stick his tongue out to look for central cyanosis. Get a quick look at the teeth and assess dental hygiene (in other words, the risk of bacterial endocarditis).

— Do not then start poking the child's neck for carotids since this will cause distress. However with prior explanation to the patient place both index and middle fingers of one hand on either side of the trachea in the suprasternal notch to determine if the trachea is in the midline. You may also be able to feel a thrill of aortic stenosis.

— Then feel for the position of the apex with the palmar aspects of your right and left hands on each side of the chest wall (a similar manoeuvre to feeling chest expansion in an older child, but with the fingers together pointing towards the sides). With this method you should pick up a dextrocardia with your left hand. Define the apical position accurately using the sternal angle as a guide (second intercostal space); usually the fifth intercostal space in the mid-clavicular line.

— Then with the ulnar border of the hand feel for thrills in all the valvular areas (mitral — apex, aortic — second intercostal space right sternal border, tricuspid — fourth intercostal space left sternal border and pulmonary — second intercostal space left sternal border).

— Then with the ulnar border of the same hand feel over the apex for a left ventricular heave and at the left sternal edge for a right ventricular heave.

— Place the bell of the stethoscope on the apex and listen (for low pitched sound such as mitral stenosis — rare in paediatrics). Next listen with the diaphragm (high pitched sounds). Listen in all the valvular areas. Place a finger on the pulse to time the heart sounds and any additional sounds, if the patient is co-operative and not getting restless. Listen specifically for the first heart sound (mitral and tricuspid closure) best heard at the apex and then the second heart sound (important in paediatrics and best heard in the pulmonary area) and then for any additional sounds. For a murmur be sure to characterise it completely: site; radiation; timing (systolic/pansystolic/continuous/diastolic); intensity (grade 1 to 6 for systolic and 1 to 4 for diastolic); and character (for example harsh, rumbling or blowing). If a systolic murmur is heard then you should also listen also over the carotids, apex and the rest of the precordium for radiation. (See later in the chapter for a method of diagnosing cardiac murmurs.)

— Use the time when auscultating to put all the clinical signs you have elicited so far together.

— Tilt the patient forward and listen over the back for the radiation of murmurs. Ask the patient to breathe deeply with the mouth open to listen for inspiratory crackles (especially at the bases). When the child is leaning forward take this opportunity to look all around for scars and don't forget to lift up both arms completely since thoracotomy scars may be hiding. This can be done earlier in the examination during initial inspection if it is easier for you to remember it at this point. Minor adjustments to the examination will be required for the smaller infant.

— Palpate the abdomen for hepatomegaly.

— Test for pitting oedema over the shins.

— Then tell the examiner that ideally you would like to:

1. Measure the blood pressure (and radiofemoral delay and four limb blood pressures if appropriate).
2. Plot the height and weight on growth charts.

Presenting to the examiner

— Do not look at the patient; look at the examiner.

— Remember that the examiner has been watching you examine the patient and does not want a detailed account of this. In all presentations of clinical findings after an examination I think that there are certain vital points of information that need to be presented followed by any relevant positive clinical findings. Thus continue:

— 'I would like to present my findings on the cardiovascular examination of [for example] Emilie' (always a good idea to remember the child's name).

— General observations. Always mention the presence or absence of cyanosis, respiratory distress at rest and dysmorphic features. Mention the following if present: scars, clubbing, pallor.

— Then mention the pulse (rate, rhythm, character), apex beat position (displaced/not displaced), heaves or thrills, first and second heart sounds (normal/abnormal). Since the second heart sound is so important in the paediatric examination one can mention that there was normal/abnormal splitting of the second heart sound. Then go on to describe the murmur as described above.

— Mention the presence or absence of signs of heart failure, in particular the liver and oedema.

— Most of your marks will now have been awarded if you have carried this out competently. But now comes the time where you have to put your clinical findings together. Simply say that these findings are consistent with (for example) a ventricular septal defect.

— If you cannot put your clinical findings together do not make one up one but say that you are unable to formulate a diagnosis.

Notes on the CVS examination

There is a useful rule for determining the likely lesions responsible for systolic murmurs in children: Divide the chest into four quadrants with a vertical line through mid-sternum and a horizontal line through the level of the nipples.

Having examined the patient, determine in which of these four quadrants the murmur was heard loudest. This is usually obvious in children.

The pansystolic murmurs are usually heard below the level of the nipples and the ejection systolic murmurs are heard above the level of the nipples.

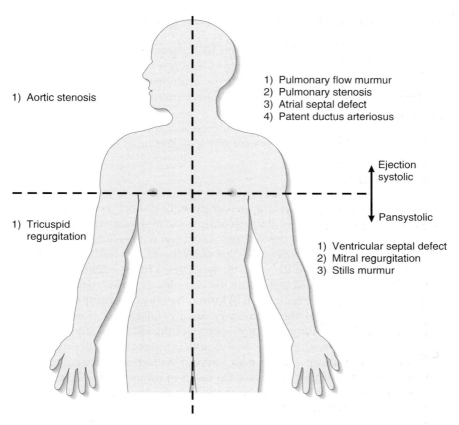

Fig. 2.3 A scheme for diagnosing the nature of heart murmur lesions in paediatrics, based on where the murmur is heard loudest.

Thus if a murmur is heard louder above the level of the nipples then it is ejection systolic and if the murmur is heard louder below the level of the nipples then it is pansystolic. This is very useful to know since the distinction is not always clear in children and infants who generally have faster heart rates (see Fig. 2.3).

— *Left upper quadrant*: pulmonary flow murmur, pulmonary stenosis, atrial septal defect and patent ductus arteriosus (the latter gives an ejection systolic murmur in younger infants and a continuous machinery murmur with systolic accentuation in older children).

— *Right upper quadrant*: aortic stenosis.

— *Right lower quadrant*: tricuspid regurgitation (rare).

— *Left lower quadrant*: ventricular septal defect, mitral regurgitation, Still's murmur (see later).

Flow murmurs are more likely in high cardiac output states such as anaemia, thyrotoxicosis, following exercise and with fever. They are best heard in the pulmonary area. Atrial septal defect causes a pulmonary ejection systolic murmur as well as a mid-diastolic murmur (if there is a large shunt) as well as fixed splitting of the second heart sound.

Continuous murmurs are the result of a combination of a systolic and diastolic murmur, caused by connections between the aorta and pulmonary artery such as occurs in a patent ductus arteriosus, arteriovenous anastamoses or over collateral vessels over the back in, for instance, coarctation of the aorta.

A third heart sound is normal in children and is caused by early diastolic filling following the aortic component of the second heart sound.

Functional murmurs

These are asymptomatic, systolic (never diastolic), short, not loud (< 3/6), heard over a limited area of the precordium, with a normally split-second heart sound, changing with posture, not associated with heaves or thrills with normal investigations such as ECG, CXR and echo. a) Venous hum (the result of blood coursing through the systemic large veins in the neck) is a blowing continuous murmur heard just below the clavicles. It varies with changes in position of the neck and respiration; b) Pulmonary flow murmur is a soft ejection systolic murmur in the pulmonary area; c) Vibratory murmur (Still's murmur) is a short buzzing murmur heard over the left lower sternal edge or apex which changes with posture and usually disappears by puberty.

If there is a murmur that is post surgical correction (that is, scars are present), then the murmur is usually the result of pulmonary or aortic stenosis (this does not obviously relate to the more complicated corrected cardiac lesion).

Thoracic scars

The other rule that is useful to know is what likely operative procedure was responsible for what thoracic scar.

Right thoracotomy scar
— Blalock–Taussig shunt
— PDA ligation.

Left thoracotomy scar
— Blalock–Taussig shunt (feel for pulses in the ipsilateral arm that may be absent)
— PDA ligation
— Coarctation of the aorta repair
— Pulmonary artery banding (listen for a murmur)
— Lung biopsy (look for other evidence of lung disease).

Mid-sternotomy scar
— Any major bypass surgery, for example valvular repair or one of the more complicated cardiac repairs.

The second heart sound

A special mention should be made of the second heart sound since it plays an important role in the paediatric cardiovascular examination. Under normal circumstances the aortic valve closes before the pulmonary valve: this is called physiological splitting of the second heart sound and increases on inspiration. Wide splitting may be caused by right bundle branch block and pulmonary stenosis. Fixed wide splitting may be caused by an atrial septal defect. Reversed splitting (pulmonary component heard before aortic component) may be caused by left bundle branch block, severe aortic stenosis and left ventricular failure. Narrow splitting of the second heart sound may be caused by pulmonary hypertension and aortic stenosis. A loud pulmonary component of the second heart sound is heard in pulmonary hypertension and a loud aortic component in systemic hypertension.

A single second heart sound may be caused by tetralogy of Fallot, pulmonary atresia, single ventricle, aortic atresia and pulmonary atresia.

Respiratory system

You should be familiar with the definitions of lung volumes and capacities. You should also know about about the spirometer tracings demonstrating the different lung volumes and capacities. This may well present itself in the form of a data interpretation question or in the viva.

OBSTRUCTIVE AND RESTRICTIVE LUNG DISEASE

You may encounter lung volumes in the data interpretation questions. Be familiar with the changes that are expected in:

— Obstructive lung diseases (such as asthma, bronchiectasis, emphysema or cystic fibrosis).
— Restrictive lung diseases (interstitial lung disease such as fibrosing alveolitis, neuromuscular disorders such as Duchenne muscular dystrophy and musculoskeletal disorders such as severe kyphoscoliosis).

Obstructive

Air trapping is the main feature.

— *Increased:* residual volume, functional residual capacity and total lung capacity.
— *Decreased:* vital capacity.

Restrictive

Usually smaller lungs which are unable to expand fully.

— *Decreased:* vital capacity, functional residual capacity, residual volume, total lung capacity, expiratory reserve volume.

BLOOD GAS INTERPRETATION

These are common questions with which you should be at ease. These questions may be in the guise of a neonate on a ventilator, or taken from a child with some respiratory disturbance, metabolic disturbance or other problem. Here we will discuss the questions that relate to respiratory problems.

The neonate on the ventilator

You should be familiar with these from clinical practice but this is a summary of the general principles.

— First look at the pH to determine if there is an acidosis or alkalosis.

— Then determine if this has a respiratory or a metabolic cause. This is done by looking at the PCO_2 for a respiratory cause (raised in respiratory acidosis and reduced in respiratory alkalosis) and the base excess/deficit and bicarbonate for a metabolic cause (low in a metabolic acidosis and raised in a metabolic alkalosis). There may of course be a mixed picture with, for example, an acidosis caused by a respiratory or metabolic cause being compensated for by a metabolic change (retaining or excreting hydrogen ions) or respiratory change (retaining or excreting CO_2) respectively. Remember that the respiratory compensatory effect in response to a metabolic disturbance may not be possible in the case of a neonate who is on a ventilator. Also remember that the premature kidney is also less efficient at acid-base homeostasis.

— A premature baby who has RDS is usually ventilated with the following initial settings that vary between units but are usually within the following ranges:

Rate	60–80/min
FiO_2	0.7–0.8
PIP	18–28 cm/H_2O
PEEP	3–5 cm H_2O
Inspiratory time	0.3–0.5 s

For pulmonary interstitial emphysema and persistent pulmonary hypertension comparatively higher rates with shorter inspiratory times are used so that lower peak inspiratory pressures can be utilised.

When considering questions that require you to alter ventilator settings in a baby with abnormal blood gases the following need to be remembered.

1. In order to increase the PO_2 the possibilities are:
   — Increase the FiO_2. This would be your first step unless the FiO_2 is already high and approaching 0.7.
   — The next step might be to increase the peak inspiratory pressure.
   — Increase the inspiratory time.
   — Then consider increasing the peak end expiratory pressure (PEEP) remembering that high PEEPs predispose to pneumothoraces and can inhibit cardiovascular function.
2. In order to decrease the PCO_2 the following are possibilities.
   — The most important manoeuvre is to increase the rate.
   — Increasing the peak inspiratory pressure (PIP) will also decrease the PCO_2.

3. In order to increase the PO$_2$ and increase the PCO$_2$ simultaneously try increasing the PEEP.

4. Another manoeuvre in order to increase the PCO$_2$ is to extubate the baby (in a baby whose ventilatory function is adequate and possibly fighting the ventilator), or if ventilation is still necessary one can increase the dead space by increasing the length of the ET tube.

Examples

1. The scenario where a previously stable premature neonate on a ventilator suddenly 'collapses' with the following blood gas picture.

pH	7.03
PCO$_2$	11.4
PO$_2$	5.9
HCO$_3$	23.7
BE	−3.5

   There is a severe respiratory acidosis of sudden onset. There are several possible causes: these include:
   - Dislodgement of the endotracheal tube (listen to the lungs and look for chest movement).
   - Blocked tube (listen to the lungs and look for chest wall movement).
   - Ventilator or generator failure (inspect the ventilator).
   - Pneumothorax (transilluminate chest +/− X-ray).
   - Intraventricular haemorrhage (exclude with cranial ultrasound).

2. A 32-week gestation baby is born with tachypnoea, grunting and intercostal recession with the following blood gas at a few hours of life.

pH	7.03
PCO$_2$	9.8
PO$_2$	7.5 (in 68% O$_2$)
HCO$_3$	13
BE	−11.1

   This shows a mixed respiratory and metabolic acidosis. This is most likely to be a result of the respiratory distress syndrome. In order to correct the acidosis the respiratory and metabolic problems should be attacked simultaneously. The metabolic acidosis can be treated with volume expansion if clinically the baby has reduced perfusion, or bicarbonate if the baby's perfusion appears adequate. Alternatively THAM can be used (advantages of this drug include no sodium load and lowering of CO$_2$ but it may cause respiratory depression). The baby will require some form of ventilation in order to control the hypercapnia and oxygen requirements.

3. A four-year-old child presents with a history of chronic middle ear effusions, snoring and failure to thrive. The arterial blood gas when asleep shows:

pH	7.40
PCO$_2$	9.1

```
PO₂      7.8
HCO₃     33
```

This child has a compensated respiratory acidosis. There is compensation since the pH is normal (and bicarbonate is high) despite the markedly raised PCO_2. The clinical history gives us a clue as to the possible aetiology which in his case was enlarged adenoids and may be part of the obstructive sleep apnoea syndrome. The child should have a formal sleep study performed looking at the oxygen saturation trace and episodes of obstructive apnoea. Remember the other possible causes of hypercapnia in a child, which may be a result of central respiratory depression (for instance, central depressant drug ingestion), respiratory neuromuscular disease (as in Guillain–Barré syndrome) and thoracic wall disorders (severe scoliosis, for example) and obesity.

4. The hyperventilation syndrome should always be considered in a child who presents with a respiratory alkalosis with no abnormal clinical or laboratory findings, especially if the PO_2 is normal. Such children are typically anxious individuals. Respiratory stimulant ingestion and the early stages of salicylate overdose should also be considered.

5. A baby born at term who is one week old is brought in to the casualty department grunting and peripherally shut down with a respiratory rate of 80/min.

```
pH       7.08
PCO₂     1.9
PO₂      7.5
HCO₃     11
BE       −18.8
```

This is caused by a severe metabolic acidosis for which the baby is attempting to compensate by hyperventilating and thus blowing off CO_2. However, the pH shows that compensation is incomplete. The most likely cause of this picture in this baby would be group B Streptococcal sepsis, congenital heart disease or a metabolic disorder.

RESPIRATORY FAILURE

Respiratory failure is defined as a PaO_2 of less than 8 kPa. It is divided into two types based upon the $PaCO_2$.

— *In type 1 respiratory failure* there is a low $PaCO_2$ usually less than 6.5 kPa. This is the result of a pure ventilation–perfusion mismatch causing a failure of gaseous exchange. The consequent hyperventilation causes the blowing off of CO_2 (which cannot occur in the case of oxygen because of the nature of its disassociation curve). Conditions causing this type of failure are: pulmonary embolus, pulmonary fibrosis, pulmonary oedema and asthma (hypercapnia in an asthmatic patient with a severe attack is a sign that suggests the child is tiring or becoming severely obstructed).

— *In type II respiratory failure* there is pure hypoventilation causing a low PaO_2 and a high $PaCO_2$ usually more than 6.5 kPa. This can be caused by central respiratory depression, neuromuscular disorders, thoracic wall disorders and pneumonia.

LUNG FUNCTION TESTS

Peak expiratory flow measurements (PEFR)

These can be measured properly only from about five years of age. They are useful for assessing the severity of asthma attacks and the response of the patient to therapy. Normal values are available and relate to height. An improvement of 20% or more following inhaled bronchodilators is diagnostic of asthma. Remember morning dips in PEFR as a sign of possible worsening of asthma.

Spirometry

This can provide a spirogram (expiratory volume as a function of time, an expiratory flow–volume curve and a flow–volume loop comprising inspiration and expiration).

Forced Vital Capacity. This is the total amount of air exhaled during maximal expiration. FEV1 is the forced expiratory volume in the first second. The FEV1/FVC ratio is useful in determining whether there is a restrictive or obstructive component. Normal values of FEV1, FVC are available for age, height and sex. Be familiar with spirometric graphs of volume against time and their interpretation.

Restrictive pattern

Here the FVC is reduced but so is the FEV1 resulting in a normal or occassionally higher FEV1/FVC (for example, 90%, usually about 75–80%).

This is caused by neuromuscular disorders, skeletal thoracic cage defects including scoliosis and interstitial lung disease (resulting from, for instance, sarcoidosis, extrinsic allergic alveolitis, pneumoconiosis, fibrosing alveolitis, post-radiation and drugs). All of the interstitial lung diseases are rare in childhood.

Obstructive pattern

Here the FEV1 is considerably reduced compared to the FVC resulting in a low FEV1/FVC (e.g. 40%).

Flow–volume loops

The diagrams in Figure 3.1 correspond to maximal flow rates measured at varying lung volumes. These loops are useful in investigating the site of possible obstruction in the respiratory tree. Proximal obstruction of the upper airway e.g. at the level of the trachea reduces the flow rate at high lung

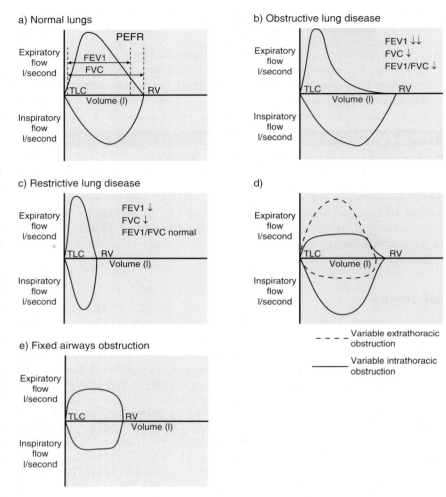

Fig. 3.1 Typical spirometric findings seen in normal children and in children with various pathological states.

volumes i.e. at the beginning of expiration whereas obstruction lower down the airway e.g. asthma reduces the flow rate after further expiration when the lung volume is low.

Arterial blood gases

These have been described earlier.

Transfer factor (TLCO)

This is a useful measure of the transfer of a gas across the alveolar/capillary interface. Basically, it involves determining the amount of carbon monoxide absorbed across the alveolar/capillary membrane following an inhaled held breath of carbon monoxide. It is dependent on a number of factors which include: (a) alveolar ventilation; (b) blood flow to lungs; (c) haemoglobin concentration; (d) lung volume/surface area; (e) age: its value increases throughout childhood.

— *Decreased TLCO:* parenchymal lung disease (inflammation, infiltration, fibrosis), reduced pulmonary blood flow (pulmonary embolus, pulmonary hypertension, emphysema), ventilation/pefusion mismatch (e.g. pneumonia, pulmonary oedema), anaemia.

— *Increased TLCO:* Polycythaemia, exercise (higher in athletes), pulmonary haemorrhage e.g. pulmonary haemosiderosis (raised initially following bleeding but with time later falls due to fibrosis). TLCO is usually normal but may be increased in asthma.

Pleural effusion aspirates

The effusion can usually be classified into a transudate or exudate depending upon the protein content of the fluid. Protein content < than 30 g/l implies a transudate and > 30 g/l implies an exudate.

— *Transudates* are usually bilateral and are caused by filtration of fluid through capillaries into the pleural space. This may be caused by right-sided heart failure, fluid overload or any condition causing hypoproteinaemia (for example, nephrotic syndrome, liver disease and protein-losing enteropathy) and also occasionally seen in hypothyroidism.

— *Exudates* are caused by inflammatory processes such as infection or neoplasia. Causes include pneumonias including tuberculosis, lymphomas and connective tissue diseases. In addition to finding a protein count in excess of 30 g/l other investigations are important in narrowing down the diagnosis and some of these are listed here: (a) microscopy, culture and sensitivities (MC&S) for micro-organisms; (b) Ziehl–Neelson stain for acid fast bacilli; (c) cytology for malignant cells; (d) differential white cell count: lymphocytosis is associated with leukaemic infiltration, viral infection, TB. Neutrophilia is associated with a purulent bacterial illness. Eosinophilia is associated with parasitic infections (which often spread to the lungs as part of their life cycle).

Remember the possibility of the effusion being a chylothorax or haemothorax. A haemothorax mainly occurs following trauma or surgery and is immediately obvious from a bloody pleural aspiration.

A chylothorax contains triglycerides which give it a milky colour (though not if the patient has not eaten for some period of time). It is caused by damage to the thoracic duct at the root of the neck usually secondary to trauma (including traumatic delivery in the newborn), surgery (most often cardiac surgery) and neoplastic disease. A purulent effusion may look the same, but if the sample is centrifuged then the white cells can usually be cleared from the liquid but this is not the case with a chylothorax which remains milky. Treatment consists of continual drainage of the chylous effusion (beware of fat-soluble vitamin deficiencies resulting as well as electrolyte and lymphocyte deficiencies if the effusion is large and drainage is prolonged). Medium chain triglycerides are given as the main source of fat as they bypass the lymphatic absorption and are transported directly into the portal vein. The effusion usually settles after a few days or weeks but if it persists surgery may become necessary.

CYSTIC FIBROSIS (CF)

As the commonest inherited disease in the Western world, cystic fibrosis comes up routinely in the written and clinical parts of the examination: exam-relevant aspects are covered below (see Table 3.1). The genetics chapter (1) discusses the genetics of cystic fibrosis, which causes a dysfunction of the exocrine glands resulting in viscous secretions affecting many organs.

Investigations

— Antenatal diagnosis. This may be performed by chorionic villous sampling (8–10 weeks) or amniocentesis at 16–18 weeks with DNA analysis.

— Sweat test. Pilocarpine ionotophoresis induces sweating (usually on a small area of skin on the forearm) and a sample of more than 100 mg is collected. A sodium concentration of more than 60 mmol/l is required on more than one sweat test to confirm the diagnosis. Values between 40–60 mmol/l should be repeated.

— DNA analysis can be performed in order to identify the most common CF mutations (see chapter 1).

— Newborn screening. Serum immunoreactive trypsin is markedly raised in newborn babies with CF. Accuracy of the test is improved with the use of monoclonal antibodies. Confirmation with other tests as above.

Table 3.1 Summary of the clinical manifestations of cystic fibrosis

Organ affected	Clinical manifestations
Respiratory tract	May present early with a raised respiratory rate, hyperexpansion of the chest, intercostal recession and cough. Later, recurrent chest infections occur (the commonest presentation) with the usual paediatric respiratory pathogens and later with *Haemophilus influenzae*, *Staph. aureus* and *Pseudomonas aeruginosa* (more rarely with *Klebsiella*, *Proteus*, *Serratia* and *Pseudomonas cepacia* — this occurs in the more debilitated older patient and may cause a rapid decline in respiratory function). Bronchiectasis develops with patchy areas of collapse and consolidation. Haemoptysis, pneumothorax, cor pulmonale and respiratory failure develop later. CF is associated with allergic bronchopulmonary aspergillosis.

Table 3.1 *Continued*

Organ affected	Clinical manifestations
Gastrointestinal tract	One of the earliest manifestations is meconium ileus (occurring in about 15% of cases) which can present with obstruction, volvulus, perforation and distal gut atresia. Pancreatic insufficiency may also be an early manifestation in the form of steatorrhoea and bulky, pale, smelly stools in a greasy film which are difficult to flush away. Malabsorption causes failure to thrive and deficiency of the fat-soluble vitamins A,D,E, and K (second commonest presentation). Failure to thrive occurs despite a very big appetite. Pancreatitis secondary to duct obstruction may occur. IDDM occurs in about 10% of cases. Bile duct obstruction leads to a secondary biliary cirrhosis in some patients with accompanying portal hypertension (with splenomegaly, hypersplenism and oesophageal varices). Gallstones occur in about 10%. Rectal prolapse occurs in up to 20% of children. Meconium ileus equivalent (distal intestinal obstruction) can occur in older children with less acute symptoms cf. meconium ileus and presents with intermittent colic, constipation and possibly vomiting caused by repeated partial bowel obstruction as a result of the viscous mucus production. A palpable mass in the lower right quadrant is sometimes found. Gastrograffin, a high osmolar contrast liquid, may dislodge the plug.
ENT	Sinusitis is common and occurs in the majority. Nasal polyps (associated with less severe chest problems) may occur in about 10–20% of cases.
Reproductive system	Delayed puberty (as with all chronic illness in children). Reduced female fertility because of abnormal cervical mucus production. Males are almost always infertile as a result of atresia of the vas deferens and epididymis.
Skeletal	Short stature (as with any chronic illness in children). Hypertrophic pulmonary osteoarthropathy (including clubbing).
Cardiovascular	Because of sweat containing excess quantities of salt, sweating — especially in hot weather — may cause heat stroke and cardiovascular collapse. Right-sided heart failure may develop secondary to pulmonary hypertension.
Metabolic	Remember that in infants CF is one of the causes of a hyponatraemic hypochloraemic metabolic alkalosis (know the others in the list).
Haematological	Anaemia of chronic disease, usually normocytic normochromic anaemia. Remember that the ferritin may be raised as it is an acute phase reactant.

Causes of a false positive sweat test
— Adrenal insufficiency
— Congenital adrenal hyperplasia

— Diabetes insipidus
— Glucose-6 phosphatase deficiency (G6PD)
— Ectodermal dysplasia
— Hypothyroidism
— Mucopolysaccharidoses.

RADIOLOGICAL FINDINGS IN RESPIRATORY DISEASE

There are a wide range of possible X-rays that you may encounter in the slide section of the written examination as well as in the clinical exam.

Radiological examination of the respiratory system may involve a plain CXR, Barium swallow, ultrasound, CT and MRI. Usually some sort of brief history is given with the slide.

Chest X-ray

A good method for looking at a CXR is the following.

1. Look at the name, date of birth and date of the examination.

2. Make sure that the orientation of the radiograph is correct (L and R). If the right mark is on the same side as the cardiac apex then think of dextrocardia (if the X-ray has been labelled correctly).

3. Determine whether the film is PA (posteroanterior) or AP (anteroposterior). PA is the routine film: an AP film will usually be labelled as such. Otherwise an AP film can be recognised firstly because the scapulae overlie the lung fields (this is not the case in a good quality PA film) and secondly the chin is usually seen on an AP. No comment can be made of the size of the heart in an AP view film and the cardiac silhouette appears larger than in a PA. AP views are usually obtained in the sicker patient who cannot stand.

4. Comment on the penetration of the film. In an over-penetrated film the lung fields appear very dark with few vascular markings. One should ideally just be able to make out the vertebrae behind the cardiac shadow.

5. Orientation: make sure that the patient is not rotated by looking at the distance between the spinous processes and the medial ends of the clavicles which should be equal on both sides.

6. Inflation: this is important in paediatrics since hyperinflation is a common finding. A normal CXR in inspiration will show the diaphragmatic level at rib 8–9 posteriorly and rib 6 anteriorly. Flattening of the diaphragm is also an important finding in hyperinflation. In 90% of children the right dome of the diaphragm is higher than the left.

7. Now you are able to go through the CXR systematically: heart, mediastinum (trace the outline of the mediastinum visually), lung fields, vascular markings (a sense of what is normal comes with experience but roughly speaking pulmonary vessels should not extend beyond two-thirds of the width of the lung fields), diaphragm, bones, soft tissue and you may

be able to see some abdominal pathology on a CXR (such as air under the diaphragm in the case of a perforated bowel). The right-heart border superiorly consists of the SVC and interiorly the right ventricle. The left-heart border consists of (from top to bottom): aortic knuckle, left pulmonary trunk, left atrium and then left ventricle.

8. Comment on the need for a lateral film which may help localise a lesion to a particular lobe or segment of the lung or pick up pathology that might be missed on a PA film (especially in the anterior mediastinum).

Always remember that an enlarged superior mediastinum in an infant less than a few months of age may be due to the thymic shadow. There is usually a characteristic sail sign. The cardiothoracic ratio in a PA film is usually 0.5 but may be slightly higher in a child under the age of two years of age. Remember that the heart diameter may vary by up to 1 cm during the cardiac cycle.

— Look for evidence of shifting of the lung or mediastinum — for example following lung collapse — by looking for movement of the hilum, trachea or fissures from their expected positions.

— Any increased density should be described as an area of *increased shadowing*. Linear shadows are described as reticular, dot-like shadows are called nodular and fluffy diffuse shadows are known as alveolar shadowing. Remember that loss of clarity of the right border of the mediastinum corresponds to right middle lobe pathology. Loss of clarity of the left border of the mediastinum corresponds to pathology in the lingula. The area above the right hemidiaphragm corresponds to the right lower lobe.

— A *pulmonary sequestration*, most common in the left lower lobe, is where a lobe of the lung receives a blood supply distinct from the pulmonary artery and in fact arises from the systemic aortic blood supply. It has a venous drainage into a pulmonary vein. Their presence is associated with an increased risk of chest infections which are often recurrent.

— The *scimitar syndrome* describes the case of a hypoplastic right lung (especially right upper lobe) which has a systemic arterial blood supply and a venous drainage into the subdiaphragmatic vena cava and is often associated with the presence of an ASD. A CXR reveals a crescent-shaped shadow next to the right heart border.

— *Cystic adenomatous malformations* are caused by irregular dilatations of the bronchi leading to variably sized air-filled cysts that are usually found in a single lobe. If widespread it may present at birth with respiratory distress and may require surgical resection.

— If they are large, *congenital lung cysts* may cause a compensatory collapse of adjacent or contralateral lung tissue. Remove because of the risk of infection and possible malignant transformation.

— *Congenital lobar emphysema* mainly affects the right or left upper lobes (and less commonly the right middle lobes). It is caused by a weakness in the wall of a lobar bronchus resulting in hyperinflation of the affected lobe or lobes (caused by a ball valve effect). The emphysema may cause respiratory distress in the neonatal period (wheeze, tachypnoea and poor feeding) with all the features of a unilateral hyperinflation (such as hyperresonance and reduced breath sounds). The CXR shows radiolucency in the region of the affected lobe together with possible compression effects such as the collapse of adjacent lobes or mediastinal shift. Treatment of symptomatic individuals involves resection of the affected lobe.

— *Respiratory distress syndrome* is a common slide. Look for hypoinflated, dense, lung fields with possible atelectasis, ground glass appearance of the lung fields and the presence of an air bronchogram (caused by the air-filled airways surrounded by dense lung tissue). Also look for the endotracheal tube (if ventilated) and other common neonatal devices such as a chest drain, UAC or UVC. Differential diagnosis of RDS is total anomalous pulmonary venous drainage (TAPVD) or bilateral pneumonia (most commonly group B *Strep.* pneumonia).

— *Meconium aspiration syndrome* causes hyperinflated lung fields with flattened depressed diaphragms and patchy areas of consolidation leading to radio-opaque lung fields as a pneumonitis develops.

— *Transient tachypnoea of the newborn* (TTN) shows streaky lung fields (especially perihilar) and fluid in the fissures.

— *Bronchopulmonary dysplasia* shows hyperinflated lung fields interspersed with areas of atelectasis, cystic changes, bronchial wall thickening and diffuse reticular shadowing.

— *Pulmonary hypoplasia* is caused mainly by (a) oligohydramnios; (b) lung compression in utero, for example diaphragmatic hernia; (c) reduced breathing activity in utero, such as Werdnig–Hoffman disease. CXR shows dense hypoinflated lung fields which often have a bell-shaped appearance. Confirm with lung function tests.

— *Tracheo-oesophageal fistula* is usually diagnosed by failure to pass a size 10 catheter into the stomach because it has become coiled up in the atretic oesophageal pouch. X-rays will confirm this as well as noting the presence of air in the stomach which can occasionally be followed to the level of the tracheo-oesophageal fistula. The presence of air in the stomach confirms the presence of a fistula between the distal oesophagus and the trachea.

— *Cystic fibrosis* may come up in a radiology question in several ways. A plain abdominal X-ray of mecomium ileus will usually show dilated proximal loops of small bowel with a ground glass appearance in the region of the caecum (a barium enema may show a distal microcolon). A CXR shows hyperinflated lung fields with patchy atelectasis. There is peribronchial thickening and areas of bronchiectasis (thickened tram-line shadows). You may be shown a bronchogram demonstrating bronchiectatic airways.

— *Asthmatics* present with hyperinflated radiolucent lung fields caused by air trapping (presenting as an increased number of ribs counted in an inspiratory film with flattened diaphragms). Look also for pneumothorax, pneumomediastinum, infection and an inhaled foreign body that may help explain the clinical presentation.

— *A pneumothorax* is seen on an X-ray (best on an expiratory film) as a radiolucent area without lung markings peripheral to the region of normal or collapsed lung. A tension pneumothorax is seen as a marked deflation of the ipsilateral lung with varying degrees of mediastinal shift (caused by air being drawn into the pleural space but unable to escape). Displacement of the trachea and apex are indicators of mediastinal shift.

— *A pneumopericardium* is seen as a thin line of air lining the pericardium, but if the line continues upwards into the neck following the borders of the mediastinal structures then it is called a pneumomediastinum.

— Causes of a *hemithorax white-out* are: unilateral pneumonia, collapse of the lung, pleural effusion (including blood-haemothorax or chyle-chylothorax) and tumour.

CLINICAL SCENARIOS

Respiratory distress

Respiratory distress in the newborn is a common problem (see Table 3.2). It presents with tachypnoea (> 60/min), nasal flaring, intercostal recession, expiratory grunt, cyanosis and poor feeding.

— A special mention should be made here regarding the respiratory distress sometimes seen in infants born to *diabetic mothers*. The possible causes include: (a) many babies are macrosomic and more likely to be delivered by caesarian section with its attendant risk of transient tachypnoea of the newborn (TTN) increase; (b) respiratory distress syndrome is more common in these babies; (c) persistent fetal circulation; and (d) polycythaemia-induced stiffness of the lungs.

— *Congenital diaphragmatic hernia* should be remembered as a cause of respiratory distress at birth especially if the question mentions that the mother had had no antenatal care (antenatal scans will usually pick it up). It is caused by failure of closure of the foramen of Bochdalek (posterolateral position). It is most common on the left because of the presence of the liver on the right. Hypoplastic lungs result from herniation of abdominal contents through the patent diaphragm compressing the ipsilateral lung (and sometimes contralateral lung). Further respiratory and cardiovascular compromise occurs after birth as a result of air entering the intestine (especially so if the condition is not suspected, and the paediatrician uses routine resuscitative measures such as bag and mask ventilation). The baby rapidly develops acidosis and pulmonary hypertension worsens.

Table 3.2 A comparison of the causes of neonatal respiratory distress

Differential diagnosis of neonatal respiratory distress	Features to look for in a question relating to respiratory distress in the newborn
Respiratory distress syndrome (RDS)	Begins within 4 hours of birth. Risk factors: prematurity, asphyxia, hypothermia, acidosis, lecithin/sphingomyelin ration < 2:1.
Sepsis/pneumonia	More likely if there has been prolonged maternal rupture of membranes, offensive liquor (green liquor is associated with listeria as is the passage of meconium by a preterm baby), maternal pyrexia, culture-positive vaginal swabs. The neonate may appear shocked, hypotensive, hypotonic, acidotic or may develop apnoea and temperature instability. The white-cell count may be elevated or depressed. Thrombocytopenia commonly accompanies sepsis in neonates.
Meconium aspiration syndrome	The baby is mature or post mature and there has been meconium-stained liquor. There may be a history of intrapartum asphyxia. At birth meconium may have been visualised beyond the vocal cords. Hyperexpanded chest. Meconium-stained liquor of long standing may cause staining of the skin and nails (possible slide question).
Pneumothorax	There may be a history of a traumatic delivery. Look for other evidence of birth trauma. Hyperresonant hyperexpanded asymmetrical chest. History of ventilation (perhaps over-vigorous resuscitation, high PEEP). Pneumothorax occurs spontaneously in about 1% of all deliveries. Remember phrenic nerve palsy as a cause of respiratory distress following a traumatic birth (diagnosed by fluoroscopic visualisation of diaphragmatic movement or ultrasound where the paralysed side moves upwards on inspiration (called paradoxical movement).
Congenital heart disease	Usually presents after the first 12 hours. Look for signs such as cyanosis, large liver, murmurs or abnormal pulses. May be history of maternal illness during pregnancy (maternal rash or fever or drug ingestion).
Pulmonary haemorrhage	History of birth asphyxia, cardiac failure, pneumonia, bleeding diathesis and in some babies the administration of some types of surfactant. History of blood (often pink and frothy) coming up from the mouth or endotracheal tube.

Clues in the clinical examination include a scaphoid abdomen, reduced breath sounds and reduced chest movement (in fact bowel sounds may be heard in the chest). Heart sounds may be displaced. Occasionally the presentation is delayed and babies present with episodes of breathlessness especially after feeds and intermittent bowel obstruction (such as colicky pain or vomiting) or as a dextrocardia. CXR appearances include tracheal and mediastinal shift, bowel in the chest, and sometimes a cystic appearance which may resemble a cystic adenomatous malformation or staphylococcal pneumonia (and possibly congenital lobar emphysema). Ideally the baby should be intubated before any inspiratory effort. Manage with the head upright, and using nasogastric suction in an attempt to deflate the intestines. Resuscitate with fluids and correct the metabolic acidosis. Pulmonary hypertension may occur and pulmonary vasodilators such as prostacyclin, tolazoline or nitric oxide should be employed to treat it. High frequency oscillation may also be used. When the baby is stable refer to a surgical centre for repair of the hernia.

— Do not forget the association of *whooping cough and a lymphocytosis* (a common data case). The question may describe the classic three-phase history, the most characteristic of these being the paroxysmal phase with paroxysms of coughs followed by a whoop in an older child. There may be large amounts of thick mucus production. Vomiting and choking attacks after the paroxysms are characteristic. Subconjunctival haemorrhages and periorbital petechiae are often seen in children with severe disease. Lymphocytosis (often > 70%) is more common in children over three years of age. Other complications include bronchopneumonia, bronchiectasis (often reversible), otitis media, convulsions (in infants more commonly) and cerebral haemorrhage with resulting mental retardation. Because of the chronic nature of the cough a rectal prolapse or umbilical hernia may be precipitated. Culture of the organism *Bordetella pertussis* can be carried out using a per-nasal swab. Alternatively IgG and IgM serology can be performed. Prophylaxis is with immunisation and erythromycin may be given (although thought to be most effective in the intial catarrhal stage).

— You may be described a history of a baby who develops respiratory distress and possibly cyanosis shortly after birth. He is intubated and ventilated but has minimal ventilatory requirements. On extubation the baby again develops respiratory distress: alternatively, the history may describe an improvement in symptoms when the baby is crying. These descriptions should lead you towards considering *choanal atresia* as a possible cause. Babies are nasal breathers and choanal atresia thus poses a particular breathing problem for them. It is most easily diagnosed by passing a feeding tube up each nostril. Insert a Magill airway (or intubate) until surgery can be carried out.

— Some questions test whether you can make a connection between respiratory symptoms such as cough, wheezing and dyspnoea and a *microcytic hypochromic anaemia*. Of course the two could be unrelated, with respiratory symptoms caused by asthma for example and the anaemia a result of poor nutrition. However you should also consider primary pulmonary haemosiderosis (which is sometimes associated with cow's milk intolerance and later on in life with Goodpasture syndrome). It is caused by repeated episodes of bleeding into the lung tissue with deposition of haemosiderin leading to progressive fibrosis. Additional symptoms may include haemoptysis with coughing up of rusty sputum. A CXR may reveal patchy shadowing caused by the presence of alveolar infiltrates. Bronchoalveolar lavage may help in the diagnosis by finding haemosiderin-filled macrophages. Treat with cow's milk protein free diet; transfusion and steroids may be of some help.

— There are questions that relate to a child with Marfan syndrome who presents with sudden onset of chest pain. The possible causes are (a) pneumothorax; (b) aortic dissection; or (c) any other cause of chest pain not associated with Marfan syndrome.

Stridor

A common paediatric problem is the child with stridor. Clues from the history should help you limit the differential diagnosis: see Table 3.3. Stridor is a noise made during inspiration as a result of airway obstruction above the level of the thoracic inlet (obstruction in the subglottic area may produce some expiratory noise in addition). Obstruction occurring below the thoracic inlet results in narrowing of the airways mainly during expiration and results in wheezing.

Other aetiologies that you should be able to list as causes of acute stridor include: retropharyngeal abscess (toxic with neck extension and cervical lymphadenopathy) treated with incision under general anaesthetic and antibiotics; angioedema (following anaphylactic reaction or rarely in hereditary angioedema); and following burns to the neck and larynx. Hypocalcaemia is a rare cause in the neonatal period.

Table 3.3 Comparison of the causes of stridor

Cause of acute stridor	History	Management
Acute laryngotracheobronchitis (croup)	Commonest in 1–3-year age group. Parainfluenza virus most common cause. Onset over a couple of days with coryzal symptoms. Mild fever, hoarse voice, barking cough, and inspiratory stridor, worse at night.	Cool steam mist vaporiser may ease breathing. Careful attention to fluid balance. Steroid nebuliser. Adrenaline nebuliser may help buy time before transferring to intensive care but should only be used as a rescue rather than as regular treatment because of its short-lived action and possible worsening of stridor when effect wears off. Intubation is needed in about 1% of cases.

Table 3.3 *Continued*

Cause of acute stridor	History	Management
Acute epiglottitis	Commonest in 2–6 year age group. *Haemophilus influenzae* type B is causative agent and results in rapid swelling of the epiglottis and aryepiglottic folds causing high fever (> 38.5°C). The child looks toxic, and is drooling with a weak muffled voice. Coughing is rare, patient adopts position with neck extended leaning forward. Lateral neck X-ray shows an enlarged epiglottis resembling a thumb.	Do not examine the throat. Nothing should be done to agitate the child since this may precipitate complete obstruction (thus no i.v. cannulation etc). An atmosphere of calm is very important. Summon an experienced ENT surgeon (emergency tracheostomy may be required at any time) and anaesthetist urgently; nebulised adrenaline may be given in the meantime. Arrange for intubation of the airway ideally in an intensive care setting (when direct laryngoscopy to confirm an inflamed cherry-red epiglottis can also be carried out). Once accomplished i.v. antibiotics should be given e.g. cefotaxime. Extubate after 1–2 days.
Bacterial tracheitis	May follow on from croup-like illness with infection by *Staphylococcus aureus*. The 'croupy child' fails to improve and develops a high fever and becomes toxic, with a productive chesty cough and stridor.	Similar to management of epiglottitis since the latter cannot be completely excluded and presentation can be similar. Intubation is usually necessary. Intravenous anti-staphylococcal antibiotics should be given after tracheal secretion swabs have been taken.

Remember that severe upper airway obstruction may not uncommonly result in acute pulmonary oedema which is thought to be brought about by the negative intrathoracic pressure resulting in the responsible hydrostatic changes.

You should be able to discuss the causes of chronic stridor. See Table 3.4.

Investigations of a child with chronic stridor consists of the following: chest X-ray (PA and lateral), neck X-rays, barium swallow, CT scan, MRI scan and possibly direct visualisation of the upper and lower airways using flexible laryngoscopy and bronchoscopy. Tracheomalacia on bronchoscopy looks U-shaped (instead of the usual circular shape) and collapses during expiration as a result of the lack of the cartilaginous rings encircling the majority of the tracheal or bronchial circumference.

Table 3.3 Continued

Cause of acute stridor	History	Management
Diphtheria	Coryzal symptoms and sore throat are followed rapidly by the development of a pseudomembrane (grey/white) which causes airway obstruction. The bacteria responsible is *Corynebacterium diphtheriae*. Release of a toxin results in carditis in week 2 (with tachycardia, heart failure), respiratory failure (secondary to diaphragmatic paralysis), palatal paralysis as well as limb paralysis in weeks 3–8.	Vaccination as prevention (Schick test checks immunity to diphtheria). For disease itself give antitoxin and antibiotic (erythromycin or penicillin). Management of airway obstruction.
Inhaled foreign body	Always suspect inhaled foreign body if the history describes an acute episode of choking or a sudden bout of coughing. The child is usually less than four years old. You should be aware that it may take several days before the features of a pneumonia may develop. Also suspect if there is unresolving pneumonia or bronchiectasis. On the other hand it may be immediately obvious by the presence of coarse stridor, fixed non-changing wheeze, aphonia, collapse or overinflation of a lobe depending on the site of lodgement of the body.	X-rays (AP + lateral) may help localise the foreign body if radio-opaque and identify hyperinflated lobe/collapse. In addition, an urgent rigid bronchoscopy under general anaesthetic should be performed in order to localise and remove the object. Remember that small objects have a predilection for the right main bronchus.

— *Vascular rings* should always be considered in the differential diagnosis of unexplained stridor, wheezing or cough, dysphagia or feeding difficulties in children. They result from congenital abnormalities in the main arteries in the thorax that cause compression of the trachea or oesophagus resulting in the above symptoms. Rings may be complete, that is completely

Table 3.4 Causes of chronic stridor

Laryngomalacia	The larynx is small with floppy aryepiglottic folds. It appears in the first month of life: mainly inspiratory stridor but some also demonstrate expiratory as well. The child grows and develops normally. The stridor appears worse when the child is supine, has an upper respiratory tract infection (URTI) or is agitated and crying. Improves spontaneously by age 1–3 years.
Subglottic stenosis	Stenosis just below the level of the cords. May be congenital or acquired (secondary to repeated or prolonged intubation, inhalation of noxious fumes or burns). Stridor worse if agitated, crying or intercurrent URTI. As the child grows the stenosis gets less severe.
Vocal cord palsy	This may result from more central CNS lesions or more peripheral lesions such as recurrent laryngeal nerve palsy secondary for example to intrathoracic pathology.
Compression leading to obstruction (intraluminal, luminal and extraluminal)	Examples include subglottic haemangioma (look for cutaneous haemangiomas that may also be present), cysts, compression of airways by vascular rings, laryngeal web, laryngeal papillomatosis (caused by HPV infection sometimes transmitted vertically via birth canal), retrosternal goitre, neoplasia and cystic hygroma.

encircling the trachea, usually producing more severe symptoms for example a double aortic arch, or incomplete, that is incomplete encircling where symptoms are less severe, such as anomalous innominate artery. Diagnosis is confirmed by CXR, barium swallow, echocardiogram, bronchogram, endoscopy, angiography and MRI. Clearly not all of these are necessary but it is not uncommon that the diagnosis will be picked up incidentally by using one of these techniques in investigating the presenting symptoms. Treatment is surgical. Remember that the long-term compression of tracheal structures may result in tracheomalacia or bronchomalacia which may persist post operatively.

— A baby who has had a *tracheo-oesophageal fistula* (TOF) repair in the past may have the following problems (essential knowledge for a possible long or short case): anastomotic leaks; strictures at the site of anastamosis (which may require intermittent balloon dilatation); gastro-oesophageal reflux; and commonly respiratory symptoms such as recurrent cough (TOF cough), bronchitis and pneumonia.

— It is possible that you may face a history of a *hypersensitivity pneumonitis* which is caused by inhalation of a type of organic dust, called extrinsic allergic alveolitis. It is thought to be caused by a combination of type 3 and 4 hypersensitivity reactions. Previous sensitisation is necessary and following re-exposure to the antigen the child develops fever, cough and dyspnea (usually 8–12 hours after contact with the antigen). Crackles may be heard on auscultation but wheezing does not occur in the majority of cases, and symptoms disappear after a few days. Eosinophilia is unusual. A chronic form occurs after severe repeated acute attacks, with pulmonary fibrosis, widespread crackles, dyspnoea on exertion and eventually respiratory failure (type 1) and cor pulmonale. Initial CXR features show patchy infiltrates leading to micronodular shadowing and later to honeycomb lung. Transfer factor is reduced. Diagnosis is also aided by estimation of precipitating antibody levels to the suspected antigen. Treatment involves prevention of allergen exposure and steroids may help reverse early disease. Examples include: Farmer's lung (exposure to mouldy hay- *Micropolyspora faeni*), Bird fancier's lung (exposure to bird droppings which contain serum avian proteins).

— Causes of pulmonary eosinophilia (combination of peripheral blood eosinophilia and eosinophillic lung infiltrates usually resulting in CXR shadows, confirmed by bronchoalveolar lavage or lung biopsy) include fungi (for example *Aspergillus fumigatus*), drugs (such as sulphonamides, NSAIDs, tetracyclines and nitrofurantoin), parasites (ascariasis and schistosomiasis), vasculitides (for example Churg–Strauss syndrome) and idiopathic causes.

— Some questions with a respiratory slant may make use of the hyponatraemia caused by SIADH (Syndrome of inappropriate ADH secretion) that occurs in some respiratory illnesses for example an acute asthma attack, pneumonia or following ventilation.

— Some questions give a history of a child — a few weeks to a few months of age — who has had feeding problems since birth, in particular choking bouts during feeds, vomiting and recurrent aspiration and chest infections. Intercurrent CXRs are normal and the baby appears to be growing and developing normally. In addition the question may also give you a history of apnoiec episodes (even in the absence of the above symptoms). Immediately you should think of two particular diagnoses to exclude: 1) *Gastro-oesophageal reflux*, excluded by a pH probe or barium study; 2) *H-type tracheoesophageal fistula* (5% of all TOFs) which can be difficult to diagnose by plain X-ray films but can be seen with a contrast barium swallow.

— The causes of lung fibrosis include sarcoidosis, extrinsic allergic alveolitis, congestive cardiac failure, fibrosing alveolitis, pneumoconiosis, sarcoidosis and drug reactions, for example busulphan, amiodarone, nitrofurantoin and methotrexate.

— *Haemoptysis* is fairly rare in children but could present as a grey case. The differential diagnosis includes: cystic fibrosis, pneumonia (including pneumococcus and TB), foreign body inhalation, bronchiectasis, bleeding diathesis, idiopathic haemosiderosis, vasculitis (e.g. Wegener granulomatosis), arteriovenous fistula and ruptured hydatid cyst.

— You may come across *allergic bronchopulmonary aspergillosis* (ABA). It occurs in long-standing asthmatic or cystic fibrosis patients as a result of an allergic reaction to *Aspergillus fumigatus* (type 1 and 4 hypersensitivity). The child will usually be in his second decade. Following sensitisation to the antigen additional exposure to the antigen results in a hypersensitivity reaction which results in recurrent episodes of fever, wheezing, crepitations, breathlessness with transient migratory pulmonary infiltrates manifest on the CXR as shadows on the lung fields. Later bronchiectasis develops (especially of the proximal airways) followed by progressive fibrosis. Investigations include: a full blood count which demonstrates the typical blood eosinophilia (also present in the sputum), increased serum IgE levels, serological tests for precipitating antibodies to *Aspergillus fumigatus* as well as a positive skin test to it (wheal and flare reaction). There are other pulmonary eosinophilias but ABA is the commonest. Avoidance of the antigen is impossible and the mainstay of treatment involves the use of steroids and bronchodilators. IgE levels fall with successful treatment. Other diseases caused by *aspergillus* include an aspergilloma forming in a lung cavity (may result in severe haemoptysis) and invasive aspergillosis.

— *Bronchiectasis* may be described in a question setting as a child who has a chronic productive cough with purulent sputum, halitosis, recurrent chest infections, episodes of haemoptysis (from a bronchial artery and thus systemic and not pulmonary blood) and clubbing. Coarse crackles and wheezing are heard on auscultation. CXR appearance shows typical tram lines caused by dilated bronchi in the affected lobe, including areas of fibrosis or evidence of the causative problem, which may be (a) obstruction e.g. an unrecognised foreign body; (b) severe viral infections, for example adenovirus, measles or pertussis; (c) allergic respiratory disorders such as allergic bronchopulmonary aspergillosis; (d) inherited disorders such as cystic fibrosis or Kartagener syndrome; and (e) in immunodeficiency syndromes. Resection is considered only for localised disease.

— You should of course be familiar with the connection between *cardiac disease and respiratory symptoms*. Cardiac failure may cause respiratory symptoms such as shortness of breath, wheezing, tachypnoea and bilateral fine crepitations on auscultation. In addition the presence of cardiac failure with pulmonary oedema predisposes to recurrent chest infections. Right-sided heart failure may cause respiratory symptoms as a result of the development of pleural effusions. Also remember the fact that respiratory diseases may cause right-sided heart failure secondary to chronically raised pulmonary hypertension (cor pulmonale).

— The causes of a bell-shaped chest include: pulmonary hypolasia, Jeune's asphyxiating thoracic dystrophy, Werdnig–Hoffman disease and bulbar palsy.

— You may be faced with a question relating to the oxygen dissociation curve in the viva. Remember the factors that shift the curve to the right (that is, the Hb releases oxygen more easily but is less good at giving it up): increased PCO_2 (mainly by an effect on pH — the Bohr effect), decreased pH, increased temperature, chronic hypoxia, anaemia, increased red cell 2,3 DPG (an end product of red-cell metabolism with increased production in chronic hypoxia, for example high altitude or chronic lung disease), HbS and polycythaemia. Factors that shift the curve to the left (good at taking up oxygen but less good less at giving it up) include a decrease in PCO_2, increased pH, decreased temperature, metHB, carboxy Hb and HbF.

— The causes of *pectus carinatum* include: Morquio syndrome, asphyxiating thoracic dystrophy, rickets and chronic respiratory problems such as obstructive airways disease.

Kartagener syndrome

Kartagener syndrome (immotile cilia syndrome) is a favourite exam topic. As the name suggests it is a disorder of cilia function and thus affects the respiratory system (as well as sperm in males). It is inherited in an AR fashion. You should be alerted to the possibility by chronic recurrent chest infections, recurrent sinus infections (that may masquerade as facial pain or headaches), nasal and sinus polyps, recurrent otitis media, bronchiectasis, clubbing and male infertility. Remember that these features are also features of cystic fibrosis (but note that in Kartagener there are no gastrointestinal features). In addition to these features situs inversus occurs in about 50% of patients (you may be shown a CXR of dextrocardia in the clinical examination or on a slide). Skull X-rays often show absent frontal sinuses. The diagnosis is made by electron microscopy of cilia obtained from nasal brushings in which structural abnormalities in the dynein arms of the cilia are demonstrated. Treatment involves management of the bronchiectasis and it is the rate of progression of bronchiectasis which determines the overall prognosis.

Your list of causes of recurrent pneumonia and persisting pneumonia should include: cystic fibrosis, Kartagener syndrome, gastro-oesophageal reflux, bronchiectasis, immunodeficiencies, foreign body and structural airway defects (these last two especially, if recurrent attacks are in the same lobe or lobes). Disorders giving rise to recurrent aspiration (such as bulbar palsy) and resistance of the organism to the antibiotic used are additional causes.

Pneumonia

Pneumonia is common in clinical practice and you should know some of the characteristics of the more prevalent ones (see Table 3.5).

NB *Haemophilus influenzae* and *Strep. pneumoniae* are encapsulated organisms and septicaemia from these organisms as a result of seeding from a pneumonia are more likely in splenectomised patients (for example, post splenectomy, sicklers) and immunocompromised patients (such as those with AIDS).

A child who has recurrent pneumonias which are slow to resolve may have bronchiectasis, obstruction of lower airways arising from any cause, presence of a foreign body, cystic fibrosis, cilia dysfunction, gastro-oesophageal reflux, cardiac failure with pulmonary oedema or the organism is not sensitive to the antibiotics used (see above). Neuromuscular disorders with bulbar palsy may have aspiration with recurrent chest infections. Pneumonias caused by *Staph.*, *Klebsiella*, and TB frequently cavitate.

Table 3.5 Comparison of the commoner organisms causing pneumonia in paediatric populations

Organism	Distinctive features
Pneumococcus (Strep. pneumoniae)	From two months of age and throughout childhood. Commonest cause of bacterial pneumonia. Patchy consolidation in younger children and lobar pattern in older children (commonest cause of lobar pneumonia). Small pleural effusions may occur. Rusty sputum or haemoptysis.
Haemophilus influenzae type B	From one month and throughout childhood but most common in under fives. Less prevalent now as a result of immunisation. Most commonly lobar and less commonly bronchopneumonia. Less acute presentation than Pneumococcus.
Mycoplasma pneumonia	From three to 15 years (most common in 10–15 year-olds). Gradual onset of symptoms. Cough, fever, headache, chest pain, sore throat are common and crepitations are heard in most. CXR highly variable but usually unilateral (often looks worse than clinical state of patient). Lower lobe bronchopneumonia is most common and hilar lymphadenopathy occurs in one third. Associations: croup, bronchiolitis, otitis media, bullous myringitis, meningoencephalitis, arthropathy and rashes, especially erythema multiforme. Postive Coombs' test with cold agglutinins in 50% of cases, some with haemolytic anaemia developing, diagnosis is by finding rising antibody titre ($\times$ 4 rise in 2–4 weeks). WCC is usually normal.
Staph. aureus	Most common in infants, also in immunocompromised children (remember chronic granulomatous disease as a cause), tracheostomy patients or prolonged intubation, post influenza and cystic fibrotics. Areas of patchy consolidation give rise to cyst and abscess formation (the result of tissue necrosis), air levels may be present in the cyst and give rise to the characteristic pneumatocoeles (*Klebsiella*, *Pseudomonas*, foreign bodies and TB may also cause abscess formation). Pneumothorax and empyema may result from abscess rupture.

You may be presented with an immunosuppressed child who develops a cough with shortness of breath. The likely possibilities include PCP pneumonia, atypical pneumonia, measles giant-cell pneumonitis (a type of pneumonitis that occurs in children with poor cell-mediated immunity) or any other type of pneumonia.

Table 3.5 *Continued*	
Organism	Distinctive features
Chlamydia trachomatis	Seen in infants up to about three months of age. It is acquired during delivery as the baby passes through the birth canal (up to 50% risk of transmission). Conjunctivitis is the most common presentation. The cough is described as a staccato pertussis-like cough with fine crepitations and an eosinophilia (in an apyrexial child). There may be a history of a conjunctivitis in preceding weeks or it may co-exist. CXR shows interstitial infiltrates. Diagnosis is by chlamydial swab from the eye (Giemsa stain showing chlamydia inclusion bodies in epithelial cells) and culture as well as serology. Treat the parents since infertility is a common complication.
Influenza virus	From infancy and throughout childhood. Typically with accompanying bronchitis and bronchiolitis. General malaise and coryzal symptoms. CXR shows interstitial pneumonia and peribronchial thickening (as with all viral pneumonias).
Parainfluenzae	Most commonly associated with croup but may cause similar picture to influenza.
Respiratory syncytial virus (RSV)	Commonest cause of bronchiolitis and common cause of pneumonia. Late autumn and winter. Half of all infants will acquire RSV infection in their first winter. Fever, cough, wheezing bilateral crackles throughout both lung fields, hyperinflated chest. CXR may show bronchopneumonic changes.
Pneumocystis carinii (PCP)	Immunocompromised children. Children in the first year of life may present with a chronic slowly progressing afebrile pneumonia. Bronchopneumonia or lobar involvement. CXR usually diffuse bilateral midzone alveolar shadowing (often looks worse than clinical findings). In older children cough, dyspnoea, tachypnoea, intercostal recession and possibly hypoxia and cyanosis are prominent features. Some HIV positive infants present in the first few months of life with a bronchiolitis-like syndrome but are RSV negative (but positive for PCP).

Tuberculosis

Tuberculosis is on the increase and thus a question topic. It is much commoner in the Asian population. Know a little about its natural history. Primary infection via inhalation of tubercle bacilli results in the Ghon focus (1–2 cm in diameter) which is subpleural and mid-zonal in position. The bacilli spread to the mediastinal and hilar lymph nodes to cause inflammation (caseous), but immunity develops quickly confining the lesion; together with the Ghon focus this forms the 'primary complex'. The primary lesion may be extrapulmonary in 25% of cases. Fibrosis or calcification may occur. Secondary or post-primary TB involves reactivation or reinfection with TB. These lesions tend to be in the posterior segment of the upper lobe or apex of the lower lobe (parts where aeration exceeds blood flow). Cell-mediated/type 4 hypersensitivity reaction takes place. In most people these lesions heal leading to calcified apical scars (Assman focus) but in a minority the disease spreads and caseating granulomas result in lung tissue necrosis leaving fibrotic and distorted lung tissue behind. This process results in haemoptysis and haematogenous spread and may result in miliary TB or in single organ involvement such as the CNS, urinary tract, bone or lymph nodes. Miliary TB may occur in primary or post-primary TB and the risk is greatest in the first year after infection, before the age of five and after puberty. Pleural involvement may result in a tuberculous empyema.

Clinical features will be dependent on the site affected.

Diagnosis

— *Microbiological*: Ziehl–Neelson stain for acid fast bacilli or culture on Lowenstein–Jensen medium. Gastric washings, early morning urine specimens and sputum if the patients is old enough provide sources.

— *Radiological*: Look for evidence of cavitating, calcified lesions.

— *Immunological*: Tuberculin test: Mantoux: Following intradermal injection of tuberculin (0.1 ml of 1 in 1000 strength PPD) cell-mediated response is read at 72 h. A positive response is induration (not just erythema) at the site of injection of more than 10 mm (< 5 mm is negative). A positive reaction (which may take 4–6 weeks to develop post infection) implies infection but immunity, that is previous infection or BCG, may also cause a positive test, although unlikely to produce induration of >10 mm (especially if 3–5 years following vaccination). If there is a large induration >15 mm this makes active infection more likely (even if low risk). A 5–10 mm wheal with an appropriate contact and clinical history should warrant a CXR and repeat test in six weeks' time (an intermediate response such as this may be the result of previous BCG or atypical mycobacterial infection).

— *Histological*: Caseating granulomas seen. Also stain for acid-fast bacilli.

— *Haematological*: ESR raised. If chronic, anaemia may develop.

— *Treatment*: Asymptomatic primary complex: Isoniazid for 6 months–1 year.

For symptomatic pulmonary disease 2 months' rifampicin, isoniazid, pyrazinamide and ethionamide and 4 months with rifampicin and isoniazid. Longer period of treatment is needed for extrapulmonary disease.

If a baby is born to a mother with TB (PPD positive) one should initially separate the baby from the mother and the baby should be given prophylaxis with isoniazid for three months; the tuberculin test and CXR should then be performed (BCG vaccination is also given by some). Isoniazid should also be given to those babies at risk of contact with infected individuals.

BCG is approximately 80% effective when given to teenagers and even more protective when given to babies in the first year of life, when it protects especially against miliary TB, TB meningitis and severe lung involvement. It should especially be offered to black and Asian babies.

A false negative tuberculin test may be the result of immunosuppression, malnutrition or severe widespread TB.

Differential diagnosis

— *Sarcoidosis*: This is rare in children but may be the basis for a grey case question. It is a non-caseating granulomatous disease which can affect any part of the body. It is most often seen in adolescents. Thoracic disease consists of bilateral hilar lymphadenopathy or may cause parenchymal lung disease with cough and dyspnoea. Skin signs include erythema nodosum, scar infiltration, raised nodules and lupus pernio. There may be generalised lymphadenopathy and hepatosplenomegaly. Eyes, heart, kidney, pituitary gland, cranial and peripheral nerves may also be affected.

Investigations include histological examination of lymph node biopsies. Bronchoalveolar lavage shows a high proportion of lymphocytes. The Kveim test is analogous to the tuberculin test in method but employs sarcoid spleen as the antigen. A positive reaction (granulomatous response within six weeks) strongly suggests sarcoidosis. Tuberculin test is negative. Hypercalcaemia, eosinophilia, serum ACE (reflecting disease activity) and immunoglobulins may all be elevated. Pulmonary function tests show a restrictive pattern and reduced diffusing capacity. Spontaneous remission may occur and active disease is treated with steroids.

— *Atypical mycobacteria*: There are several types of organisms in this category but *Mycobacterium avium-intracellulare* is the most common in the Western world. There is no history of exposure to TB and the child presents with a unilateral hard non-painful swelling (lymphadenitis) most commonly affecting the submandibular and cervical regions. Rarely lung disease resembling TB may occur and widespread disease is a feature of immuno-compromised patients such as those with AIDS. Diagnosis is by biopsy, histology and culture, and treatment involves surgical removal.

Asthma

Differential diagnoses of asthma include: viral-induced wheeze, cystic fibrosis, inhaled foreign body, heart failure, post-infectious wheeze, recurrent aspiration due to gastro-oesophageal reflux, airway compression caused by a cyst, tumour, adenopathy and cardiomegaly, immunodeficiency, Kartagener syndrome, congenital lung disease (as described above) and bronchomalacia.

Cough, wheeze and shortness of breath are the hallmarks of asthma. PEFR readings are a possible data question and you should be familiar with some commoner patterns such as the PEFR morning dipper, or reduction of PEFR by more than 15% following exercise challenge which may be reversed by bronchodilator administration.

A typical CXR during an asthmatic attack shows hyperinflated lung fields with flat diaphragms and increased bronchial markings.

Some children present with a troublesome nocturnal cough without any wheezing (common outpatient dilemma). These children may have post-nasal drip syndrome, asthma (especially house dust mite allergy-related exacerbations), sinusitis, inhaled foreign body, immunodeficiency or cystic fibrosis.

EXAMINATION OF THE RESPIRATORY SYSTEM

There are several chronic stable paediatric respiratory diseases and these conditions are highly likely to be called up in the clinical examinations. With the respiratory system you will have to tailor your examination to the age of the child: a number of examination procedures in the older child will not only be extremely difficult to perform in the younger child but more often than not will be uninformative.

— Introduce yourself to the child and parents.

— Undress the child's top half (to the waist) and stand back. Ideally the child should be at 45° and in the case of a baby on his back or in whatever position the infant is most comfortable at rest.

— *Inspection*: The younger the patient is the more important this part of the examination. Is the child in respiratory distress? Is the child using the accessory muscles of respiration? You should measure the respiratory rate (over 10 s and multiply by six for 1 min). Look for dysmorphic features; does the child look well/unwell, is he thriving? Are there any structural chest deformities (pectus excavatum/carinatum) or chest expansion? Look for abdominal wall movement, since children under the age of five are essentially diaphragmatic breathers and thus increased abdominal movements implies increased respiratory effort (in addition to other signs).

Look for Harrision's sulci (evidence of long-standing respiratory distress), cyanosis, nasal flaring, pursed lip breathing, tracheal tug, oxygen administration, intercostal recession or scars (from previous surgery, chest drain or tracheostomy). Look all round the chest including under the axillae. If you suspect cystic fibrosis glance at the abdomen looking for evidence of bowel surgery for a possible previous meconium ileus. Look for features of Cushing disease (as a result of steroid therapy for the respiratory disease). Look for the presence of haemangiomas in the presence of stridor. Listen for any audible breathing noises such as wheezing, stridor or cough.

— Take both hands and look specifically for clubbing, anaemia, cyanosis and tremor (ask the child to hold out his hands to look for the fine tremor of salbutamol administration or with their fingers widely separated for the flapping tremor of CO_2 retention).

— Ask the child to stick his or her tongue out to look for central cyanosis.

— Examine the cervical lymph nodes. At this stage of the examination this is done from the front, although of course it is ideally performed bimanually from the back when the patient is sitting forwards as you auscultate the back of the chest (if you remember to do it then) — the reason for doing it now is simply so that you do not forget it.

— Examine the trachea by gently putting your index finger in the gap between the trachea and the sternal head of sternocleidomastoid on each side and seeing if the gap on both sides is equal. Perform this on one side and then the other to avoid alarm to the child (who may be frightened or ticklish).

— Palpate the apex beat with the palm of your hand feeling for the most peripheral point that you can feel the apical heart beat. Define its position from the sternal angle which corresponds to the second intercostal space. Depending on whether the trachea or the apex beat or both have deviated will indicate whether the upper or lower mediastinum has shifted to a greater or lesser degree.

— *In an infant*: you should leave out palpation and percussion of the chest and go straight to auscultation at this point.

— *In an older child*: you should now palpate the chest. Spread your fingers out widely place both your hands on each side of the child's chest so that your fingertips are fixed tight against the lateral parts of the child's thorax and your thumbs meet in the midline over the sternum. As the child breathes your thumb movements should act as a gauge of chest expansion on each side of the chest.

— The next stage of palpation is tactile vocal fremitus (TVF). Place the palms of both hands on each side of the chest and ask the child to say 99. Feel for the vibratory sensation in your palms and assess if it is equal on both sides. This should be done on the upper, middle and lower parts of the chest wall. TVF is increased when there is underlying consolidation and reduced over a pneumothorax, pleural effusion or area of collapse.

— Now percussion. Warn the child that you are going to tap on his chest ('like a drum' many use). Start percussing in the supraclavicular fossa and work your way down the chest (top, middle and bottom) comparing right with left as you descend. Percuss additionally in the mid-axillary line on each side. Hyperresonance is seen in hyperinflation or pneumothorax and reduced in pleural effusion (stony dull), collapse, consolidation and over the liver and heart. Remember the liver will usually be at the level of the nipples in most cases (sixth intercostal space anteriorly).

— *Auscultation*: If the child is compliant then ask him to open his mouth and breathe in and out. Show them first and demonstrate how to do this properly. Listen with your stethoscope to the top, middle and bottom parts of the lung fields and then in the mid-axillary line, comparing right and left at each level. At each site listen for one cycle of inspiration and expiration:

you should be listening for the nature of the inspiration and expiration. Normal vesicular sounds consist of inspiration and the start of expiration with no break in between. Additional sounds such as crepitations, wheeze, pleural rubs, bronchial breathing (the same sound heard when the stethoscope is placed over the trachea: inspiration time = expiration time with a pause in between). Listen for a prolonged expiratory phase as seen in bronchial airway obstruction. If wheezing is present is it monophonic (implying obstruction of a single larger airway) or polyphonic (many airways). If crepitations are present, are they fine (for example, pulmonary oedema) or coarse (bronchiectasis, pneumonia).

— Now sit the child forwards. Now repeat TVF and percussion (though these two not in an infant) and auscultation over the back in the same fashion as you did over the front. As you come to auscultation use this time for bringing your clinical signs that you have found together.

— Sit the child back again and turning to the examiner say that to complete the respiratory examination you would like to perform an ENT examination, measure PEFR (if the child has evidence of bronchial obstruction) and plot the height and weight on a growth centile chart.

You may want to feel for a right ventricular heave (at the left sternal edge), listen for a loud P2 and ask to feel for liver enlargement and peripheral oedema if you suspect cor pulmonale.

Presentation to the examiner

On examination of the child:

— *Always mention*: whether the child was in respiratory distress or not at rest, whether the child was cyanosed, whether the child was clubbed or not, and the respiratory rate.

— *Mention only if present*: dysmorphology, scars, mediastinal shift, and lymphadenopathy.

— *Then*: describe your findings on palpation (TVF and expansion), percussion and auscultation (breath sounds and any additional sounds).

Then say that these findings are consistent with whatever you think the diagnosis is.

Nephrology

Renal questions are common in the examination. You should have a grasp of the basic physiology of renal function since some basic science knowledge is required. The clinical examination section is incorporated with the clinical section of the gastroenterology chapter since it is usually examined as part of the abdominal examination.

BASIC RENAL PHYSIOLOGY

The functions of the kidney are as follows:

1. Fluid and electrolyte homeostasis.
2. Excretion of waste products and drugs.
3. Hormonal: Vitamin D metabolism (1-alpha hydroxylation of 25-hydroxycholecalciferol), erythropoietin production, renin production and prostaglandin production.
4. Acid-base homeostasis.

Renal blood flow accounts for about 20% of the cardiac output. Most of this (approximately 90%) is carried to the renal cortex (that is, the glomeruli). Urine begins to be produced by about the third month of gestation. The fetus does not rely on the kidneys for waste product excretion since this is performed by the placenta (it does, however, produce a very dilute urine which is a major component of the amniotic fluid). All the nephrons have been formed by birth (approximately 1 million in each kidney). There can be no further increase in the number of the nephrons after birth (although compensatory hypertrophy is possible following damage). Although the total number of nephrons is complete at birth the glomerular filtration rate (GFR) at birth is only 20 ml/min/1.73 m^2 (compared to adult values of about 120 ml/min/1.73 m^2). Adult values are reached between the first and second years of life.

In the cortex ultrafiltration occurs at the glomerulus and the filtrate enters Bowman's capsule. Ultrafiltration is dependent upon renal blood flow, hydrostatic pressure and plasma oncotic pressure (similar to Starling's forces in the capillary). The glomerular ultrafiltrate is then mostly reabsorbed (two-thirds) from the proximal convoluted tubule (PCT). Sodium is reabsorbed actively and is followed passively by water. In addition glucose, potassium (almost complete absorption), bicarbonate, phosphate and amino acids are absorbed in the PCT. The straight portion of the PCT secretes some organic acids such as penicillin.

In the loop of Henle that protrudes into the medulla about 20–25% of the water and sodium are absorbed. The fluid entering the loop is isotonic but leaves hypotonic. There is a counter current multiplier present with active chloride transported from the thick (water impermeable) ascending limb of the loop of Henle. The result of this process is that the medullary interstitium becomes very hypertonic and this is extremely important for urinary concentration (remembering that the collecting ducts pass in very close proximity to the tips of the loops of Henle). The hypotonic filtrate reaches the distal convoluted tubule (DCT) whose walls are impermeable to water. In its wall there is, however, a pump that reabsorbs a sodium cation in exchange for a potassium or hydrogen ion: it is controlled by aldosterone. Thus in the DCT sodium chloride reabsorption, potassium excretion and urinary acidification occur. In the last part of the journey through the nephron the urine passes through the collecting ducts which as mentioned before pass close to the tips of the loops of Henle deep in the medulla. The concentration of the urine is under the control of the hormone ADH (secreted from the posterior pituitary) which increases the permeability of the collecting ducts and thus allows the concentration of urine to occur.

The concentrating ability of the kidney increases during gestation: however, the newborn term baby still has a reduced ability to conserve sodium (compared to older children). Other tubular functions are also reduced, such as the excretion of phosphate, which results in higher phosphate levels. A reduced bicarbonate threshold and ability for hydrogen ion excretion means that neonates may tolerate acidic insults less well.

Various hormones have an influence on kidney function. An increase in plasma osmolality causes an increase in thirst and the release of ADH from the posterior pituitary gland (which as described above affects urinary concentration via collecting duct permeability). Reduced renal perfusion results in the production of renin from renin substrate (renin release is also controlled by sympathetic stimulation). Renin is produced from the juxtaglomerular apparatus that is located on the afferent arteriole that enters the glomerulus. Renin release subsequently activates the conversion of angiotensinogen to angiotensin I which is then converted by angiotensin converting enzyme (ACE) to angiotensin II. Angiotensin II increases thirst, produces marked vasoconstriction and increases the production of aldosterone from the zona glomerulosa in the adrenal cortex. Aldosterone has its main action on the DCT where it promotes the reabsorption of sodium and water (in exchange for potassium and hydrogen ions) thus completing the feedback loop by increasing the vascular extracellular volume. Atrial natriuretic peptide found in atrial tissue (released in conditions of fluid overload) is a vasodilator and promotes natriuresis. Prostaglandins are important in the distribution of blood flow within the kidney itself.

PRESENTATION OF RENAL DISEASE

Renal disease presents in a limited number of ways.

— Flank mass
— Haematuria
— Pain (loin pain, suprapubic pain, groin pain)
— Oedema
— Polyuria/oliguria
— Hypertension
— Metabolic consequences of renal disease such as rickets
— A single umbilical artery in the umbilical cord is associated with renal anomalies and the baby should have an ultrasound performed (and possibly a karyotype).

RENAL INVESTIGATIONS

Renal failure

A common clinical scenario is the child who presents with oliguria. Questions will often present you with a few laboratory investigations and ask you to determine the particular type of renal failure (that is, prerenal, renal or post-renal). Know a list of causes of each type of renal failure. Remember that it is of extreme importance to differentiate these types since rapid correction of pre-renal failure caused by hypoperfusion will reduce the risk of progression to acute tubular necrosis, and in turn to the more serious acute cortical necrosis which damages glomeruli permanently. In prerenal failure the kidneys are still functioning to conserve sodium and water (thus urinary sodium will be low).

The question may guide you to the suspicion of acute renal failure (ARF) by describing a lethargic child who may be dehydrated or fluid overloaded, oliguric (less than 1.0 ml/kg/hour), oedematous, or with features of acidosis (Kussmaul breathing) or comatose as a result of hypertensive encephalopathy. You should be able to distinguish between prerenal and renal failure with appropriate laboratory investigations (see Table 4.1).

In post-renal failure the indices are extremely variable and thus not useful: you must therefore place importance on your history and examination. Unless the onset was acute there may be a history of reduced urinary stream for some time, abdominal or flank pain, UTIs, passage of renal stones or a history of a disease associated with renal outflow obstruction such as renal tubular acidosis (which predisposes to stones). Examine for a flank mass. A palpable bladder is associated with urethral obstruction. In every patient with unexplained acute renal failure an ultrasound scan is vital to exclude obstruction.

Measuring GFR

Ideally a substance is required that is freely filtered by the glomerulus but that is neither reabsorbed or secreted (e.g. insulin). Clinically creatinine clearance is used as an approximation to GFR (creatinine is only minimally reabsorbed

Table 4.1 Comparison of laboratory investigations in prerenal and renal failure

	Prerenal failure	Renal failure
Urine osmolality (mOsmol/l)	> 500	< 350 (inability to concentrate urine)
Urine sodium (mmol/l)	< 10 (remember in fluid depletion kidneys retain sodium and water)	> 20
Urine/plasma urea ratio	> 5	< 5
Urine/plasma osmolality	> 1.3	< 1.3
Fluid challenge +/– frusemide	Diuresis	No change
Urinalysis	Usually normal	Haematuria, proteinuria, WCC, casts
Ultrasound scan	Normal	Normal, enlarged or increased echogenicity
Clinical features	History of precipitant e.g. severe gastroenteritis. Signs of fluid depletion. Cold extremities. Reduced capillary return, reduced skin turgor, sunken eyes, tachycardia, orthostatic, hypertension.	History of precipitant e.g. haemolytic uraemic syndrome. May have fluid overload with periorbital and pedal oedema, hypertension, bounding pulses, CCF. Visible neck veins.

in the tubules). Plasma creatinine alone is not an ideal measurement of renal function. Remember that creatinine concentration changes with body composition, age and sex and during renal insufficiency creatinine is reabsorbed to varying degrees. Neonatal creatinine concentrations reflect maternal concentrations at birth, however the true neonatal values are reached in the first few days of life.

GFR = U × V/P (U = urine creatinine concentration (mg/dl); V = volume of urine collected over period of time (ml/min); P = serum creatinine (mg/dl)).

This must be corrected for surface area by multiplying by 1.73/SA. Since collecting 24 h urine specimens can be a difficult process in children, GFR is sometimes measured by determining the rate of fall of concentration of an injected radioactive isotope (for example, Cr51 EDTA with radiation measurements of blood samples taken at 2 and 4 h post-injection).

Urea

The plasma urea concentration depends on the GFR and the urea production rate. Its level may be increased by a high protein diet, catabolic states such as infection, trauma and surgery, steroid use, glomerular disease, hypotension and renal obstructive disease. Its level may be decreased by a low protein diet or high GFR in hyperdynamic states. It is important to remember that the large reserve of renal function means that the plasma, urea and creatinine concentrations will not rise until there is about a 50% reduction in the GFR. Once kidney disease has produced a rise in their concentrations it is more useful to follow the progression of disease with plasma creatinine compared to plasma urea.

Complement levels

Measuring complement levels is useful in various renal diseases. Reduced complement levels are seen in lupus nephritis, post-streptococcal glomerulonephritis, mesangio-capillary glomerulonephritis (associated with C-3 nephritic factor), cryoglobulinaemia, infective endocarditis and chronically infected atrioventricular shunts.

Urinary microscopy

— Red cells imply haematuria. Know a list of causes starting from the top and working your way down the urinary tract, dividing the causes into painful and painless causes.

— White cells are seen in any inflammatory infective disorder affecting the urinary tract (more than 10 WCC/mm^3 is considered abnormal).

— Casts are cylindrical in shape and are moulded into the shape of the distal renal tubule.

— Hyaline casts are transparent and do not indicate renal disease on their own.

— Granular casts which look more granular because of precipitated protein on their surface are seen in glomerular and tubular disease although finely granular casts may be seen in normal children.

— White cell casts are typically seen in acute pyelonephritis and interstitial nephritis. Thus if a child with a UTI is found to have white cell casts, suspect acute pyelonephritis.

— Red cell casts are always pathological and indicate renal disease — almost always glomerulonephritis.

— Provided that the urine has been collected in an aseptic fashion the demonstration of bacteria after Gram stain indicates infection and is a useful indicator until more confirmatory tests of culture are available.

Renal biochemistry

These are a good source of questions for the data interpretation and grey cases and you must therefore have a grasp of the commoner patterns.

Acute renal failure

To some extent this has already been dealt with but know the typical biochemistry picture.

Sodium: high if volume depleted but low if fluid overload
Potassium: raised
Phosphate: raised
Hydrogen ions: raised (low pH)
Urea: raised
Creatinine: raised
Urate: raised
Calcium: low
Bicarbonate: low.

Chronic renal failure

Here there is a slow and irreversible reduction in the number of functioning nephrons resulting in reduced glomerular and tubular dysfunction. This results in a gradual onset of uraemia as a result of declining GFR. Urinary osmolality will eventually equal the osmolality of filtered plasma.

— Urea is raised and will also reflect the degree of hydration of the patient. Creatinine clearance will indicate the degree of renal dysfunction.

— Plasma sodium will generally reflect the degree of hydration of the patient: there is, however, overall sodium retention partly caused by renin release.

— Potassium is raised.

— Phosphate is raised secondary to phosphate retention by the kidneys.

— Calcium: In chronic renal failure vitamin D metabolism is affected by lack of 1-alpha hydroxylation. Thus a lowering of plasma calcium levels results in osteomalacia (lack of bone mineralisation) and a secondary hyperparathyroidism which results in bone resorption and thus osteoporosis (loss of bone density). These effects along with phosphate retention contribute to the picture of renal osteodystrophy.

— Acidosis helps prevent the patient from tetany as the hydrogen ions displace plasma protein-bound calcium increasing the total amount of ionised calcium in the blood.

— Urate is raised.

— For completeness erythropoietin production declines and results in a normochromic normocytic anaemia.

Renal tubular acidosis (RTA)

This is a much hated topic for candidates revising for the examination but a very common question! I will therefore give it a disproportionate amount of space compared to its clinical incidence, so that I cover all of the salient points necessary to answer any questions relating to it. A comparison of proximal and distal renal tubular acidosis is found in Table 4.2.

— *Normal urinary acidification*: plasma acid-base homeostasis is achieved predominantly by the kidneys controlling the amount of bicarbonate in the

Table 4.2 Comparison of proximal and distal renal tubular acidosis

	Distal RTA (Type 1)	Proximal RTA (Type 2)
Age at presentation	Childhood or adolescence	Infancy
Incidence	Commoner	Rarer
Main pathology	Failure of distal tubular hydrogen ion excretion	Failure of proximal tubular bicarbonate reabsorption
Metabolic picture	Normal anion gap Hyperchloraemic metabolic acidosis with inappropriately high urinary pH	Normal anion gap Hyperchloraemic metabolic acidosis with inappropriately high urinary pH
Urinary pH	Urinary pH never below 5.5–6.0	Urine pH can fall below 5.5
Typical presentation (in addition to features of precipitating/causative disease)	Classically with failure to thrive from infancy. Hypokalaemia presents as muscle weakness, hyporeflexia, polyuria, polydipsia etc. Renal stones and nephrocalcinosis are common cf. proximal RTA. Rickets secondary to bone buffering the acidosis.	Classically with growth failure and vomiting. Hypokalaemia presents as muscle weakness, hyporeflexia, polyuria, polydipsia. In addition features of Fanconi syndrome may be present (see below). No nephrocalcinosis.
Hypokalaemia	++	+
Treatment	Aim to correct acidosis to allow normal growth and prevent nephrocalcinosis; potassium and bicarbonate supplements. Beware of correcting acidosis before potassium supplementation because of possible life threatening hypokalaemia.	Aim to correct acidosis to allow normal growth; potassium and bicarbonate supplements
Bicarbonate replacement	Smaller doses such as 1–3 mmol/kg/day	Large doses such as 10 mmol/kg/day
Prognosis	Variable	Good

plasma. Usually 85% of filtered bicarbonate is reabsorbed in the proximal convoluted tubule in exchange for hydrogen ion excretion (at normal plasma bicarbonate concentrations). The remaining 15% of the filtered bicarbonate is reabsorbed by the distal convoluted tubule again in exchange for hydrogen ion excretion. The secreted H+ ions combine with the urine buffers ammonia (NH_3) and H_2PO_4. Renal tubular acidosis occurs when the kidneys are unable to maintain a normal plasma bicarbonate concentration.

Distal renal tubular acidosis: Type 1 RTA
— Pathophysiology: There is an inability of the distal nephron to secrete hydrogen ions (resulting in failure to reabsorb the remaining 15% of

filtered bicarbonate and also a failure to acidify the urine). Thus metabolic acidosis occurs. Since there is no hydrogen ion excretion the sodium fails to be reabsorbed (via the Na/K/H pump) and as a result of the intravascular depletion that ensues aldosterone release increases and promotes potassium loss.

Causes include:

— Idiopathic

— Familial

— Drugs e.g. amphotericin toxicity

— Inherited diseases: sickle cell disease, osteopetrosis

— Systemic diseases: Sjogren disease, SLE, chronic active hepatitis

— Diseases causing nephrocalcinosis: hyperparathyroidism, hypercalciuria, vitamin D intoxication, medullary sponge kidney

— Interstitial renal disease: chronic pyelonephritis, obstructive nephropathy.

Proximal renal tubular acidosis: Type 2 RTA

— *Pathophysiology*: There is reduced proximal tubular reabsorption of bicarbonate. The extra bicarbonate in the tubular fluid reaches the DCT and here there is some compensatory reabsorption of bicarbonate ions. Eventually this capacity is exceeded and bicarbonate spills into the urine and the plasma bicarbonate falls until an equilibrium is reached between the plasma and tubular fluid, that is all the filtered bicarbonate is reabsorbed (this occurs when the plasma bicarbonate is usually between 15 and 20 mmol/l). Urine can be acidified since distal hydrogen ion excretion is normal. In an attempt to hold on to hydrogen ions, potassium is lost in the DCT in exchange for sodium ions at the Na/K/H pump. Proximal RTA can occur in isolation but is usually part of a more global proximal renal tubular dysfunction called Fanconi syndrome (see later).

Causes include:

— Primary/idiopathic

— As part of Fanconi syndrome

— Familial disease: cystinosis, Lowe syndrome, galactosaemia, Wilson disease, hereditary fructose intolerance, tyrosinaemia

— Drugs and toxins: heavy metal poisoning (lead, cadmium, mercury), acetazolamide (carbonic anhydrase inhibitor), out of date tetracyclines

— Others: renal transplantation, renal vein thrombosis and interstitial nephritis.

In order to distinguish between the two types of renal tubular acidosis firstly demonstrate that the child has a normal anion gap metabolic acidosis (by performing a serum urea and electrolytes and blood gas), and an inappropriately high urinary pH (a pH > 6 in the presence of metabolic acidosis is always abnormal). Next you must demonstrate whether the child can acidify their urine by lowering the urine pH < 5.5. This can be achieved by using the NH_4CL loading test. If the urinary pH falls below 5.5 then the diagnosis is likely to be proximal RTA; if the urinary pH stays above 5.5 the diagnosis is likely to be distal RTA.

Normal urinary pH values vary during the day and are affected by diet but are usually between 5–6 (with a range between 4.6–8.0).

Renal tubular acidosis: Type 4

Type 4 RTA is caused by a reduced production or unresponsiveness to aldosterone, leading to a metabolic acidosis with hyperkalaemia. Urine pH can fall below 5.5 during acidotic states. It occurs in a number of conditions:

a. Aldosterone deficiency: congenital adrenal hyperplasia, Addison disease, tubulointerstitial disease (hyporeninaemia)
b. Aldosterone resistance: tubulointerstitial disease, drugs (spironolactone, amiloride, triamterine)
c. Others: post renal transplant, chronic pyelonephritis.

Whenever you are given biochemical data with a low plasma sodium and high potassium level consider aldosterone deficiency/resistance.

Fanconi syndrome

This is an inherited or acquired syndrome associated with a defect of proximal tubular function with characteristic impaired reabsorption of glucose, phosphate, generalised amino aciduria, bicarbonate, potassium, sodium and water loss.

Clinically it presents with failure to thrive, polyuria, polydipsia, hypophosphataemic rickets, hypokalaemia (weakness, constipation) and proximal RTA. Of course the features of the precipitating disease will also be among the clinical features.

The causes are similar to those described above causing proximal renal tubular acidosis.

Bartter syndrome

This is another common question that you should recognise. The pathophysiology is not fully understood. There is a defect in chloride (and thus sodium) reabsorption in the ascending loop of Henle. There is juxtaglomerular apparatus hyperplasia. This results in raised renin levels and consequently raised aldosterone levels. There is a normal blood pressure (and no peripheral oedema) despite raised renin and aldosterone levels (and reduced pressor response to infused angiotensin). There is raised urinary excretion of prostaglandin E2. Bartter can be distinguished from other causes of hyperaldosteronism by the absence of hypertension.

— *Metabolic picture:* There are decreased sodium, potassium and chloride levels; metabolic alkalosis; and increased urinary chloride excretion. **NB** You must have a list of other causes of hypochloraemic hypokalaemic metabolic alkalosis in your differential diagnosis. They include: diuretic abuse and extra renal causes of chloride loss such as pyloric stenosis, persisting diarrhoea or vomiting, cystic fibrosis and chloridhorrhea.

— *Clinically:* Failure to thrive, polyuria, polydipsia, muscle weakness, constipation (last four secondary to hypokalaemia), salt craving and tetany (secondary to reduced ionised calcium concentration due to alkalosis).

— *Treatment:* Potassium supplements, sodium supplements and diuretics such as spironolactone (an aldosterone antagonist) and amiloride (blocking distal K secretion). Prostaglandin synthesis inhibitors for example indomethacin are also used. This will improve the majority of biochemical abnormalities to normal: however potassium depletion persists to some extent.

Renal hypertension

You may be given some data for a hypertensive child as follows.

Sodium: 143 mmol/l
Potassium: 2.8 mmol/l
Bicarbonate: 32 mmol/l
Urea: 2.6 mmol/l
Creatinine: 35 µmol/l.

As mentioned above the presence of a high sodium and low potassium pattern should trigger thoughts of hyperaldosteronism. The converse is also true, in other words a low sodium and high potassium should make you think of hypoaldosteronism: the metabolic alkalosis adds strength to the diagnosis.

Remember that in terms of hyperaldosterone hypertensive conditions relating to the kidney, you have to distinguish between renal artery stenosis (usually caused by fibromuscular dysplasia in the paediatric population) and primary hyperaldosteronism (Conn syndrome) — see Table 4.3. In Conn syndrome a useful screening test is to check the plasma and urinary electrolytes. Plasma K is usually less than 3.5 mmol/l and urinary excretion is usually in excess of 30 mmol/day (provided the child has not received diuretics or had a high salt intake). Both cases will of course give a hypokalaemic alkalosis.

In the case of primary hyperaldosteronism two-thirds are the result of an aldosterone-secreting adenoma and one-third of adrenal hyperplasia and only rarely adrenal carcinoma. The increased blood pressure will inhibit renin secretion. Interestingly in adrenal hyperplasia serum aldosterone levels increase on ambulation whereas they decrease on ambulation in the case of an adenoma.

Table 4.3 A comparison of renal artery stenosis and primary hyperaldosteronism

	Renal artery stenosis	Primary hyperaldosteronism
Serum renin	High	Low
Serum aldosterone	High	High

Using catheter studies it is possible to sample blood from various sites, and in the case of renal artery stenosis the blood renin level in the lower inferior vena cava will of course be lower than in the upper IVC. The actual side of the stenosis can be determined by sampling the blood from both renal veins (renin levels will of course be higher on the affected side). By similar methods adrenal vein sampling will help determine the affected side in Conn syndrome. Sodium/potassium urinary concentration ratios may also be helpful. Renal arteriography may be used to identify the anatomy of a stenosis more clearly. Other methods include a renal doppler ultrasound scan and a captopril renal scan.

You should also know the other renal causes of hypertension such as chronic renal failure and renal tumours.

Any initial investigation in a child found to be hypertensive must include urinalysis, urine MC&S, serum U&Es and a renal ultrasound. Further investigations will of course be guided by the results of these.

Cystinuria

This topic comes up in various forms in the examination. You should know that it is caused by impaired renal and gastrointestinal transport of the dibasic amino acids cystine, ornithine, arginine and lysine (COAL). It is inherited in an AR fashion. The only clinical effect of this is the production of cystine renal stones (in about 3% of sufferers) because of its low solubility. This can go on to produce repeated infections, haematuria, obstructive nephropathy and ultimately renal failure. In data interpretation questions the condition may be recognised by the following:

— *Urinalysis:* Yellow/brown hexagonal crystals

— *Positive urine cyanide nitroprusside test.* Also positive in Fanconi syndrome, homocystinuria, generalised amino aciduria and other rarer disorders.

The diagnosis can be confirmed by urine chromatography or electrophoresis.

Radiological studies may show stones which are typically bilateral and staghorn in appearance. Treatment consists of a high fluid intake, alkani-sation of the urine with bicarbonate/citrate (keeping the urinary pH over 7.5). Stone dissolution can sometimes be achieved with captopril or D-penicillamine.

URINE TESTS

Urine colour

— **Red urine:** Haematuria, haemoglobinuria, myoglobinuria, beeturia, acute intermittent porphyria, urates especially in neonates (with concentrated urine). Serratia marcessans can form a reddish pigment causing a nappy to look red.

— **Black urine:** This may be caused by alkaptonuria after urinary exposure to air (caused by homogentisic acid excretion). It is also seen in melanotic sarcomas resulting from melanin excretion in the urine.

— *Urine that darkens on standing:* The urine could contain either porphobilinogen or urobilinogen. These are colourless, but on standing exposed to the air are converted to porphobilin and urobilin respectively both of which are orange-brown.

Clinitest and Clinistix

Knowledge of these will be expected. See chapter 10. Clinistix is a urine dipstick test that is specific for glucose. Clinitest is a urine dipstick test that detects reducing sugars including glucose, for example lactose, fructose and galactose (useful for galactosaemia), not sucrose. Note the false positives seen with ascorbic acid and homogentisic acid.

See above for urine microscopy description.

RENAL STONES

These can usually be seen on a plain abdominal X-ray. Only pure uric acid, xanthine and oxalate stones will appear radiolucent, they may however be detected on ultrasound scan.

— *Calcium-containing stones* (85%): Calcium oxalate, calcium phosphate, mixed. Causes: idiopathic, primary hyperparathyroidism, renal tubular acidosis, hyperoxaluria and the milk-alkali syndrome.

— *Triple stones* (magnesium ammonium phosphate) 10%. Associated with infection (especially *Proteus* infection). Their formation is favoured by high urinary pH.

— *Uric acid stones* (5%): increased uric acid excretion, for example tumour lysis syndrome. Their formation is favoured by a low urinary pH.

— *Cystine stones* (1%) Cystinuria. Their formation is favoured by low urinary pH.

Investigations

— 24 h urinary calcium, phosphate, oxalate, uric acid and amino acid urine collection. Urinary pH. Calcium: creatinine ratio (usually < 0.2). Urine microscopy and crystal examination.

— Urine MC&S

— Plasma electrolytes, uric acid and blood gas

— Renal imaging to exclude obstruction or reflux.

Hyperuricaemia may be seen in gout, Lesch–Nyhan syndrome, myeloproliferative disorders, tumour lysis syndrome, high purine diet, hyperparathyroidism, lead poisoning, Down syndrome, exercise, starvation, drugs (low dose salicylates, thiazide diuretics) and alcohol ingestion.

RENAL RADIOGRAPHY

There are many radiological methods of visualising the renal tract and they are all potential slides, parts of data interpretation questions, grey cases or topics for discussion in the clinical examination.

Plain abdominal X-rays

These can be used to look for calcification in the kidneys. Nephrocalcinosis is characterised by the presence of pyramidal deposits of calcium found within the kidney parenchyma itself. The causes include renal tubular acidosis (distal mainly), hyperparathyroidism, sarcoidosis, hyperoxaluria, idiopathic hypercalciuria and the milk-alkali syndrome. Other causes of calcification in the renal tract are calcium-containing stones, calcified tumour, TB, calcified hydatid cyst, calcified haemorrhage, infarct or cyst.

The renal shadow can usually be seen on a plain abdominal X-ray and renal size can thus be estimated. Note that the long axes of the kidneys are not vertical but oblique and parallel to the psoas muscle. The right kidney is usually lower than the left kidney (a result of liver displacement).

Intravenous urography (IVU)

Following intravenous administration of dye serial X-rays are taken of the renal tract. Always compare the films with a control film taken with no dye. The kidney outline should always be smooth and if it is irregular you should consider renal scarring. The dye is first taken up by the kidney within 5 min post-injection. Renal outline and size can be identified as well as the presence of space occupying lesions. Following this so-called nephrogram, the pelvis followed by the ureters and bladder are outlined, and you should look for strictures and stones.

A common slide is of duplication of the renal collecting system. It is common (F > M) with 30% of cases being bilateral. Here the kidney has two ureters leaving it, one from the upper pole and one from the lower. The ureter from the upper pole is usually associated with obstruction and the ureter from the lower pole with vesicoureteric reflux.

A horseshoe kidney (usually asymptomatic) shows loss of the normal long axis lie of the kidneys. It can present as a midline mass.

Micturating cystourethrogram (MCUG)

In this investigation the bladder is filled (via a urinary catheter) with contrast dye and the child is X-rayed during voiding. The main indication for this investigation is following UTIs in children in order to exclude vesicoureteric reflux. Be familiar with the grading system for vesicoureteric reflux. A posterior urethral valve can be easily demonstrated with an MCUG. There is usually a markedly dilated proximal urethra. In some slides an MCUG and IVU may look surprisingly similar but you should look for the dye-introducing catheter (in an MCUG) to help you distinguish them.

Ultrasound

Extremely useful in diagnosing renal masses, renal obstruction, renal size and renal cystic disease.

CT scan

Useful for looking at the retroperitoneal space that is not easily accessible with other types of scanning.

DMSA, DTPA and MAG3 scans

These scans are included in data interpretation questions. DMSA (dimercaptosuccinic acid) is taken up and retained by the tubular cells in the kidney. The scan is a static scan. It is used to determine renal shape and size, and renal function. It picks up areas of functioning renal tissue and uptake is proportional to function. It will thus show the shape and size of the kidneys and will pick up areas of kidney scarring. It has a higher sensitivity and specificity for detecting scars as compared to IVU. Function is usually split fairly evenly between the two kidneys, approximately 45–55% upper limit of normal. It should be performed at least six weeks post UTI for accurate results.

A DTPA (diethylene triamine pentacetic acid) scan is a dynamic scan, excreted by glomerular filtration following venous injection. A Tc99m MAG3 scan (Tc-mercaptoacetyltriglycerine) is another type of dynamic scan and is excreted from the kidney by tubular secretion. MAG3 scans generally give better pictures of the tract when there is impaired renal function compared to DTPA scans. Following intravenous injection the patient is scanned for emissions by the tracer and a time/activity curve is produced. Thus the function of the kidney, from tracer filtration through to tracer excretion from the collecting system is assessed. We can thus assess renal blood flow, renal obstruction, bladder voiding (including assessing vesicoureteric reflux) and determine GFR. Frusemide is sometimes injected to help distinguish outflow obstruction from a dilated non-obstructed tract (which may appear obstructed because of tracer stasis). In the case of a dilated non-obstructed outflow tract frusemide will help wash out the isotope from the kidneys, but in the case of a truly obstructed tract there will be no washout. See Fig. 4.1.

Understanding the DTPA scan (Fig. 4.1)

The letters (a), (b) and (c) correspond to the letters on the graph in Fig. 4.1.

a. A normal kidney.
b. An obstructed kidney.
c. A kidney with hydronephrosis (non-obstructed).
1. In the normal kidney initially the count of tracer will increase sharply from 0 as the DTPA is injected, followed by a slower rise as the tracer is taken up by the kidneys. This reaches a peak at around 3–4 min.
2. As DTPA begins to be excreted from the kidney we can see the count gradually fall as the tracer leaves the kidney and enters the outflow tract.

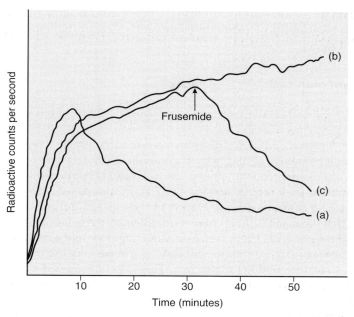

Fig. 4.1 A typical DTPA scan result from a normal and an obstructed kidney.

3. In the case of the obstructed kidney we can see that DTPA is taken up by the kidney but fails to be excreted, shown by the failure of the tracer count falling. We can see that injection of frusemide has no effect on curve (b) but results in excretion of tracer in curve (c) simply implying that there is a true obstruction rather than a dilated non-obstructed system in case (b) and the converse in curve (c).

CLINICAL SCENARIOS

Hypertension

Hypertension is a common presentation of renal disease in the child population. In severe cases the child may present with hypertensive encephalopathy. There may be a past history of abnormal urinalysis such as proteinuria or haematuria. Plasma U&Es may have been failed to be taken in response to these urinary results, and the renal disease may have progressed until the child presents in chronic renal failure. Look for specific clues such as a family history of hypertension, previous UTIs or drug ingestion. Examination clues include looking for syndromes, especially Cushing syndrome, William syndrome (hypercalcaemia), neurofibromatosis (renal artery stenosis) and phaeocromocytoma, listening for renal artery bruits, differential blood pressure in arms and legs (coarctation of the aorta), signs of raised intracranial hypertension (Cushing reflex), obesity, abdominal masses (for example, nephroblastoma or hydronephrosis) and virilisation (congenital adrenal hyperplasia). Retinal hypertensive changes are indicative of chronicity of the hypertension. As in adult hypertensive disease examination and investigations will be geared to looking for cause and effects of the hypertension on various systems.

History of skin rash

A common clinical scenario is the child who presents in renal failure who has had a history of a skin rash. The possibilities are:

1. *Henoch–Schönlein purpura.* This is an allergic vasculitis (IgA mediated with the same pathological findings as IgA nephropathy). It may be proceeded by a viral or streptococcal illness. The M:F ratio is 2:1, peaking in the winter months. It is usually first noticed as maculopapular urticarial-type lesions over extensor surfaces mainly of the legs and buttocks. In addition there may be some diffuse cutaneous oedema on the face and dorsum of the hands and feet. There is then a fairly rapid progression of the lesion into the classic non-thrombocytopaenic purpuric rash. At the time of the skin lesions the child is usually well. This may be followed by abdominal pain which is classically colicky because of gastrointestinal involvement causing oedema and haemorrhage into the gut wall (GI haemorrhage may cause malaena, fresh rectal or occult bleeding). The vasculitis may act as an apex for intussusception. Abdominal symptoms may precede the onset of the rash. Arthritis occurs most commonly in the ankles, knees and hips (referred hip pain may be responsible for abdominal pain). Renal involvement occurs in one-half to two-thirds of cases, with microscopic haematuria occurring in about 50–70%. About a quarter of cases may demonstrate varying severities of nephrotic syndrome, nephritic syndrome and may be responsible for end-stage renal disease in about 1% of all cases of HSP. There are no confirmatory tests for HSP. Treatment involves observation, analgesics and follow-up. Steroids may be useful in abdominal pain. The condition remits after about a month with a good prognosis, however patients must be followed up since in some of these patients there will be a progression of the renal lesions. Other conditions that can produce a vasculitic rash, nephritis, arthritis and abdominal pain include the connective tissue diseases such as SLE, polyarteritis nodosa and Wegener granulomatosis. You should thus consider an autoantibody screen and further additional tests if your diagnosis is uncertain.

2. *Streptococcal disease.* Post-streptococcal glomerulonephritis occurs 1–3 weeks following a group A Streptococcal infection of the throat or skin. The onset of nephritis is heralded by the onset of periorbital oedema and a smokey/tea/coca cola-coloured urine. Oliguria occurs and this is followed by hypertension. Most cases are mild and often are not even noticed; severe disease can however occur and require dialysis. Nephrosis can also occur but this is rare. AntiDNAse B titres of antibodies are more specific for Streptococcal skin infections whereas antistreptolysin antibodies are more specific for throat infections caused by *Streptococcus*. C3 and C4 levels are reduced. Also reduced in SLE nephritis, mesangiocapillary glomerulonephitis, shunt nephritis and SBE.

3. *Systemic lupus erythematosus* affection of the kidney occurs in about 50% of cases and severity varies from very mild to very severe. Nephritis is the commonest presentation of lupus in children. Proteinuria is common. Skin lesions consist of the classic malar butterfly rash, maculopapular lesions, alopecia, nail fold infarcts and telangiectasias. In lupus nephritis there are reduced C3 and C4 levels.

Haemolytic uraemic syndrome

A typical picture might include: Hb 7.1 g/dl, WCC 9.6, platelets 64; fibrin degradation products are increased; sodium — 146; potassium — 6.4, urea — 25, creatinine — 223.

The classic triad that you should be looking for in the questions is of (1) acute renal failure; (2) microangiopathic haemolytic anaemia (on a blood film this is identified as schistocytes — red cell fragments shred through the fibrin meshwork — which is Coombs' negative and other features of haemolytic anaemia such as reticulocytosis or possible unconjugated hyperbilirubinaemia; (3) thrombocytopenia, which is variable.

Two main groups of disease are seen: (a) epidemic/typical (most common) seen in younger children; (b) sporadic/epidemic — rarer and seen in older children.

In the epidemic form the children tend to be younger and present with features of gastroenteritis (vomiting and diarrhoea, often bloody). The acute renal failure is usually of acute onset. The most common causative organisms are the verotoxin from *E. Coli* (serotype O157:H7 strain), *Salmonella, Shigella, Campylobacter* and *Strep. pneumoniae*. It is commoner in the summer months. The sporadic type tends to have no such prodrome. It tends to affect older children. Renal damage is more severe but of more insidious onset.

Other forms include hereditary and secondary causes, for example drugs (cyclosporin), malignancy and post-renal transplant. These secondary causes are however commoner among adults.

A proposed mechanism is that an initial insult causes damage to the microvasculature causing activation of prostaglandins and coagulation pathways leading to the development of microthrombi in the glomeruli. Histologically there is a linear fibrin deposit in the glomerular capillaries. It is speculated that there may be a deficiency of prostacyclin (a platelet inhibitor) in the circulation (in the sporadic form).

Questions may make use of the large number of complications.

Complications of haemolytic uraemic syndrome (HUS)

— *Gastrointestinal:* Abdominal pain, perforation and strictures.
— *CNS:* Encephalitis-like features. Persisent neurological sequelae may occur.
— *Cardiovascular:* Myocarditis, cardiomyopathy.
— *Pancreatic involvement:* IDDM, pancreatitis.
— *Liver involvement:* Hepatitis.
— *Eye:* Retinal haemorrhages occur in about a third of cases.

Treatment is conservative and symptomatic consisting of: transfusion of blood and platelets; treatment of hypertension; careful fluid and electrolyte balance; treatment of renal failure with dialysis for severe electrolyte disturbance or fluid overload; and antibiotics to treat a possible bacterial trigger. In addition dipyridamole (an antiplatelet drug), heparin, prostacyclin infusions, steroids and other immunosuppressive agents have been used with varying success.

Prognosis appears to be better with the epidemic forms. The overall mortality in the acute disease is about 5–10%. The extent and duration of renal involvement affect prognosis. The degree of CNS involvement is also an important determiner of prognosis. About 5% of cases may progress to chronic renal failure.

Hypochloraemic hypokalaemic metabolic alkalosis

Several questions refer to the conditions that produce a metabolic alkalosis with low sodium, potassium and chloride. The list is as follows:

— Pyloric stenosis or other conditions that result in significant gastric juice loss
— Chloridhorrhoea
— Cystic fibrosis
— Barrter syndrome
— Use of diuretics.

The individual cause will be dictated by the clinical history and further investigations, for example the sweat test for CF.

Cyclosporin

Cyclosporin is commonly used in paediatric disease and you should be aware of its toxicity and side effects. It is nephrotoxic (sometimes reducing difficulty in differentiating from rejection in renal transplant children), results in hypertension, increases low density lipoprotein (LDL) and triglycerides, and may result in tremor, gingival hypertrophy, hypertrichosis, liver enzyme disturbance and immunosuppression.

Polycystic kidney disease

Questions occasionally come up on polycystic kidney disease. There are AD and AR forms, both of which may occur in infancy and adulthood. In the AR/infantile type the baby typically presents with very enlarged kidneys resulting from the presence of numerous cysts (dilated collecting ducts). Renal failure is usually present at birth and is of rapid onset. As a result of the reduction in urinary flow, pulmonary hypoplasia is often present leading to respiratory distress. Congenital hepatic fibrosis is also often present leading to hepatomegaly and impaired liver function and there may be bile duct ectasia (Caroli disease) leading to portal hypertension. Ultrasound shows a lack of differentiation between the renal medulla and cortex with the presence of microcysts. Babies generally have a poor prognosis but some may be suitable for renal transplant. Sodium replacement is important because of ongoing sodium leakage.

Although commoner in adulthood, the AD type may also occur in the paediatric population. Children present in a similar fashion to adults with an abdominal mass, hypertension and progressive renal failure. There is cystic dilatation of the nephrons which gradually enlarge, compressing adjacent renal parenchyma and causing parenchymal ischaemia. About 30% have hepatic cysts (less commonly seen in the pancreas, lungs and spleen), and Berry aneurysms are present in about 15% (about 15% of these die from the resulting subarachnoid haemorrhage). Treatment involves managing the hypertension, renal failure and considering renal transplant.

Posterior urethral valves

Any male child who has a history of renal outflow tract obstruction should have posterior urethral values excluded as a possible cause. The age of presentation in the questions may vary from birth to 4–5 years of age depending on the severity of the obstruction caused by the valves. Indeed the valves may have caused urinary obstruction to such a degree as to have caused dysplastic kidneys and pulmonary hypoplasia at birth. In the more severe cases that present earlier there will usually be a bilateral hydronephrosis presenting as bilateral flank masses and renal failure of varying degrees. Older children may present to paediatricians because of parental concern about poor urinary stream, urinary tract infections or abdominal pain. An MCUG provides the diagnosis by finding a dilated urethra proximal to the valves. The bladder wall is thickened as a result of secondary bladder wall hypertrophy. Remember that between 50–60% of cases are associated with vesicoureteric reflux. Treatment involves initial relief obstruction (for example with vesicostomy) initially followed by ablation of the valves +/– treatment of the reflux.

Combined renal and neurological signs

The combination of renal signs and neurological signs is a pattern with which you should be familiar.

— *Wilson disease:* proximal renal tubular acidosis, Fanconi syndrome. Basal ganglia features and peripheral neuropathy may be seen (see chapters 5 and 6).

— *Renal hypertension:* any cause of acute or chronic renal failure resulting in hypertension may result in neurological features as well as seizures and hypertensive encephalopathy.

— *Renal biochemical disturbance:* by alteration of the normal biochemistry and in particular plasma sodium concentration, seizures may be precipitated.

— *Haemolytic uraemic syndrome* (see above).

— *Alport syndrome:* this causes a glomerulonephritis (with thickened split basement membrane), sensorineural deafness especially in the high frequency range (may appear in later childhood) and ocular changes.

Microscopic haematuria is common and males are more often affected than females. They may have recurrent macroscopic haematuria and onset of renal failure in the early twenties.

— *AD polycystic kidney disease* and the association with Berry aneurysms (see above).

— *Sickle cell disease* can cause acute papillary necrosis and neurological features.

— *Lead poisoning:* Fanconi syndrome and signs of raised intracranial pressure.

— *Shunt nephritis:* the association of a ventriculo-peritoneal shunt with nephritis.

— *Tuberous sclerosis:* angiomyolipoma (often misdiagnosed as polycystic kidney disease in the absence of other features of the syndrome) may lead to hypertension and renal insufficiency. CNS features are a result of the presence of intracranial tubers (see chapter 5).

— *Drug ingestion* must never be excluded from the differential diagnosis.

Haematuria

Be familiar with a list of the causes, investigations and management of haematuria and proteinuria, available in most paediatric textbooks.

Haematuria is a common clinical condition in paediatrics. The causes can be divided up as either painful or painless. The causes include: UTI, pyelonephritis, stones, hydronephrosis, trauma, bleeding diathesis, sickle cell disease, strenuous exercise, vascular malformations (such as hereditary telangiectasia) and tumours (for example Wilm tumour). Glomerular causes of blood loss include vasculitis (e.g. Henoch-Schönlein purpura), any cause of glomerulonephritis, benign familial haematuria, Alport syndrome, connective tissue diseases e.g. SLE, Berger disease (associated with viral illnesses) and SBE.

In the history one should determine the presence, site and nature of any pain, history of trauma, recent upper respiratory tract infections (including sore throats) or skin rashes (especially Streptococcal-like skin rashes) and recent medications causing a possible interstitial nephritis (e.g. penicillins). You should ask about a family history of haematuria, renal stones or sensorineural deafness (Alport syndrome). You should examine for oedema, hypertension and renal masses (such as hydronephrosis) and look for rashes.

Investigations for haematuria should include: MC&S of the urine, FBC, U&E, ASOT, antinuclear factor (ANF), C3, C4, CH50. In painful haematuria include calcium, phosphate and urate levels. Send urine for Ca/Cr ratio, and 24 h collection for calcium, urate and phosphate. Abdominal X-ray, renal ultrasound (preferable) and possibly renal biopsy.

— *IgA nephropathy* (Berger disease) is the commonest glomerulonephritis in children. Males are twice as commonly affected as females. Gross haematuria (and more rarely microscopic haematuria) occurs shortly after an upper respiratory tract infection (or during) cf. post Streptococcal disease where haematuria occurs generally 10–14 days after infection. There may be associated loin pain. It is self limiting. Between 10–30% of children will go on to develop renal failure. Renal biopsy (rarely required) shows identical features as those of Henoch–Schönlein purpura.

— *Benign familial haematuria* occurs in children with persistent microscopic haematuria usually without proteinuria. It is a benign condition with no deterioration of renal function over time. It tends to run in families so you should test other family members' urine. Definitive diagnosis involves renal biopsy where a reduced thickness of the glomerular basement membrane may be found.

— *Idiopathic hypercalciuria* describes the condition where calcium excretion/day exceeds >4 mg/kg. It can be found in approximately 2% of children. It produces macroscopic or microscopic haematuria which is usually painless. However the development of calcium-containing stones (a potential complication) will be associated with pain. A random urine sample may be tested for the Ca/Cr ratio which in normal individuals is less than 0.2. If > 0.2, then perform a 24 h urinary collection to determine daily calcium excretion. Treatment is conservative with a reduced salt and calcium diet (not to the extent that growth is affected), high fluid intake and occasionally the use of thiazide diuretics that reduce renal calcium excretion.

Polyuria

This may be caused by excessive drinking (for example, psychogenic polydipsia), hyperglycaemia — diabetes mellitis, diabetes insipidus (central or nephrogenic) — Fanconi syndrome, following prolonged obstruction to the urinary tract, chronic renal failure and any cause of hypokalaemia that induces a nephrogenic diabetes insipidus.

Drugs and the kidney

Know a list of the commoner drugs that are associated with nephrotoxicity.

— *Membranous GN:* gold, penicillamine, captopril.
— *Interstitial nephritis:* penicillin, cephalosporin, NSAIDs.
— *Renal tubular damage:* amphotericin, heavy metals (gold and mercury), cytotoxics and aminoglycosides.

Nephroblastoma

The pattern of an abdominal mass, haematuria as well as hypertension in a child aged between about one and four should suggest the diagnosis of nephroblastoma (Wilm tumour). It is derived from mesonephric mesodermal tissue. M > F. It is inherited in about one-fifth of cases with the remainder being sporadic. It is bilateral in 5–10% of cases (more common in familial cases). It presents as a smooth unilateral mass in the flank which may enlarge rapidly. Pain may be present. Hypertension occurs due to pressure on the renal artery causing renin production. Microscopic haematuria (in a third of patients) is usually seen as opposed to gross haematuria. Generalised features such as fever, weight loss and anorexia may be seen. Do not forget the rare presentation of heart failure in Wilm tumour as a result of proximal spread of the tumour through the renal vein and IVC into the heart which can cause tricuspid regurgitation. Blockage of the IVC can cause distended veins over the skin of the abdomen. Pulmonary metastases are present in about 10% of cases at diagnosis (often seen as cannon ball metastases).

It spreads by direct extension, blood spread and via the lymphatics. Metastases are found in about 15% at presentation (mostly cannon ball metastases in the lungs). Investigations include intravenous pyelogram, CT scan and biopsy. The IVP shows characteristic distortion of the calyceal system or collecting system with however no change in the axis of the kidney.

Know the associations:

— Gastrointestinal abnormalities
— Beckwith–Wiedemann syndrome
— Hemihypertrophy
— Aniridia in association with 11p13 deletion
— Genitourinary abnormalities such as adrenal hypoplasia and horseshoe kidney.

Treatment consists of radical nephrectomy +/− radiotherapy and chemotherapy.

Neuroblastoma

The other common intra-abdominal tumour of infancy is neuroblastoma. It occurs most commonly before the age of two and a half (one-quarter before one year). It is associated with Beckwith–Wiedemann syndrome, nesidioblastosis and neurofibromatosis. It may occur anywhere along the sympathetic nervous system, most commonly in the adrenal gland but is also seen in the mediastinum (posterior thorax with throacic cord invasion), neck and pelvis. It presents with an irregular mass arising from the flank and unlike Wilm tumour it crosses the midline. It often presents late when metastases are present (in about 70% of cases). Metastases are most commonly found in bone, bone marrow, lymphatics, liver and subcutaneous tissues. Thoracic involvement may cause a Horner syndrome or tracheal or vascular compression. There may be heterochromia iridis present. Skin involvement, common in infants, may cause raised bluish non-tender nodules. Bony metastases produce bone pain, proptosis and 'raccoon eyes' — periorbital bruising caused by invasion of the sphenoid bone or periorbital tissues. The bone marrow may be invaded in about half of the cases. In children less than one year of age a syndrome consisting of an undetectable primary tumour, most often in the adrenal gland, with metastases to skin, bone marrow and liver (however not involving the bone) may be seen. This form of neuroblastoma often undergoes a spontaneous remission without treatment. It is seen in about one-tenth of all cases. The opsoclonus-polyclonus syndrome consists of acute cerebellar and truncal ataxia with 'rapid dancing' eye movements. Occasionally chronic watery diarrhoea may be seen (Verner–Morrison syndrome) due to vasoactive intestinal peptide (VIP) secretion. Olfactory neuroblastomas may cause recurrent nose bleeds and obstruction. The investigation involves IVP, CT scan and biopsy. The IVP demonstrates the classical 'drooping lily sign' as the kidney is pushed down and laterally by the tumour. Unlike Wilm tumour, the calyceal architecture is maintained. On a plain AXR calcification may be seen in about half of all cases.

Congenital nephrotic syndrome

There are two types:

— *Finnish type* (the most common form). There is a raised maternal serum and amniotic fluid antenatal AFP, large placenta (usually more than 25% of the birthweight) with early proteinuria and normal renal function. It presents in the first few days to weeks of life. There is a gradual onset of the nephrotic picture with recurrent infections, and declining renal function with death by 4–5 years of age.

— *Diffuse mesangiosclerosis*. There is a normal maternal antenatal serum AFP and proteinuria presents at birth. There is a more rapid decline in renal function than compared to the Finnish type.

Treatment is supportive with dialysis; transplant will be considered when the baby is big enough. Unlike adult nephrotics steroids and immunosuppressives are of no therapeutic value.

Nephrotic syndrome

Nephrotic syndrome is said to occur when the following are present:

— Proteinuria > 40 mg/m^2/h. In normal children one expects < 4 mg/m^2/h
— Hypoalbuminaemia
— Peripheral oedema
— Possibly hyperlipidaemia.

The causes can be listed as:

1. Primary structural glomerular disease
2. Systemic causes such as SLE, HSP
3. Drugs and toxins: gold, penicillinamine and heavy metals.

The commonest forms of nephrotic syndrome are those with primary structural damage. Eighty-five per cent are caused by minimal change glomerulonephritis, 10% by focal segmental glomerulosclerosis and 3% by mesangiocapillary glomerulonephritis (the others such as membranous and membranoproliferative make up the remainder).

The patterns of clinical signs with which you may be presented in the exam include: the onset of oedema (which may occur following a viral illness) which will be periorbital in the mornings, and pitting and dependent a few hours after getting up (especially pedal, legs and genitalia). Abdominal pain is a relatively common symptom and is caused by splanchnic ischaemia. There may be a history of frothy urine. As severity increases, there may be signs of hypovolaemia with an increased core–peripheral temperature gap, tachycardia and hypotension. Don't forget that hypertension as opposed to hypotension may also be seen (secondary to reduced renal perfusion leading to increase in renin production) which is surprisingly reversed following administration of fluid. Be aware of the vicious cycle of reduced oncotic pressure→oedema→decreased intravascular volume→thirst, ADH secretion and renin production→salt and water retention→ increased extravascular space→oedema: and so the cycle continues.

Complications of nephrotic syndrome

a) Plasma immunoglobulin loss (including IgG), complement components and others result in increased susceptibility to encapsulated bacterial infections such as *Pneumococcus* and *Haemophilus influenzae*. Pneumococcal sepsis is a particularly important problem and vaccination with Pneumovax should be offered. Peritonitis can occur either because of *Pneumococcus* or Gram-negative organisms.

b) There is an acquired thrombophilia because of the loss of clotting factors such as antithrombin III in the urine. Thrombosis can occur in the renal vein, pulmonary and peripheral vasculature.

c) Plasma protein loss may result in rickets secondary to urinary loss of vitamin D binding globulin. Hypothyroidism may occur secondary to thyroid binding globulin loss.

It is beyond the scope of this book to go into treatment options but these are readily available in most paediatric texts. General measures include (a) salt restriction; (b) if fluid depleted, the use of albumin i.v. or if fluid overloaded, then diuretics are given; (c) steroids or immunosuppressives; (d) prophylactic penicillin.

Hepatorenal syndrome

Renal failure (marked by the onset of oliguria — distinguish from prerenal failure secondary to dehydration) may develop in a child with severe liver disease and is called the hepatorenal syndrome. There is reduced cortical perfusion as a result of the accumulation of vasoactive substances that are thought to be usually cleared by the functioning liver. The urinary sodium excretion is low with a normal tubular function. Improvement in renal failure will only occur if the liver failure improves drastically: the prognosis otherwise is poor.

Renal vein thrombosis

It is essential that you are familiar with the clinical presentation of RVT. It will occur in a state of severe dehydration (such as a newborn baby who is febrile and not having sufficient fluid intake) or a hypercoagulable state (such as nephrotic syndrome, in polycythaemia or protein C deficiency). Clinically there may be renal enlargement, flank pain, irritability (in a baby), haematuria (microscopic or macroscopic) and declining renal function. Renal ultrasound will help make the diagnosis. Beware the progression to breathlessness or respiratory distress indicating the possibility of a secondary pulmonary embolus. Treatment is with hydration and anticoagulation.

Prune belly syndrome

This comes up in the slides so be familiar with a picture of it. In addition you may be asked further questions relating to it. Ninety-seven per cent occurs in males. There is (1) absent anterior wall musculature; (2) genitourinary abnormalities: bilateral cryptorchidism, non-obstructive dilatation of the renal tract (the ureters are often tortuously dilated), vesicoureteric reflux (in 75%) and cystic renal dysplasia which may lead to chronic renal failure. Antenatal oligohydramnios may lead to varying degrees of pulmonary hypoplasia. Recurrent urinary tract infections are common as a result of stasis; (3) cardiac abnormalities (4) musculoskeletal abnormalities.

Prognosis is related to the severity of renal involvement.

Neurology   5

Neurology has a significant presence in all the sections of the Part 2 examination, as neurological cases are especially good at discriminating clinical proficiency and confidence. In paediatrics, where neurological signs and symptoms may result from a diversity of causes, they also test the candidates' wider knowledge.

CEREBROSPINAL FLUID PATHOPHYSIOLOGY

This would be a good basic science topic since many disease states cause a disruption of normal function and this in turn leads to disorders with which you should be familiar.

Cerebrospinal fluid is continually produced as an ultrafiltrate of plasma from the choroid plexuses in both lateral ventricles. The CSF from the right and left lateral ventricles then flows into the third ventricle through the foramen of Monro and then into the fourth ventricle via the aqueduct of Sylvius. The CSF then passes through a central foramena of Magendie and two lateral foramina of Luschka into the subarachnoid space to surround the brain and spinal cord. It is then absorbed mainly by the arachnoid granulations that project into the dural venous sinuses. The normal opening pressure of the CSF is 7–18 cm H_2O and at any one time in an older child there will be between 80–150 ml fluid.

Hydrocephalus

You should be familiar with the causes of hydrocephalus – defined as an increased amount of CSF, usually under increased pressure and usually with some degree of dilatation of the ventricular system.

In paediatrics it is useful to classify the types as follows.

1. Obstructive
2. Decreased absorption of CSF
3. Increased production of CSF.

Alternatively a different classification of communicating and non-communicating hydrocephalus exists. Communicating implies that CSF can flow through the fourth ventricular foramina into the subarachnoid space but cannot be absorbed by the arachnoid granulations. Non-communicating implies that there is little or no communication between the ventricles and subarachnoid space.

Aetiological factors

— *Obstruction to CSF flow*: this can occur at the level of the foramen of Monro, third ventricle, aqueduct of Sylvius, and foramina of Luschka and Magendie of the fourth ventricle. Any of these obstructions can be caused by:
1. Tumours
2. Congenital abnormalities, such as the following:
    — *Dandy–Walker cyst*. This describes the absence or deficiency of the cerebellar vermis and fourth ventricle foramina outlets together with subsequent cystic dilatation of the fourth ventricle leading to hydrocephalus (in 80% of cases), and can sometimes be seen with posterior fossa transillumination.
    — *The Arnold–Chiari malformation*. This describes a small posterior fossa and downward displacement of the cerebellar tonsils and medulla into the foramen magnum often associated with spina bifida.
    — *Aqueduct stenosis* (which may be X-linked or sporadic). In the rarer X-linked form the thumb is commonly flexed in opposition and the first metacarpal is short. A possible slide of a child with a large head and overlapping fingers should alert you to the possibility of X-linked hydrocephalus. Sporadic cases of aqueduct stenosis account for the vast majority.
    — *Aneurysm of the vein of Galen* (causing obstruction at the level of the aqueduct).
    — *Achondroplasia* where bony abnormalities result in obstruction.

— *Decreased absorption*. (a) Infection: meningitis or encephalitis including intrauterine infections with toxoplasmosis; CMV; (b) Intraventricular or intracranial bleeds; (c) Sagittal sinus thrombosis with resulting increased pressure and reduced CSF absorption; (d) Arachnoid villi hypoplasia.

— *Overproduction of CSF*. Rare and usually caused by a choroid plexus papilloma.

INTERPRETATION OF CSF DATA

Many questions in the exam will ask you to discuss the causes of abnormal CSF results. In order to do this you will need to know the normal values (see Table 5.1). Table 5.2 describes the expected findings with different types of meningitides that you are likely to encounter in the examination.

Additional important notes on CSF values

— Remember that if you are given CSF values with the presence of erythrocytes and white cells and you want to determine whether their presence is

Table 5.1 Normal CSF values for different age groups

	Premature	Neonate	Infant	Child
appearance	Clear	Clear	Clear	Clear
white cells/µl	0–100	0–15	0–10	0–5
polymorphs/µl	0	0	0	0
lymphocytes/µl	0–100	0–15	0–10	0–5
red cells/µl	0–1000	0–500	0	0
protein g/l	1–4	0.3–2	0.2–1	0.2–0.4
glucose mmol/l	2/3 of blood glucose in all cases			

NB A neonatal lumbar puncture is more likely to be traumatic with more erythrocytes on microscopy and does not necessarily indicate intraventricular haemorrhage (IVH). Neonatal CSF may be incorrectly reported as xanthochromic if there is co-existing jaundice.

Table 5.2 Abnormal CSF findings found with different types of meningitis

	Bacterial meningitis	Partially treated meningitis	Viral meningitis	TB meningitis
appearance	Often turbid	Often clear	Usually clear	Not clear. Fibrin web occasionally seen.
polymorphs/µl	Up to 50 000	Up to 1000	Few	Up to 1000
lymphocytes/µl	Few	Up to 1000. (i.e mixed picture or with lymphocyte predominance)	Up to 1000. (i.e. lymphocytes predominate)	Up to 1000
MC&S	Organisms often seen	Often sterile culture	No organisms seen or grown	ZN stain for acid-fast bacilli
protein g/l	1–5	1–2	< 1.5	1–6
glucose	< 2/3 blood	Normal or low	Approximately same as plasma (except mumps and herpes simplex, see below)	Very low

caused by a bloody tap or intraventricular haemorrhage, or CSF inflammation then calculate the ratio of white: red cells. In peripheral blood the ratio is 1:500. Thus a relative excess of white cells in this ratio implies that there is some meningeal inflammation present.

— A cerebral abscess can give a sterile tap but there is sometimes a raised protein count and a lymphocytosis.

— Don't forget leukaemia in your differential diagnosis of a CSF lymphocytosis. Check the blood film! (CSF glucose is usually less than two-thirds blood glucose).

— In herpes simplex encephalitis there is a haemorrhagic encephalitis and the CSF is often bloodstained (increased erythrocytes). The WCC is increased as is the protein count and the glucose may be low in 20% of cases. Remember that clinical features may include strange behaviour (e.g. lip smacking) because of involvement of the temporal and frontal lobes.

— Mumps meningitis is an exception to the viral meningitides and CSF glucose is often low.

— Occasionally TB meningitis can be confused with a cerebral abscess by looking at the clinical history and CSF values alone, since both have a long indolent history of several weeks of fever, headache and other non-specific symptoms. Both also give a raised CSF protein count and sterile cultures; TB meningitis however gives a low CSF glucose.

— The causes of a CSF with a raised protein count include: Guillain–Barré syndrome, spinal block, TB, fungal, bacterial and viral meningitis, cerebral abscess, neurosyphilis, subdural haematoma, cerebral malignancy and acoustic neuroma.

— The presence of oligoclonal bands in the CSF may be caused by sarcoidosis, multiple sclerosis, SLE, SSPE, subarachnoid haemorrhage (also low glucose) and neurosyphilis.

CSF microbiology

The commonest organisms causing meningitis in the neonatal period reflect maternal vaginal colonisation.

— Group B *Streptococcus*
— *E. coli*
— *Listeria monocytogenes*

After the neonatal period:

— *Staphylococcus aureus*
— *Staphylococcus epidermidis* (especially if there are indwelling prostheses such as shunts)
— *Haemopilus influenzae* type B
— *Neisseria meningitidis*
— *Streptococcus pneumoniae* (sicklers at increased risk)
— *Pseudomonas*
— *Klebsiella*
— Tuberculosis
— *Salmonella* (sicklers at increased risk).

Neurological sequelae following meningitis are most common in pneumococcal meningitis, less common in meningococcal and least common (but still a significant problem) in *Haemophilus influenzae* meningitis. However you should remember that the effect of reducing subsequent neurological sequelae with dexamethasone is greatest with *Haemophilus* meningitis.

In general all cocci are Gram +ve except *Neisseria*. All bacilli tend to be Gram −ve except the bacilli *Clostridia, Corynebacterium, Lactobacillus* and *Listeria*.

EEG INTERPRETATION

This comes up in the data interpretation questions and you should be familiar with the commoner patterns: it can be a complicated topic but you are only expected to recognise the commoner patterns. It is usual in the questions that you will be given a montage or map of where the leads are attached to the scalp. The traces from the odd number leads are usually from the left side of the head and the even number traces from the right side.

Sometimes a scale/amplitude or time marker is included as well.

Basic rules of interpretation

1. Make yourself familiar with what a normal EEG should look like (see Fig. 5.1).

2. Look at all the traces from the EEG. Now determine whether the EEG is normal or abnormal.

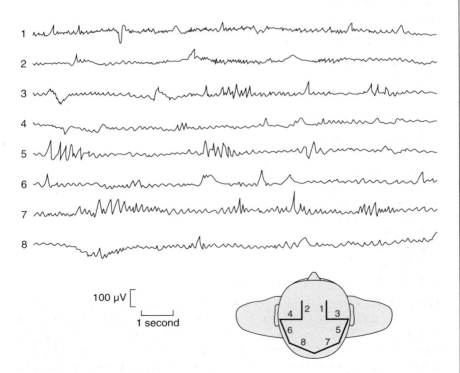

Fig. 5.1 The normal EEG.

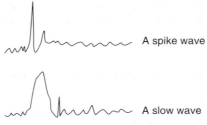

Fig. 5.2 Spike and slow waves.

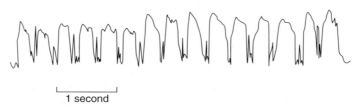

Fig. 5.3 Petit mal epilepsy.

3. Then find out whether this abnormality is generalised: that is, occurring in all the traces, or limited to particular traces (localised to a particular part of the brain).
4. Determine the nature of the wave abnormalities — spike waves or slow waves (see Fig. 5.2).
5. Now look at the amplitude of the EEG waves (high or low voltage).

Petit mal epilepsy (Fig. 5.3)
The EEG shows typical three spike-wave complex cycles per second (3 Hz). The changes are synchronous in all the leads, and may be accompanied by an absence attack which may be precipitated by hyperventilation (family history in 20%).

Hypsarrythmia
(This is an EEG description and not a clinical diagnosis). (Fig 5.4.) Here we can see a chaotic pattern of high voltage slow waves and multifocal spike waves with no constant pattern associated with infantile spasms (in about 50% of all cases). The slow waves and spike activity disappear with the onset of an infantile spasm. Hypsarrhythmia is enhanced by sleep and drowsiness.

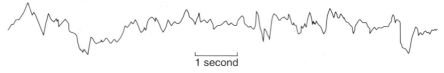

Fig. 5.4 Hypsarrhythmia.

Peak age of onset 3–12 months. Strongly associated with mental retardation, delayed motor development and loss of acquired skills. Know a list of causes of infantile spasms:

— 30% idiopathic
— *Prenatal*: tuberous sclerosis (25%), congenital infection
— *Perinatal*: birth asphyxia
— *Post natal*: meningitis, encephalitis, head injury, severe hypoglycaemia, PKU and other aminoacidopathies.

Appropriate investigations will include examination of the skin under Wood's light for ash-leaf macules, skull X-ray for calcification (see later), CT scan (for calcification, atrophy and congenital anomalies such as agenesis of the corpus callosum). An abnormal CT scan is associated with a poorer prognosis. Various serological and metabolic screens might also be indicated.

— *Treatment of infantile spasms*: ACTH/prednisolone/vigabatrin. Be familiar with the classic infantile spasm (often described as the opening and closing of a book repetitively). Mothers may occasionally misinterpret the child bringing their legs up to the abdomen repetitively as colic or constipation. Fifty per cent will go on to develop other types of seizures especially of the grand mal type.

Subacute sclerosing panencephalitis (SSPE) (Fig. 5.5)

Here we see an EEG with relatively normal EEG activity punctuated by recurrent paroxysmal bursts of high voltage slow waves occurring at regular intervals (periodic complexes). These occur synchronously in all the leads. These periodic complexes may be associated with myoclonic jerks. Diagnosis is confirmed by finding high antimeasles antibody titre in the serum and CSF.

Herpes simplex encephalitis

As in the previous example, here we see the presence of periodic complexes. Importantly, however, they do not occur in all the leads but in those over the temporal lobe. This is highly suggestive of *Herpes simplex* encephalitis. Other confirmatory tests are described later. If one suspects *Herpes simplex* encephalitis one should perform a lumbar puncture, viral titres (especially herpetic + PCR), restrict fluid to two-thirds maintenance, start i.v. acyclovir and consider steroids and anticonvulsants. Periodic complexes are also seen in Creutzfeld–Jakob disease.

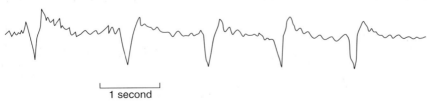

Fig. 5.5 Subacute sclerosing panencephalitis (SSPE).

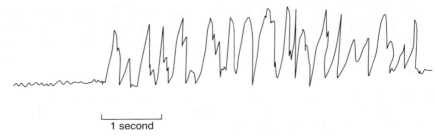

Fig. 5.6 Grand mal epilepsy.

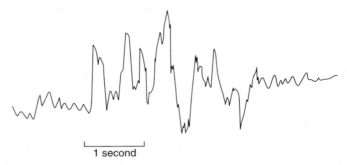

Fig. 5.7 Myoclonic epilepsy.

Grand mal epilepsy (Fig. 5.6)

Patients with grand mal epilepsy may have normal interictal EEGs. During an attack there will be spike waves and polyspikes that usually occur at the start of the episode. These are bilateral, synchronous in all leads and generally symmetrical over both hemispheres.

Myoclonic epilepsy (Fig. 5.7)

Myoclonic epilepsy is associated with synchronous periodic polyspikes (at about 3 Hz) with a normal interictal EEG. It accounts for about 10% of childhood epilepsy. Attacks, which usually begin around puberty, can be precipitated by sleep deprivation or alcohol. Attacks may consist of a sudden jerking of limbs usually symmetrically and bilaterally often affecting the arms. They may proceed to generalised fits. Fits are usually in the morning within a few hours of waking. A sleep-deprived EEG is useful in making the diagnosis. Treatment is with sodium valproate.

Other patterns:

— Focal abnormalities can often be detected with the aid of EEGs. There is usually high amplitude slow wave activity seen over space-occupying lesions. Also seen after substantial vascular lesions or advanced neurodegenerative diseases. Not uncommonly the focal abnormality may become generalised.

— Onset of epileptic EEG activity with a photic stimulus is diagnostic of photosensitive epilepsy. It usually remits in adult life.

— Benign Rolandic epilepsy (peak at 5–10 years of age). The EEG shows high amplitude spikes in the Rolandic area (centrotemporal region) in contrast to temporal lobe epilepsy (anterior temporal region). M > F. Usually nocturnal onset and may become generalised. Spontaneous remission in later life (see later).

— Lennox–Gastaut-type epilepsy peaks between 1–4 years of age and has a similar list of causes to infantile spasms. The EEG shows slow and spike waves with multiple abnormalities.

— An acute encephalopathy will show generalised irregular slow wave activity which is independent of the cause. This phenomenon is also seen in the post-ictal EEG.

Optic pathway lesions

This is a possible data interpretation question. See Fig. 5.8: this diagram looks at the brain from the top.

— A lesion at the level of 1 will result in a blindness in the ipsilateral eye (optic nerve lesion, optic atrophy).

— A lesion at the level of 2 (the optic chiasm, often secondary to pituitary pathology) will lead to a bilateral hemianopia usually resulting from a pituitary tumour.

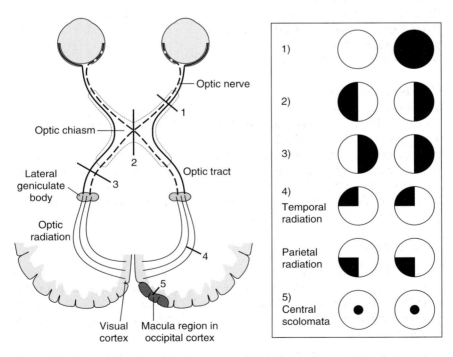

Fig. 5.8 A diagram showing the effect on visual fields of various optic pathway lesions.

— A lesion at the level of 3 (the optic tract) will result in an homonymous hemianopia. **NB**: The visual field defects are described according to what the patient actually sees. Thus a right-sided hemianopia will be caused by a left-sided lesion.

— A lesion at the level of 4 (the optic radiation) beyond the lateral geniculate nucleus will result in an homonymous quadrantic field loss. If the lesion is in the temporal lobe radiation then there will be an homonymous upper quadrantic field loss and if the lesion is in the parietal lobe radiation then there will be lower homonymous quadrantic visual field loss.

— A lesion at the macular region of the visual cortex (occasionally secondary to trauma) will result in central scotomata. The macular region is supplied by the middle and posterior cerebral arteries and thus a posterior cerebral infarction will result in a homonymous hemianopia with macular sparing.

RADIOLOGICAL APPEARANCES IN NEUROLOGY

The aim here is to cover the more commonly asked questions that relate to neurology. Radiological slides occur frequently in the examination and knowledge of the basics of X-rays, ultrasound, CT and MRI are expected for the slides and the clinical part of the examination.

Skull X-rays

These should only be requested in certain circumstances which include:

— If a skull fracture is suspected. Large force/area impact. Suspicious mechanism of injury. Possibility of presence of foreign body in laceration.

— If one is looking for the presence of intracranial calcification (see later for causes).

— Enlargement or destruction of the sella turcica by raised intracranial calcification or by a tumour.

— Possibility of craniosynostosis. The expected suture lines are absent on the SXR.

— Multiple punched out lesions in the skull can be caused by histiocytosis, leukaemia and neuroblastoma.

— Wormian bones are seen in cleidocranial dysostosis, hypothyroidism and Down syndrome.

— Increased density. Osteopetrosis (marble bone disease, Albers–Schönberg disease) shows generalised increased density in all bones but is especially well seen in the skull (common slide). Remember the hair-on-end appearance of beta thalassaemia major.

Intracranial calcification

You should be familiar with the causes of intracranial calcification in paediatrics since a slide is likely in the exam or for discussion in the clinical section.

1. Choroid plexus calcification in the lateral ventricles.

2. Secondary to an intracranial bleed.

3. Infectious causes:
    — Toxoplasmosis: diffuse calcification (remember typical triad of hydrocephalus, bilateral chorioretinitis and intracranial calcification).
    — CMV: periventricular calcification
    — TB meningitis, cerebral abscess, cysticercosis.

4. Tuberous sclerosis. Calcification (often seen as nodules) is periventricular and subependymal especially around the foramen of Monro. The subependymal tubers can sometimes be seen as 'candle dripping' into the ventricles.

5. Sturge–Weber syndrome. There is a characteristic 'tram-line' configuration on plain X-ray with a linear parallel configuration. This is commonest in the parieto–occipital region. It is not usually seen before 2 years of age.

6. Hypo- and hyperparathyroidism.

7. Tumours. Craniopharyngioma, astrocytoma and others.

8. Vascular. Subdural haematoma, extradural haematoma.

Features of raised intracranial hypertension on SXR:

— 'Copper beating' of the skull.
— Widening of cranial sutures.
— Thinning of the vault.
— Erosion of the clinoid processes.

Basic neonatal cranial ultrasonography

This is expected knowledge. It is performed through the anterior fontanelle. Look at coronal and sagittal scans in the neonatal unit to be familiar with the normal anatomy.

Know the classification of peri/intraventricular haemorrhage (IVH and its consequences are the commonest examination slides).

— *Grade 1*: Haemorrhage confined to the germinal matrix.
— *Grade 2*: Extension of grade 1 with blood in the lateral ventricle without ventricular enlargement.
— *Grade 3*: Extension of grade 2 with ventricular dilatation.
— *Grade 4*: Parenchymal involvement.

IVH bleeds occur in the subependymal germinal matrix immediately anterolateral to the lateral ventricle. Ninety per cent of bleeds occur in the first four days of life. Post-haemorrhagic ventricular dilatation occurs in up to 40% of cases (see hydrocephalus above).

Periventricular leucomalacia describes the progression of previously echodense lesions into periventricular echolucent cystic lesions not usually visible until after the second week of life. It is associated with cerebral palsy. There may be no evidence of abnormality on earlier scans. The cysts may coalesce.

Other cranial ultrasounds

Other cranial ultrasounds to be familiar with:

— *Hydranencephaly*: Here almost all the brain substance (with the exception of brainstem, thalamus and minimal cortex) is replaced with CSF often with a normal head circumference. Babies die soon after birth. **NB**: In the exam there may be a slide with transillumination of a baby's skull to demonstrate this. In this case there will be gross transillumination of the entire skull. Alternatively other imaging may be used.

— *Porencephaly*: These are cystic cavities in one or other cerebral hemispheres. There may be in continuity with the lateral ventricles and are most common following an intraparenchymal haemorrhage.

CT scans

Remember the orientation: the image is seen as if one is looking from the bottom of the patient to the top. Differences in X-ray attenuation mean that it is possible to distinguish between normal, infarcted tissue, bleeds, tumour and oedema. CT scans are especially good at detecting blood. Contrast can be injected to show areas of increased/decreased blood supply and oedema.

The common views that you should use in your description of a slide are (1) sagittal; (2) coronal; and (3) transaxial. Other descriptions that you should use when referring to CT scans are areas of high or low attenuation, referring to darker or lighter regions respectively. High CT attenuation is caused by blood, bone or calcium. Comment also on the use of contrast enhanced/unenhanced (in contrast films the blood vessels can be seen clearly and contrast is indicated on the film).

MRI scans

These can be distinguished from CT scans by the greater definition of anatomy in the MRI scan. In contrast to CT scans lighter areas and darker areas are referred to respectively as areas of high and low signal: T1 weighting used more for anatomy, T2 for pathology. T2 weighted scans show the CSF as white.

The particular advantages of MRI over CT of the head is the greater ability to distinguish between grey and white matter and for imaging the posterior fossa. CT scan is often preferred for looking at the chest and abdomen and MRI for the head and limbs.

Examples to be familiar with:

— All the examples of calcification above will be viewed better with CT or MRI.
— *Lissencephaly*: here the brain appears smooth without the usual sulci. These children present with microcephaly, microphthalmia, seizures and severe developmental delay. There is a problem with neuronal migration and the normal six-layered cortex is not formed.
— *Macrogyria*: the sulci are broader than usual and consequently fewer in number.
— *Microgyria*: the sulci are narrow and greater in number.
— *Schizencephaly*: there are symmetrical clefts in the hemisphere that extend from the cortex to the ventricle.
— Be familiar with the classic CT or MRI coronal sections of a subdural and extradural haemorrhage (in an extradural haematoma look for air bubbles in the haematoma as evidence of a skull fracture).
— When there is a space-occupying lesion define its location and determine if there is any midline shift. Remember that loss of tissue in one hemisphere may cause compensatory ventricular dilatation in the other.
— A scan of raised intracranial pressure will have a lack of differentiation between grey and white matter (as in cerebral oedema), loss of gyri, and reduced space between the skull and brain. The ventricles may also be compressed.
— Cerebral atrophy may be confused with hydrocephalus since in cerebral atrophy there is compensatory ventricular enlargement.

CLINICAL SCENARIOS

Many related questions are asked and a wide knowledge of paediatric neurology is expected. Here are the commoner patterns that you should recognise; these should help you answer many of the questions encountered.

— A child who presents with *meningism* (neck stiffness, positive Kernig sign and Brudzinski sign) should alert you to the possibility of meningitis or subarachnoid haemorrhage, but also be aware that in paediatrics there are several other possibilities. They include: acute tonsillitis, otitis media, upper lobe pneumonia and pyelonephritis.
   Don't forget other causes of a stiff neck which include: torticollis, juvenile chronic arthritis and dermatomyositis.
— A commonly asked question relates to the young child with *lead poisoning* who presents with one or more of the following: ataxia, convulsions, features of raised intracranial pressure such as papilloedema and sixth nerve palsy, mental retardation, behavioural disorders, peripheral neuropathy and coma. In addition there may be abdominal pain, anaemia (microcytic with basophilic stippling) and evidence of Fanconi syndrome. There may

be a clue in the history: do the family live in an old house? This relates to the possibility of old paint flake ingestion (old paint had high concentrations of lead). Lead is also found in some Asian cosmetics (surma) and imported medicines. The neurological features are secondary to cerebral oedema, increased capillary permeability and vasculitis. Avoid a lumbar puncture (the CSF is normal but the pressure may be raised significantly). A serum lead level is diagnostic. Lead poisoning is discussed in more detail in chapters 6 and 8. Treatment centres on reducing the cerebral oedema, preventing fits with anticonvulsants, and using a lead chelator such as Ca EDTA.

— The list of causes of *neurological regression* in the older child is not as long as the number of causes in the younger child (see later). The list includes SSPE, Wilson disease (discussed in chapter 6 and often presenting in questions as reduced school performance, rigidity etc.), acute psychosis, Huntington chorea and late onset metachromatic leukodystrophy.

— A child who presents with hyponatraemia and has evidence of intracranial pathology must be considered to be suffering from syndrome of inappropriate ADH secretion (*SIADH*) until proven otherwise (bear in mind that fits and cerebral oedema among other conditions can be caused by hyponatraemia *per se*). The possible neurological causes include meningitis, encephalitis, head injury, cerebral abscess and intracranial bleeds. The investigation and treatment is discussed in chapter 10.

— You may face a question that relates to a floppy infant and be given clues which will help you narrow down your differential diagnosis. The list includes the following (the non-neurological causes are noted first): birth asphyxia, acute illness (e.g. sepsis), neonatal chromosomal abnormalities (for example, Down, Prader–Willi syndromes), congenital hypothyroidism, osteogenesis imperfecta, cervical cord trauma/pathology, metabolic problems, benign hypotonia. The purely neurological causes include congenital myotonic dystrophy, congenital myaesthenia and congenital myopathy (for instance myotubular myopathy and mitochondrial myopathies).

— Beware the child who presents with *headache and vomiting* having been to the GP two days' earlier and been given antibiotics. The CSF shows a normal protein count, normal glucose and a mixed white cell pleocytosis. The answer is most likely to be a partially treated meningitis. The differential diagnosis is viral meningitis or brain abscess. Remember that it is possible to identify polysaccharide cell walls from the killed bacteria using latex agglutination studies despite the fact that antibiotics have been given.

— *Neonatal fits* are common and you should know a differential diagnosis (found in most paediatric textbooks). Don't forget babies born to mothers who are drug abusers. Other signs of drug withdrawl include irritability, tremulousness, nasal congestion and sneezing, poor feeding, jitteriness, a high-pitched cry and diarrhoea as well as seizures.

— Poor prognostic features in *spina bifida*: Presence of hydrocephalus, incontinence of urine or faeces, paralysis of legs, lumbar kyphosis.

— *Delay in walking* (usually achieved between 12 and 18 months) can be caused by a whole host of causes. Bottom shuffling (often with a family history) and familial delay are the commonest causes. Abnormalities such as congenital dislocation of the hip, weakness (cerebral palsy, muscular dystrophies), failure to thrive and part of global developmental delay are other possibilities.

— Clinical features of *hypothalamic disorders* include hyperphagia, anorexia, sleep disturbance, hyper- hypopyrexia and thirst.

— Benign essential tremor is a familial condition that occurs at rest and is not worsened by movement. It is improved with alcohol and propranolol.

— Some questions will make use of the fact that some *anticonvulsant drugs* (such as phenytoin) can induce liver enzymes. You should be aware of the fact that children treated with drugs such as phenytoin may develop (a) megaloblastic anaemia secondary to enhanced folate metabolism; and (b) rickets secondary to vitamin D metabolism. Be familiar with the reduced efficacy of certain drugs given concurrently with hepatic enzyme inducers as well.

— *Fasciculations* are seen in anterior horn cell damage (LMN) with Werdnig–Hoffman disease, poliomyelitis, syringomyelia, cervical spondylosis, edrophonium test, partial denervation of a nerve root and hyponatraemia and hypomagnesaemia.

— Neurological consequences of *vitamin B12 deficiency* include subacute combined degeneration of the spinal cord (pyramidal tracts and dorsal column involvement); peripheral neuropathy; optic neuritis; and dementia.

— The causes of the clinical pattern of absent ankle jerks and extensor plantar responses (that is, a mixture of UMN and LMN signs) may be seen in: Vitamin B12 deficiency, Werdnig–Hoffman disease, Friedreich ataxia, a lesion at the conus medullaris and taboparesis.

— The following drugs are associated with *peripheral neuropathy*: metronidazole, isoniazid, nitrofurantoin, vincristine, vinblastine, amiodarone, phenytoin, cisplatin and AZT.

— You may be shown a picture of a newborn baby with a *sacrococcygeal teratoma* which looks like a large skin-covered mass arising from the coccyx. It may cause an obstructed labour. They are usually benign and can usually be excised uneventfully.

SSPE

Another rare clinical scenario but relatively common exam question relates to the rare neurological sequela of measles called subacute sclerosing panencephalitis (SSPE). It must be considered in any child/adolescent who shows progressive mental deterioration and myoclonic jerks or seizures. Be familiar with the four clinical stages.

— *Stage 1*: Diminished performance in school work, behavioural changes, intellectual deterioration, small involuntary movements and sometimes falling backwards are described.

— *Stage 2*: Further intellectual decline, worsening involuntary movements and myoclonic jerks, speech and swallowing difficulties, muscular rigidity, fits, focal choroidoretinitis and cortical blindness.

— *Stage 3*: Increasing rigidity and worsening dementia.

— *Stage 4*: Coma and death in 1–3 years secondary to bronchopneumonia. There may be some intermittent remissions during the course.

Onset is usually before the age of 20 (usually 4–10 years following infection with measles). Diagnosis is made clinically as well as by finding raised levels of measles antibody in the patients serum and CSF. The classic EEG is described above. The CT scan may show some cortical atrophy or low density lesions in the white matter. Treatment is symptomatic.

Myotonic dystrophy

This has two forms. One presents at birth (neonatal myotonic dystrophy) and the other classic form presents in adolescence. The congenital form should be recognised in questions by the following features. One parent — almost invariably the mother — is affected. It is inherited as AD. Remember it is one of the diseases which displays genetic anticipation (see chapter 1). There may have been reduced fetal movements during pregnancy (indeed there may be polyhydramnios secondary to reduced swallowing in utero). Hypotonic at birth, patients may need ventilatory assistance after birth, show impaired sucking and swallowing and may need NGT feeds. Facial diplegia, joint contractures and talipes are not uncommon. Unlike the older form, myotonia is uncommon in neonates. Questions will sometimes make a note of the presence of reflexes to distinguish it from Werdnig–Hoffman disease. If you suspect neonatal myotonic dystrophy you must examine the mother for facial weakness, myotonic handshake (slow to release) and consider an EMG (dive bomber noise) and muscle biopsy (diagnostic).

The older form of myotonic dystrophy is characterised by weakness, wasting and myotonia, especially of the face and neck (worsened by the cold). Mental retardation, myopathic facies, ptosis, cataracts, frontal balding, delayed release of grasp (manifestation of myotonia), testicular atrophy, IDDM and cardiomyopathy (most die from arrhythmias). Some improve with quinine, procainamide and phenytoin.

Myotonia congenita describes a condition in which generalised muscular hypertrophy (cf. Duchenne that affects just the calves and is a pseudohypertrophy) develops during early childhood: the children often resemble body builders (possible slide question). The muscles are however weak. Myotonia is present. These children remain clinically stable for many years.

Myaesthenis gravis

In neonates there are two clinical forms that exist. They are (1) neonatal and (2) congenital form.

The neonatal form occurs in about 10% of all babies born to mothers with myaesthenia gravis and about 50% will be floppy at birth. In addition they may also demonstrate weakness of facial and bulbar muscles, ophthalmoplegia, a weak cry and weak sucking reflexes. The transfer of antiacetylcholinesterase antibodies are responsible for the features. The babies improve over about 4–8 weeks and show a clinical improvement in response to anticholinesterase drugs (basis of the intramuscular neostigmine test).

The congenital form of the disease may occur in babies born to mothers who do not have the disease. There is a a defect in the neuromuscular junction. The condition tends to be less severe than the neonatal form of the disease but is less responsive to treatment. Antiacetylcholine receptor antibodies are not detected. A juvenile form also exists and resembles that of adult MG with fluctuating fatiguability of muscles (muscle weakness worse after exercise). Females are affected more commonly. Ocular involvement (ptosis and ophthalmoplegia) and bulbar involvement are common (and may be the only presentation) but may extend to the trunk and elsewhere (including respiratory involvement). Muscle weakness tends to worsen during the day. Diagnosis may be confirmed by the edrophonium test (given i.v. it improves muscle strength within a couple of minutes for up to 5 min). In addition look for the presence of antibodies. Treatment involves longer-acting anticholinesterases (such as pyridostigmine), steroids, plasmapharesis and thymectomy (thymomas are less common in juvenile myaesthenia cf. the adult form).

Werdnig–Hoffmann disease or spinal muscular atrophy

This is an AR disease that causes progressive destruction of the anterior horn cells. The presentation is very variable and may start in intrauterine life (manifest as reduced fetal movements and polyhydramnios) or after birth (breathing difficulties and poor feeding) and has a variable rate of progression. The earlier the onset is the quicker the decline in function. Proximal muscle weakness, hypotonia, muscle wasting, reduced facial expression (facial diplegia) with a characteristic alert look, flaccid quadriplegia with early loss of reflexes (cf. myotonic dystrophy), bulbar palsy, predominantly abdominal breathing (see-sawing) and a bell-shaped chest. Fasciculations may be seen especially in the tongue and later respiratory failure with death occurs in the first year of life.

A milder form exists and starts during late childhood and is called Kugelberg–Welander syndrome. There is a proximal weakness of the legs which progresses slowly over years. Normal mental function is maintained throughout. EMG abnormalities include spontaneous fasciculations and fibrillations and muscle biopsy demonstrates group atrophy. Treatment is supportive.

Duchenne muscular dystrophy

This is a common question. Remember that these children may be completely normal until the age of two or even three. Points in the history to look out for are the following: proximal muscle weakness (as in most myopathies) with characteristic sparing of the facial, bulbar and hand muscles; these children may have been late to start walking, or demonstrate a waddling gait (Trendelenburg gait); frequent falls; gluteal weakness manifested as the Gower sign (getting into the upright position from lying by climbing up their own legs – also seen in dermatomyositis). They have generalised wasting but may have prominent calves (pseudohypertrophy) caused by degenerated skeletal muscle being replaced by fat (a common slide question). Kyphosis, scoliosis and lumbar lordosis are also common as is bilateral pes cavus and achilles shortening leading to walking on tiptoe. The children are wheelchair bound usually by puberty and death results from respiratory complications or myocardial involvement. They may have absent knee jerks. Increasing loss of weight is a poor prognostic sign and progression of weakness occurs rapidly thereafter. The IQ is less than 75 in about a third of cases. It is an X-linked disorder with a spontaneous mutation rate of approximately 30%. There is a defect in the gene encoding for the dystrophin protein. Diagnosis is by finding a markedly elevated CPK enzyme level (highest at disease onset and decreases subsequently) and muscle biopsy. There are no characteristic EMG findings. Becker muscular dystrophy is milder than Duchenne and has a slower progression (also X-linked).

Fascioscapulohumeral dystrophy is AD and starts at any time from childhood to adulthood: you should look in particular for facial weakness, especially an inability to close the eyes tightly, whistle or smile and proximal arm weakness and wasting with winging of the scapula as the commoner signs.

For completeness, the limb-girdle type of dystrophy affects the shoulder and pelvic girdle regions with proximal arm and leg weakness. It is inherited as AR.

Guillain–Barré and poliomyelitis

An important clinical distinction is that between Guillain–Barré syndrome and poliomyelitis. It comes up in questions and you should be armed with the knowledge to be able to differentiate the two (see Table 5.2). Both conditions appear between 7–10 days following a respiratory or gastrointestinal infectious illness. Guillain–Barré syndrome is the commonest acquired peripheral neuropathy in the paediatric population and you should be familiar with its presentation.

Investigations will include throat swab, stool culture, lumbar puncture and acute and convalescent serology samples two weeks apart for rising polio antibody titres.

In Guillain–Barré syndrome treatment is supportive including nursing and physiotherapy (to prevent DVT and contractures), careful feeding and fluid regimens, ventilatory assessment (for example, FVC 4–6 hourly) and

Table 5.3 Comparison of Guillain–Barré syndrome and poliomyelitis

Guillain–Barré syndrome	Poliomyelitis
Sensory symptoms may be a feature	No sensory symptoms
Symmetrical	Asymmetrical
Paraesthesiae, numbness in toes and muscle pain precede onset of flaccid paralysis which then ascends. Rarer proximal type affects cranial nerves, upper limbs and proximal muscles initially. Miller–Fisher syndrome presents with ophthalmoplegia, areflexia and ataxia.	Muscle pain often precedes the onset of flaccid paralysis. Paralysis most commonly affects the legs.
Paralysis usually over 1–2 weeks, but may be much more rapid.	Paralysis is usually over 1–2 days.
Autonomic involvement can occur including urinary problems and cardiac arrhythmias.	No autonomic involvement.
Motor nerve conduction studies are slow.	Motor nerve conduction studies are normal.
CSF findings show a very high protein count (3–10 g/l) with minimal white cells.	CSF as for other types of viral meningitis (see earlier). Protein normal and increased lymphocytes. Also carry out paired viral titres.
Pathology involves inflammation, oedema and demyelination of spinal nerves near nerve root junction.	Pathology involves destruction of anterior horn cells.
No virus isolated	Virus can be isolated from stool, throat and CSF.

plasmaphoresis. Steroids have no use in this condition. Recovery over several weeks to months usually occurs but residual disability may continue.

In poliomyelitis immunisation is the best prevention. Isolation, ventilatory assessment and careful nursing initially; subsequently, following the pyrexia, slow rehabilitation and physiotherapy.

If a clearly defined motor and sensory level is noted then consider transverse myelitis. Here at the level of the lesion there are lower motor neurone (LMN) signs and dermatomal involvement, and below the level of lesion upper motor neurone (UMN) signs. Other differentials to think about are botulism and myopathies.

Landau–Kleffner syndrome

If a question gives a history of a child whose development including speech and language has been normal but between the age of 3–10 years develops an abrupt deterioration in speech to the extent that the child may become mute then you must consider Landau–Kleffner syndrome. This may be associated with partial or generalised seizures (in about 70% of cases). The EEG aids diagnosis and shows post-temporal and parietal continuous spikes and slow waves during sleep. In addition to the acquired receptive dysphasia there are also behavioural and psychomotor developmental problems. Treatment with carbamazepine and other anticonvulsants is disappointing and steroids may be used in the short term.

Remember in your differential diagnosis of a mute child the following: psychiatric illness, deafness, neurodegenerative disease, autism (younger age than Landau–Kleffner) and fragile X syndrome.

Focal frontal seizures

You may be described a child who is having episodes of abusive, violent and shouting behaviour that are self-limited, unusual and atypical for the child. He appears distant though conscious during the attacks. You should consider focal frontal seizures. Similarly temporal lobe epilepsy can present as a periodic behavioural problem. The onset of psychotic features in a child may be caused by the onset of schizophrenia, manic depressive psychosis or an acute confusional state induced by major anxiety in the child's life or drug ingestion. One should also consider some type of epilepsy-induced confusional state.

Benign Rolandic epilepsy

This has a characteristic history and could thus be a possible grey case. It accounts for about 20% of all cases of childhood epilepsy and occurs between three and 13 years of age (peak 7–10). A family history is present in about 15% of cases. Seizures are nocturnal but may occur on waking. They often start with tonic contractions of the tongue, cheek and lips on one side associated with drooling and grunting but if awake there may be slurred speech. It is the grunting during sleep that might first alert the parents or siblings to the fits. There may be progression to a generalised fit. EEG abnormalities consist of high amplitude spikes in the left centrotemporal region (Rolandic spikes). Intelligence is normal and spontaneous remission occurs by 16 years of age. Treatment is with carbamazepine.

Acute paraplegia

A child who presents with acute paraplegia is an important case. Remember that in the case of trauma to the spinal cord a period of spinal shock ensues where there will be predominantly lower motor neurone signs. This is replaced slowly by upper motor neurone signs (weakness, hypertonia, hyper-reflexia, upgoing plantars, loss of anal sphincter tone and possible urinary retention or incontinence).

Spinal cord involvement by any pathology may be manifested by back pain and stiffness with a dragging gait, clumsiness of walking, possibly urinary incontinence and constipation. Look for a sensory and motor level. Remember that upper motor signs in the legs are more likely to be a result of thoracic lesions: lumbar lesions are more likely to produce lower motor signs in the legs.

Cord compression is usually caused by tumour, abscess, bone (for example following trauma) or the result of a syndrome such as Down. These may be spinal–intramedullary, intradural, extradural or epidural. Consider a myelogram or MRI scan. Other causes include infectious transverse myelitis (see above) following a viral illness such as chicken pox (treated with steroids), discitis, Guillain-Barré syndrome, hysterical paraplegia (often can define a precipitating emotional trauma). In the latter there will usually be some incongruity in neurological signs elicited. Other causes include multiple sclerosis, subacute combined degeneration of the cord, sagittal sinus thrombosis, anterior spinal artery thrombosis and Friedreich ataxia.

Hemiplegia

An important and common question that may be asked is the child who presents acutely with hemiplegia. You should have a differential diagnosis.

1. Vascular malformation/bleed. Arteriovenous malformation, aneurysm, angioma. Generalised bleeding disorder. Look for a predisposing factor such as hypertension.

2. Migraine. Hemipleia is usually temporary: it may also be associated with sensory changes, dysarthria and dysphasia, and often a family history.

3. Space-occupying lesion. Subdural haematoma, extradural (remember that trauma is the commonest cause of hemiplegia in children — consider non-accidental injury), abscess (including spread from middle ear infection), tumour — a sudden bleed into a tumour may cause acute hemiplegia.

4. Arterial occlusive disease. Thromoboembolic, hypertensive, arteritis, atheromatous, traumatic. Venous thrombosis may be secondary to dehydration, congenital heart disease (polycythaemia). Plasma protein deficiencies (such as protein C deficiency) may also cause a hypercoagulable state. Collagen vascular disease (SLE, PAN), sickle cell disease, Moya Moya disease — which causes progressive arterial occlusion leading to acute hemiplegia — seizures, dysphasia and recurrent TIAs. It is sporadic and half of all cases are less than 10 years of age.

5. Cerebral disease. Meningitis (secondary to cortical vein/artery thrombosis), encephalitis (e.g. *herpes simplex*) or post-infectious encephalitis and post-ictal states (Todd palsy).

    Your investigations will include an urgent CT scan of the brain, and depending on the results, FBC, clotting, blood cultures, possibly EEG and cerebral angiography.

Acute and chronic encephalopathies

Remember that neurological signs are a common presentation of a number of metabolic disorders in neonates and infants. They can be descriptively divided into acute and chronic encephalopathies. Acute signs to look out for are seizures, poor feeding, vomiting, lethargy and irritability. More chronic ones are developmental delay and mental retardation which may be periodically punctuated by acute symptoms. There may be a relationship between the onset of symptoms and signs, and the ingestion of fat, protein or carbohydrate. Additional precipitating factors include stress and infection. (A fuller description of metabolic disorders is found in chapter 10).

Whenever you are dealing with a question that relates to an acute encephalopathy of sudden onset, with or without focal signs, you should have a list of causes, but never forget the possibility of drug or solvent abuse. In paediatrics the population may be divided up into older children/adolescents and younger children. Fifty per cent of teenager poisoning is considered accidental and 50% intentional (experimentation or suicidal gestures). Accidental poisoning is seen mainly under the age of five years. Anything leading to poorly supervised children such as a recent move, a new pregnancy or the absence of one parent will predispose to accidental poisoning (are the family known to social services?) You should look for such clues in the grey case. The commonest drugs ingested that are fatal are analgesics, antidepressants and sedatives. The commonest neurological signs are confusion, sleepiness, lethargy, headache, vomiting, extensor plantars, focal neurological signs, seizures and varying levels of coma. In addition psychiatric features may be present such as psychosis or agitation (see chapter 10 for other features of drug ingestion). The differential diagnoses of encephalopathy in a child are numerous but the commoner ones are viral encephalitis, head trauma, drug ingestion, intracranial bleed, space-occupying lesion, metabolic disorder — for example Reye syndrome — and remember also that urea cycle defects can present in older age groups. In a case such as this drug screens from blood and urine will take time; the history may not yield a cause and you will therefore have to investigate the patient accordingly. This investigation may include taking blood cultures, FBC, U&Es, drug screen (urine and plasma), blood ammonia, CT scan and EEG. Treat the patient cautiously with broad-spectrum antibiotics, acyclovir, possibly dexamethasone (before antibiotics — it can help reduce cerebral oedema), fluid restriction and anticonvulsants (prophylactically or therapeutically).

Failure to reach developmental milestones

There will be questions describing a normal infant who has been developing normally who may gradually be failing to reach developmental milestones or regressing. In addition there may be personality changes, dementia and convulsions (associated with grey matter involvement — poliodystrophy) and there may be weakness with spasticity, ataxia, peripheral neuropathy, dysphasia and cortical blindness (associated with white matter involvement — leukodystrophy).

Causes

— *Metabolic*: (a) metachromatic leukodystrophy, adrenal leukodystrophy; (b) Tay–Sachs, Niemann–Pick disease, Gaucher (poliodystrophies); (c) mucopolysaccharidoses in those where there is neurological involvement e.g. Hurler syndrome; (d) abnormal copper metabolism, Wilson disease, Menkes syndrome; (e) Lesch–Nyhan syndrome; (f) lead poisoning.

— *Infection*: HIV, encephalopathy, subacute sclerosing panencephalitis (SSPE) (see earlier in this chapter).

— *Immunological*: ataxia telangiectasia.

— *Miscellaneous*: Huntington chorea, Rett syndrome, Batten disease.

Some of the causes named above are associated with characteristic fundoscopic appearances which may be helpful in clinical diagnosis. Therefore pay attention to the fundi in examining these children.

— HIV: CMV retinitis 'cottage cheese and ketchup'.
— Batten disease: optic atrophy, increased pigmentation and attenuated vessels (also have abnormal EEG and electroretinogram (ERG)).
— Tay–Sachs and Niemann–Pick: cherry red spot.
— Lead poisoning: papilloedema, –/+ exudates, haemorrhage.

In addition urine must be sent for glycosaminoglycans and various blood tests should be ordered (for Tay–Sachs: hexosaminidase levels; for Lesch–Nyhan: uric acid levels; caeruloplasmin levels for Wilson disease; carnitine levels for fatty acid oxidation defects). Skin fibroblast culture studies looking for various enzyme deficiencies, muscle biopsy, EEG and MRI scan are other investigations.

Movement disorders: chorea

There are many movement disorders in paediatrics but there is one in particular that you should be familiar with for the purpose of exams, and that is chorea. Chorea describes rapid and non-sustained, non-purposeful movements that are usually jerky and flit from one limb or part to another. They may come to the attention of the parents or teacher, and the child is characteristically described as 'fidgety' or 'clumsy' in the cases of Sydenham chorea. There may be a description of difficulty in getting dressed or eating (look for these clues in the question). The causes are as follows: Sydenham chorea (St. Vitus' dance): a Jones' major manifestation of rheumatic fever. It may be as long as six months after the acute rheumatic fever before the chorea begins (but usually before) and therefore antistreptococcal lysins may be completely normal. F > M. There is often a period of inattentiveness before the onset of chorea. There may be 'milkmaid's sign' felt when the child squeezes the examiner's fingers (early sign). The chorea disappears during sleep and is often made worse by excitement. Recovery occurs spontaneously over weeks to months. Other causes include Huntington chorea (commoner in adults with a positive family history, dementia), benign familial chorea, kernicterus, Wilson disease, during pregnancy or oral contraceptive use, drugs (such as those that increase dopamine for example L-dopa and decrease dopamine, such as metoclopramide), acanthocytosis, thyrotoxicosis and SLE (antinuclear antibodies usually positive). Athetoid movements are slow, involuntary writhing movements often affecting proximal limbs caused by disease of the basal ganglia and most commonly by cerebral palsy.

Ataxia

Another movement disorder that you should be familiar with is ataxia. It describes an inco-ordination of movement brought about by altered sensory input or altered processing in the cerebellum. In paediatrics ataxia is divided up into acute, chronic and intermittent forms. Remember that in the clinical examination weakness and loss of muscle bulk may give movements an appearance of ataxia and therefore check muscle power first.

Acute ataxia

— Drug/toxin ingestion. Alcohol or solvent abuse. Phenytoin, piperazine neuroleptics, various pesticides.

— Head injury.

— Infection. Acute cerebellar ataxia of childhood. Implicated agents include Cocksackie, Echo and influenza viruses. It starts suddenly usually 1–3 weeks following the infection, and resolves spontaneously after 1–2 months. Recent *Varicella* infection implies varicella encephalitis. It is rare (< 1:1000 cases), and occurs at the end or 1–2 weeks after the disease. Prognosis for recovery is generally good cf. measles encephalitis.

— Cerebellar lesions: Infarct, tumour, abscess or haemorrhage. Other cerebral tumours such as brainstem tumours. Hydrocephalus.

— Hypoglycaemia.

— Labyrinthitis.

Episodic ataxia

— Basilar artery migraine. F > M. Family history.
— Seizures. Post-ictal state, minor motor status.
— Metabolic causes. Maple syrup urine disease, porphyria, Hartnup disease, urea cycle disorders.

Chronic ataxia

— Ataxic cerebral palsy. 10% of all CP. Static.

— Degenerative. Friedreich ataxia, ataxia telangiectasia, Wilson disease, Refsum disease, Batten disease and metachromatic leukodystrophy.

— Neoplastic. Astrocytoma, medulloblastoma and haemangioblastoma of the cerebellum.

— Other diseases. Hypothyroidism, multiple sclerosis (a rare condition of childhood but may present with ataxia). Abetolipoproteinaemia is important to pick up since it is potentially reversible with a low fat diet (see gastroenterology chapter).

Friedreich ataxia (may come up in a grey case). Degeneration occurs mainly in the dorsal tracts, lateral corticospinal tracts of the spinal cord and spinocerebellar tracts. AR inheritance. The typical clinical features are that at age 5–15 years cerebellar ataxia develops affecting the lower limbs first followed by the upper limbs. There is a broad-based gait. The lateral corticospinal tracts cause spasticity in the legs with upward going plantars and dorsal column involvement causes sensory changes and absent ankle jerks. Scoliosis and pes cavus is common. Cardiomyopathy causes heart failure and arrhythmias. Optic atrophy may occur. Dementia and death occur in middle age.

Ataxia telangiectasia (see chapter 9). Usually normal motor development until onset of the ataxia which usually begins in the first few years of life. Oculomotor apraxia is common. Consider this in a child who in addition has had recurrent sinopulmonary tract infections.

Neurofibromatosis

This is a common examination question on slides or in the clinical examination. It is inherited in an AD fashion with a 50% mutation rate. Neurofibromatosis type 1 (90% of cases) and neurofibromatosis type 2 (10%). In order to diagnose NF-1 two or more of the following features must be present.

— Six or more café au lait patches (greater than 5 mm or 15 mm in the prepubertal and post-pubertal child respectively). Café au lait patches are often present at birth but may also appear later. Scalp, palms and soles are spared. Remember the differential diagnosis of café au lait macules (see chapter 12).

— Axillary freckling. Freckling may also be seen in the groin.

— Two or more neurofibromas or one plexiform neurofibroma. Neurofibromas may be seen anywhere along the length of a nerve. They appear as smooth flesh-coloured polyp-like swellings. Plexiform neurofibromas are found on the face and neck and tend to be more diffuse.

— Optic glioma are found in about one-fifth of cases.

— Two or more Lisch nodules (melanocytic iris hamartomas) seen in about one-quarter of children with neurofibromatosis.

— Fibrous dysplasia of bone (often sphenoid, tibia or fibula).

— First-degree relative with neurofibromatosis.

Other skin features include: molluscum fibrosum (skin tags) commonly seen over the trunk. Additional ocular features include astrocytic hamartomas (seen as white dots on the retina) and congenital glaucoma. Additional skeletal involvement includes short stature, kyphoscoliosis, macrocephaly and spinal stenosis.

Neurofibromatosis predisposes to the development of many tumours. These include astrocytomas (most commonly), medulloblastomas, ependymomas and meningiomas. Phaeochromocytomas, neuroblastomas and Wilm tumour are also more common as is medullary thyroid carcinoma. Neurological involvement may be caused by compression effects of neurofibromas on the spinal cord or nerves. Mental retardation may occur. Renal artery stenosis may be seen (and thus hypertension). The rare NF type 2 is associated with bilateral acoustic neuromas.

Tuberous sclerosis

This is inherited as AD (chromosome 9) with 70% new mutation rate. CNS involvement is the result of the presence of sclerotic tubers which can be found throughout the brain tissue. It causes seizures in infancy manifest mainly as infantile spasms later developing other seizure types (for example myoclonic seizures). Mental retardation and developmental delay is common. Hydrocephalus may develop secondary to tuberous obstruction. The skin manifests adenoma sebaceum, ash-leaf macules, shagreen patches, subungual fibromas and café au lait macules are sometimes seen (see chapter 12). In the eyes retinal phakomas (retinal astrocytomas) are seen as round white outgrowths from the optic disc. In the kidney cysts and angiomyolipomas are seen. In the heart rhabdomyomas may occur. See the radiology section for a description of radiological findings. Management involves control of seizures.

Blocked shunt

A common question and clinical scenario is the child who has a ventriculo-atrial or ventriculo-peritoneal shunt in situ for management of their hydrocephalus. They may present with feeling generally unwell and have a fever, headache, vomiting and papilloedema on fundoscopy. The answer is a blocked shunt (with signs of acute hydrocephalus) which often goes along with infection and an accompanying ventriculitis (*Staph. epidermidis*, *Corynebacterium*). Contact the neurosurgeons who will be able to tap the shunt (+ CT scan). One variation in the question/clinical scenario is to add the clinical features of hypertension, haematuria and splenomegaly which will lead you to a diagnosis of shunt nephritis which occurs when there has been a shunt in place for a long period of time (*Staph. epidermidis*). C3 and C4 are usually low.

Pes cavus

There are a number of neurological conditions that give rise to pes cavus (a possible slide question). They are as follows:

— Idiopathic
— Friedreich ataxia
— Duchenne muscular dystrophy
— Spina bifida
— Charcot–Marie–Tooth
— Tethered spinal cord syndrome.

Raised CPK

You may be given results from a child with a raised CPK and you should know the differential diagnosis. Remember the three isoenzymes: BB — brain, MM — skeletal muscle (the predominant plasma form) and MB — cardiac origin. The differential diagnosis of raised MM–CPK includes: rhabdomyolysis, following surgery, following muscle trauma (including following intramuscular injection), following seizures, myositis, muscular dystrophies, hypothyroidism (caused by the enzyme's reduced catabolism) and sometimes raised after birth for a few days.

Self-mutilation

Self-mutilation is seen in lead poisoning, familial dysautonomia, leprosy, congenital sensory neuropathy and in Lesch–Nyhan syndrome (lip biting, head banging and fingertip biting usually after a couple of years). Self-mutilation is usually seen in a setting of global developmental delay and not on its own (and thus isolated head banging is rarely cause for concern).

Encephalocoele

A common slide in the exam is an encephalocoele. It is a protrusion of the brain and meninges through a skull defect. It is in the midline usually and occipital or nasal in position. It may be mistaken for a cephalhaematoma or haemangioma. CT scan is required for confirmation. Treatment involves surgical removal. An occipital encephalocoele is associated with the Meckel–Gruber syndrome (see chapter 14).

Benign paroxysmal vertigo

A possible clinical scenario is the child aged between 1–3 years who has sudden unexplained episodes of going pale, clammy, unsteady and falling to the floor. The child is often fearful and may cling on to the mother or nearby furniture. There may be vomiting following such as episode. Consciousness is maintained throughout. The whole episode lasts about five minutes. This condition is called benign paroxysmal vertigo. It may recur several times a month. Video recording by the parents may help in diagnosis. Differential diagnosis would include arrhythmia and syncope (therefore consider a 24 h tape, ECG and echo cardiogram).

Raised intracranial pressure

Recognise the pattern of raised intracranial pressure in the absence of a mass lesion — benign intracranial hypertension (pseudotumour cerebri). There may be headache, vomiting and possible diplopia from a sixth nerve palsy. There is a normal neurological examination apart from papilloedema and a normal CT scan (the CSF pressure is distributed uniformly thus normal sulci and ventricles). The CSF is normal apart from a high opening pressure. It is caused by impaired absorption from the arachnoid villi. Lumbar puncture is associated with a low risk of coning caused by the absence of a pressure gradient. Ninety per cent of cases are idiopathic but it is associated with drugs (tetracycline, corticosteroids), obesity, Cushing, Addison disease and in children following acute otitis media. The main danger is of visual loss as the blind spot enlarges. Treatment involves removal of any precipitating cause, for example weight loss. Acetazolomide (a carbonic anhydrase inhibitor) may be given and repeated CSF drainage may be performed. Finally a shunt may be required.

Dermatomyositis

Usually presents with an insidious proximal muscle weakness (however weakness can be of relatively sudden onset). There may be a positive Gower sign. Neck pain is common. The rash occurs early and is characteristically a purple heliotrope over the eyelids which may spread down over the upper trunk (shawl distribution). Collodion patches (scaly erythematous lesions) may be found on the extensor surfaces of elbows, knuckles, knees and ankles. There are characteristic nailbed telangiectasia. There can be calcinosis and calcific extrusion and nodules in the skin and subcutaneous tissues. As opposed to adult DMT there is no relationship with neoplasia. The vasculitic process is generalised and gastrointestinal haemorrhage is a potentially life-threatening complication. CPK is raised. An EMG and muscle biopsy should be performed. Treatment is with steroids, immunosuppressives and physiotherapy.

Tethered cord syndrome

You should be able to recognise the features of the tethered cord syndrome. At three months of intrauterine life the end of the spinal cord (conus medullaris) lies at the same level as the end of the spinal canal. However as a result of differential growth patterns, by birth the end of the spinal cord lies at L3. At three months of age, because of increased growth, the end of the spinal cord lies at the level between L1 and L2 (adult position). Thus any process that interferes with the ascent of the spinal cord up the spinal canal will result in tethering of the spinal cord (between the site of tethering and the base of the brain). Lesions that may cause tethering are usually found in the lumbosacral region and result from spinal dysraphism (interference in the process of neurulation or fusion of the neural tube). Non-skin covered lesions include myelomeningocoele and there is an array of skin-covered lesions including tight filum terminale syndrome, diastomatomyelia and intradural lipoma.

Occult spinal dysraphism describes the common disorder where the spinal processes are absent in a vertebra most commonly seen in L5 and S1 vertebrae in approximately 15–30% of the population (usually found as an incidental finding on AXR), often with an overlying skin lesion (see later). Symptoms usually develop after a period of rapid growth and may be exacerbated by exercise or deformity causing increased stretching of the cord, which is already under tension. Skin lesions such as hypertrichosis (commonest), dimple, lipoma and haemangioma may overlie the spinal dysraphism in about half of the cases. Weakness of the legs with spasticity and abnormal gait may occur. Sensory problems with paraesthesiae and numbness may also be seen. Structural deformities such as club foot and pes cavus are seen commonly. Sudden or gradual onset of loss of bladder and bowel control, with urinary or faecal incontinence or voiding problems and constipation may be seen. There may be reduced anal sphincter tone. Diagnosis involves the use of ultrasound (best under the age of two) and ideally MRI scan which will pick up the abnormally low lying cord, and will also determine the pathology causing the tethering. Urodynamic studies will be helpful for assessing the degree of urinary dysfunction. Treatment involves untethering and the success of this is inversely proportional to the duration of time from onset of the symptoms.

Headaches

Headaches are extremely common in clinical practice but relatively rare in examinations. However you should be able to look for and elicit the important discriminating details in the history and examination. The classic migraine consists of recurrent episodes of headache which may be preceded by an aura which is most commonly visual in nature such as flashing lights, scotomas and shimmering lights. The headache is often unilateral and described as throbbing. In younger children the headache is more often than not bilateral, nausea and vomiting are more common and an aura is not usually described. The migraine is called complicated if there is presence of neurological features such as hemiplegia or basilar features such as vertigo or ataxia. Remember that migraine may have been preceded by recurrent unexplained attacks of abdominal pain earlier in life. In children the sex incidence is equal but in adolescents females are more commonly affected. A positive family history of migraine is often found. Children often describe relief following sleep. The EEG characteristically shows slow wave activity.

Headaches that are present on awakening, or awaken the child during sleep, that increase in severity and frequency over time, where there is nausea or vomiting, or are aggravated by coughing and straining are indicative of raised intracranial pressure and require urgent investigation. Features on examination that should ring alarm bells are bradycardia with hypertension (Cushing reflex), neck stiffness, other signs of meningism and papilloedema on fundoscopy.

Reflex sympathetic dystrophy

You may be given a clinical history of a child who presents with a continuous burning sensation in a part of the body with possible hyperaesthesia which does not correlate to the distribution of a peripheral nerve. There may be a history of previous trauma in the area of the pain (fracture or contusion). The pain may be worsened by movement. This should lead you towards the diagnosis of reflex sympathetic dystrophy. There may be in addition autonomic features such as localised increased temperature, sweating or erythema caused by vasodilatation. In the long term skin atrophy and underlying disuse atrophy may be seen. The initial injury appears to provoke a localised overactivity of the autonomic nervous system. Treatment involves physiotherapy and possibly sympathetic blockade. Many patients improve with time.

Erb palsy and Klumpke palsy

A common brachial plexus injury following birth is the Erb palsy. It involves damage to the fifth and sixth cervical nerve roots. This results in the upper arm held adducted with the elbow extended, the forearm pronated, wrist flexed and fingers extended. This is the so-called 'waiter's tip' sign. It will cause an asymmetrical moro reflex with absent biceps reflex. Klumpke palsy (rare) involves damage to the seventh and eighth cervical nerve roots and presents with weakness of the forearm and hand with an absent grasp reflex. Both these types of brachial injury improve with time usually before the end of the first year. Physiotherapy will play an important role in preventing contractures (passive stretching exercises).

Developmental milestones

You should be familiar with the important developmental milestones under the headings of (a) gross motor skills; (b) fine motor skills; (c) vision; (d) hearing and speech; and (e) social skills. You may sometimes be given a description of a child's abilities in a data interpretation question and be expected to give an estimate of the child's age or you may be given a child in the clinical exam and be expected to perform a developmental assessment. One particular data question relates to the child's drawing ability: you must know the approximate ages at which you would expect a child to copy different images. See Fig. 5.9.

CLINICAL SECTION

Neurological cases are very common in the Part 2 examination. This is partly because of the fact that there are many patients with chronic neurological conditions who are stable enough to be brought back time after time for examination purposes. They also usually have excellent clinical signs.

You will never be asked to perform a complete neurological examination in the short cases. You will, however, be asked to perform examinations of parts of it. It is important that you have a system that makes you look confident in front of the examiners and enables you to pick up the clinical signs. In paediatrics the neurological signs are usually not difficult to elicit.

More than any other assessment, the neurological examination has been compared to an art form. Practice it often, since if you are not fluent in it, it has the potential of looking fragmented and messy. Here follows a description of various parts of the examination: I have assumed that the child is old enough and co-operative enough to understand the requests made of them. The examination will obviously have to be tailored to the age and co-operativity of the child concerned. A description of a typical neonatal neurological evaluation is included.

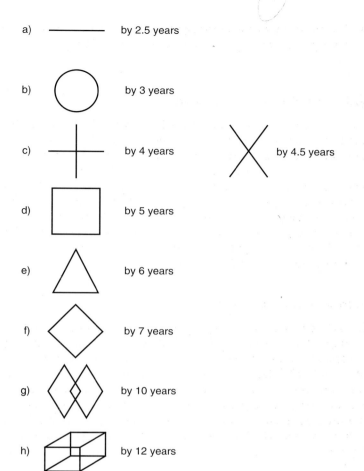

Fig. 5.9 The approximate ages by which a child should be able to draw or copy the following shapes.

Because of the wide variation in clinical signs such as reflexes and power, it is important that throughout your neurological examination you compare the left side with the right.

General inspection

— Look for syndromes, dysmorphology head size, head shape and posture.

— Look for visual clues around the bed such as wheelchairs or callipers.

— Look at the skin for any stigmata of neurocutaneous syndromes. Ataxia telangiectasia (bulbar and elsewhere), neurofibromatosis (axillary freckles, café au lait patches, neurofibromas). Tuberous sclerosis (ash-leaf macules, adenoma sebaceum, shagreen patches and subungual fibromas), Sturge–Weber syndrome (port wine stain in the distribution of the sensory divisions (mainly first) of the trigeminal nerve).

Examination of the cranial nerves

Introduce yourself to the child and parent. Observe the face for obvious abnormalities.

I: Olfactory nerve

Usually not formally tested unless there is a complaint of anosmia or frontal lobe pathology. Occlude each nostril in turn and ask the patient (who has his eyes closed) to tell you when he can smell — for example — a Polo mint when brought into the vicinity of the nostril.

II: The optic nerve

— *Visual acuity*: This will depend on the age of the child. Remember to put any glasses on before testing. From the age of five Snellen charts may be used. Normal acuity should be 6/6 to 6/9 in both eyes.

— *Visual fields*: In a younger child this can be done by moving a small toy from the periphery into the line of vision until the child reacts to this. Be careful to be at an appropriate distance so as not to elicit a blink response. Over the age of five the visual fields can be tested by confrontation. Sit with your face at exactly the same level as the child's. Then with your left hand cover his right eye. Now with your right hand wiggle your index finger (alternatively a red pin) as you bring it in from the top right and top left extremities towards the centre of vision (the finger should be equidistant between you and the child). Ask the child to tell you when he can see the finger moving. In order to check the other half of the visual field swap hands, that is, cover the left eye with your right hand and this time your index finger of your left hand will be the visual stimulus. Then test the right eye. You will assess normality by simultaneously seeing when you see your index finger move in from the periphery (your non-tested eye will be closed). This method will obviously only pick up gross visual field defects.

— *Fundoscopy*: You may be brought to a child with pupils already pharmacologically dilated. If not you should ask the examiner if you can dim the lights. Depending on the child's age explain to him that he should look at an object in the distance and keep looking at it even if you come in front of them: that is, to look through you. Your right eye should look through the lens of the scope to examine the child's right eye and the reverse for the left eye. Approach the child from the periphery and at about 20–30° from the midline and you should be able to see the optic disc. If you are unable to do so focus on a vessel and follow it in the direction it gets larger. If in order to focus on the retina you need a red (positive) lens: this implies hypermetropia (long sightedness); a black lens (negative) implies short sightedness.

III, IV, VI: Oculomotor, trochlear and abducens nerves

These nerves are examined together. Hold the child's forehead with your left hand and then ask the child to look at the tip of your right index finger. Ask the child to follow your finger as you move it in the directions that make a letter H. At each stop ask the child how many fingers he can see (testing for diplopia). Also look for nystagmus. Remember nystagmus is normal at extremes of gaze. It is the fast phase of nystagmus that defines its direction. (If nystagmus is demonstrated then also check hearing, check the optic fundus and do a cerebellar examination). If diplopia is found two important rules need to be applied to determine the pathology (for a paralytic squint): (a) diplopia is maximal when looking in the direction of pull of the affected muscle; (b) the peripheral image is always from the affected eye.

Now look at the pupils and see if they are equal in size. Using a torch, shine the light into one eye to look for constriction (direct reflex). Afferents pass via the second nerve to the lateral geniculate nucleus and efferents pass from the Edinger–Westphal nucleus through the third nerve to the ciliary ganglion and subsequently to the pupil. Then shine the light in the same eye but look for constriction in the contralateral pupil (consensual reflex).

The convergence reflex is performed by asking the child to focus on an object in the midline which is gradually brought closer to the eyes. This is accompanied by convergence of the eyes and pupillary constriction.

V: Trigeminal nerve

— *Sensation:* Test light touch using a wisp of cotton wool. Ask the child to close his eyes and to tell you every time you touch them. Now on each side of the face touch (and not stroke) the skin of the ophthalmic, maxillary and mandibular divisions of the trigeminal nerve. The corneal reflex is tested again using a clean wisp of cotton wool while asking the child to look away. Quickly from the periphery (away from the child's vision) touch the cornea to elicit a blink. (Always consult the examiner before doing this. They will usually tell you to skip this check as it will cause unnecessary distress to the child).

— *Motor:* Ask the child to open his mouth while at the same time applying pressure to the chin to keep it closed. The jaw deviates towards the side of the lesion. Next ask the child to bite together and then feel the bulk of the temporalis and masseter muscles.

VII: Facial nerve

— *Sensation:* You will not be expected to test this in the exam, but you should know that the facial nerve supplies taste to the anterior two-thirds of the tongue via the chorda tympani branch. A parasympathetic component supplies the lacrimal gland.

— *Motor:* Ask the child to raise his eyebrows while at the same time looking for symmetrical wrinkling of the forehead. Then ask the child to close his eyes tight while you try and force the eyelids open gently. Ask the child to show you his teeth and to smile (a normal side can smile, the weak side usually has flattening of the nasolabial fold with drooping of that side of the mouth). Again look for symmetry. A sensitive test of function is to ask the child to blow out his cheeks and to hold them blown out while you press on each cheek in turn to see if they can indeed hold in the air.

You must know the theory behind facial nerve palsies.

Essentially the upper part of the face (above the eyebrows) receives bilateral innervation from the cortex. Thus an UMN lesion will cause contralateral weakness below the level of the eyebrows (remember that eye closure and blinking are not affected). An LMN lesion will cause ipsilateral weakness of all the muscles of facial expression (including those above the eyebrow). Remember that there is no ptosis since the facial nerve controls eye closure and not opening. Thus there may be a widening of the palpebral fissure on the affected side. Eye opening is under control of the third nerve and sympathetic nervous system. If you detect an LMN facial nerve palsy always look behind the ears for scars or other pathology. Also look at the pinna, external auditory meatus and tympanic membrane for vesicles of herpes zoster that occasionally affect the geniculate ganglion (Ramsey Hunt syndrome). Remember that an important differential diagnosis of facial nerve palsy is that of congenital absence of depressor anguli oris.

— *Causes of facial nerve palsies*:
- UMN: cerebral palsy, cerebral tumour, bleed
- LMN: Bell's palsy, mastoiditis or mastoid surgery, Guillain–Barré syndrome, trauma
- Bell's palsy is associated with oedema of the facial nerve in its intraosseous route. About 80% make a complete recovery. It may be preceded by aching behind the ear during the previous 24 h. Chorda tympani and stapedius muscle may be involved leading to loss of taste on the anterior two-thirds of the tongue and hyperaccusis respectively. Complete facial paralysis at the outset is a poor prognostic factor. Neurophysiological studies may be of prognostic value (looking particularly at evidence of denervation) and nerve conduction studies are normal in 70%. Steroids may improve the outcome if given early. Hypromellose eye drops may be used if eye closure is incomplete (to prevent corneal drying). In UMN lesions of the facial nerve, emotion-related movement of muscles may be less affected than voluntary movement.

VIII: Vestibulocochlear nerve
There are two components: the acoustic and vestibular parts.

By the bedside this is most easily carried out by asking the child's parent if there have been any concerns about their child's hearing or by asking the child himself if he can hear the ticking of your watch. If you suspect a hearing deficit look in both external auditory canals for wax, foreign bodies or a perforated ear drum and perform the Weber and Rinne tests to confirm whether there is sensorineural or conductive hearing loss (see chapter 13).

Vestibular problems may be elicited by asking the child if he experiences any dizziness. Also check for nystagmus.

IX and X: Glossopharyngeal and vagus nerves
These two nerves are intimately associated. It is extremely rare that one of them is affected without the other. Ask the child to open his mouth and to say

'Ah'. The uvula should move straight up. If there is a weakness on one side the uvula will move away from the weaker side.

Next you should formally check the gag reflex; you should not, however, do this in the exam but tell the examiner that under normal circumstances this is what you would do.

XI: Accessory nerve
Ask the child to shrug his shoulders; feel the bulk of trapezius on both sides. Then put the palm of your hand on one side of the child's face and ask him to force his face against your hand. Feel the contraction of the contralateral sternocleidomastoid muscle. Repeat on the other side.

XII: Hypoglossal nerve
Ask the child to open his mouth and observe for bulk and fasciculation of the tongue. Then ask the child to stick his tongue out. It should of course point straight out. A deviation of the tongue will however be towards the side of the lesion.

The motor and sensory systems

One important rule in the examination is never to cause pain to the child. Before any test that you carry out, always ask the child if the limb hurts at all. Then in a careful and caring manner perform your test, looking frequently at the patient's face to make sure that he is not holding himself from screaming. Commonly the examiner says 'examine the arms' or 'examine the neurological system in the arms'. If you are asked to examine the arms, and if nothing is immediately obvious on inspection, I would then move on to a neurological examination followed by a rheumatological examination.

I. The arms

— *Inspection*: Look for wasting, abnormal posture, contractures, scars or involuntary movements. An extremely discriminatory test for an upper motor neurone lesion is to ask the patient to hold both arms out in front with the palms facing upwards and the eyes closed. In an upper motor neurone lesion the affected limb will gradually drift downwards and pronate. This immediately gives you important information and will guide you as to what you might expect in the rest of the examination. Indeed the lesion may be severe enough so that the child may not even lift his arms up.

— *Tone*: Hold the child's hand, and extend and flex the elbow several times. Clasp-knife spasticity will usually be easy to feel (initial stiffness followed by giving way). Then still grasping the hand alternate between pronation and supination. You may find it difficult for the child to relax completely and this may affect your tone assessment. Therefore try to distract the child and perform the tests in an unexpected, irregular fashion.

— *Power*: The easiest way to do this is to put the child's arms into the position of the muscle strength you are testing. For example, if you are testing shoulder abduction then put the shoulders into an abducted position. Then tell the child to hold the position and resist while you apply pressure against the positioned limb. Know your root values for the different muscle actions. Test shoulder abduction, shoulder adduction, elbow flexion and extension, wrist flexion and extension, fist making ('squeeze my fingers as strongly as you can'), finger abduction and thumb abduction (testing flexor pollicis brevis, median nerve). In a pyramidal lesion the flexors are stronger than the extensors (the reverse from the legs), the typical hemiplegic posture. There is a scale: 0 — no muscle contraction; 1 — flicker; 2 — movement (gravitational effects removed); 3 — movement against gravity; 4 — reduced power to resistance; 5 — normal power against resistance.

— *Reflexes:* It is important that you look confident otherwise the testing of reflexes can become a messy affair. Hold the tendon hammer at the base of the stick part, so that there is a reasonable swing phase before the hammer part hits the tendon. You may repeat the swings a couple of times (but not endlessly) in order to observe the reflex, but be uniform in the strength of swings. If you are unable to elicit a particular reflex then you can try reinforcement just before testing by asking the child to bite his teeth together or by pulling his hands apart with the fingers interlocked.

— *Co-ordination:*

  a. Finger–nose test. Ask the child to put his index fingertip on their nose and then on your index finger. Ask him to continue doing this alternatively as you move your index finger around a plane in front of the child (midway between yourself and the child). Look for intention tremor (more marked when the child has to stretch to reach your finger), ataxia and past-pointing. Remember that weakness of the muscles of the arm may make these movements look unsteady and resemble or be mistaken for past-pointing or ataxia.

  b. Dysdiadochonesis. Rapidly alternate putting the palmar and dorsal aspects of your hand on the palm of the other. Ask the child to copy what you do.

  c. Fine movements. Ask the child to put his thumb tip on the tips of each of his fingers in turn and to increase speed as he does this. This is a useful test of co-ordination and function.

— *Sensation:* This is rarely tested in the exam. You should, however, be able to demonstrate light touch (use the technique described when testing sensation in the face), two-point discrimination, pinprick (offer only!), position sense (remember to hold the distal phalanx on the sides only since otherwise you will be testing pressure and touch) and vibration sense.

2. The legs

The examiner will ask you to 'examine the neurology in the legs' or simply 'examine the legs'. The latter request is more vague and sometimes the diagnosis is made on simple inspection. However if this is not the case then perform a neurological examination followed by rheumatological examination (as in the arms).

— *Inspection:* Carry out a brief general inspection including the surroundings of the child since this may give you some clues (such as the presence of a wheelchair or callipers). Look for abnormal posture, abnormal involuntary movements such as fasciculaions in the legs, wasting, or the scars of previous operations. Under inspection it is always a good idea to get the child to walk a few steps since this will give useful information about gait, weakness and co-ordination. A useful test is Fog's test in which you ask the child to walk quickly in a straight line on inverted feet. This may bring out a hemiplegic posture in the upper limbs of the affected side (as he walks) and will thus give you information about which side the UMN lesion is. Then check the child's back before he sits down again for any stigmata of occult spina bifida.

— *Tone:* This is tested in three ways with the patient supine. (a) One can roll his legs from side to side (a good indicator of rigidity); (b) By placing your hand under each knee abruptly lift it upwards. The heel should remain on the bed. If the heel raises with this movement this infers increased tone; (c) Place one hand on the knee and the other hand around the foot and unpredictably flex and extend the knee. This is a good test of clasp-knife spasticity (initial hypertonia that gives way).

— *Power:* Test the power of hip flexion/extension, knee flexion/extension, ankle dorsiflexion/plantar flexion, foot inversion/eversion. The easiest way of doing this without confusing the child (or you) is to put the limb in the position that you are testing (for example if you are testing hip flexion then flex the hip and tell the child to keep it there while you push against it). Do this for all the muscle groups. Know your definition of muscle strengths from 1–5 (see above). Also learn the root values for these movements. Remember that in UMN lesions of the leg the extensors are stronger than the flexors (giving rise to the typical hemiplegic posture). If the child can walk on tiptoes and on heels successfully and without difficulty, then this implies 5/5 power in the leg muscles.

— *Reflexes:*
  1. The use of a reflex hammer is described above. Test both knees while they are in the flexed position. Then with the knees at right angles, hips externally rotated and ankle at right angles test the ankle reflex by tapping on the Achilles tendon.
  2. Plantar reflex/Babinski sign. This may be extremely uncomfortable so warn the child first 'I am just going to tickle your feet'. Using a sterile orange stick run it along the lateral border of the sole until you reach the ball of the foot and the stroke it medially towards the base of the big toe. A normal response is a downward movement of the big toe. An upward movement implies an UMN lesion. Do not keep on repeating this if you unsuccessful at first since this will not impress the examiner or the child! Upgoing plantars may be seen in infants up to a year of age.
  3. Clonus. Do not forget this vital sign. This can be performed by suddenly forcing the patella downwards: that is, towards the foot with the knee

extended, or more routinely by flexing the knee, flexing and externally rotating the hip (frog-like) and then rapidly dorsiflexing the ankle. More than three beats of clonus is pathological.

— *Co-ordination:* This will have been tested to some degree by observing the child walking. The heel shin test is, however, the most common leg co-ordination test and consists of asking the patient to rub his or her heel up and down the contralateral shin as carefully as possible. Also test walking heel to toe, ideally along a straight line.

— *Sensation:* This will rarely be asked for in the exam but you should be proficient in light touch (know your dermatomes), two-point discrimination, pinprick (offer only!), position sense (remember to hold the toe on the sides otherwise you will also be testing pressure) and vibration (tested on bony peripheries such as malleoli). Sensation will be particularly more difficult to test in the younger child.

Presenting to the examiners

Whichever limb you are examining start your presentation as follows:

— General observations such as presence of dysmorphic features, cutaneous signs, posture, wasting, involuntary movements and gait.

— Describe the tone as normal, reduced or increased.

— Describe the power in each limb as normal or reduced (or absent). There may be a differential difference in each limb. Don't mention each muscle group tested in turn since this sounds laborious but mention in particular any weaknesses, for example hip flexion power was weak.

— Although reflexes have a scale between 1–3 you should describe them as normal, reduced or absent, or present only with reinforcement.

— Co-ordination is either normal or abnormal as shown by the tests performed.

— Sensation. Mention only deficiencies in sensation.

Then you should summarise your findings by saying 'these findings are consistent with… .

Examination of the cerebellar system

It is important to have a system of examining the cerebellar system practised before the exam.

— Start at the hands and test tone (as described earlier). You would expect to find hypotonia, but this will be difficult to elicit in a child and is included only for completeness.

— Test for co-ordination as described above (finger–nose test, dysdiadochonesis and fine-finger movements).

— Examine the eyes for nystagmus (as described above). Typically nystagmus is horizontal in cerebellar lesions.

— Ask the child to speak and possibly to repeat several words such as 'hippopotamus' in order to demonstrate dysarthria. In cerebellar disease the child's speech sounds drunk and explosive at times.

— Ask the child to walk. In cerebellar disease there is typically a wide-based gait with the arms held out wide. The gait is ataxic and the child will tend to stagger towards the side of the lesion. This may be accentuated by the heel-to-toe test. Inco-ordination may be caused by cerebellar disease or posterior column disease. The posterior columns carry information about vibration, position sense and touch. The spinothalamic tract carries information about pain and temperature.

— Romberg's test is a test of cerebellar dysfunction and posterior column disease. Ask the child to stand with his feet together and then to close his eyes. In cerebellar disease there may be truncal ataxia with the trunk swaying in an attempt to stay upright with the feet together (even with the eyes open). However in posterior column disease the patient will become unsteady only when you ask him to close his eyes, thereby removing any visual clues that he is using to stay upright (since proprioceptive input has been lost). For causes of cerebellar disease see before.

Proximal myopathy

There are a number of important hereditary muscular dystrophies and myopathies that present with proximal myopathy. Have a screen for testing for its presence.

— Ask the child to put his hands in the air (in the history they may complain of not being able to comb their hair).
— Ask the child to stand up from the sitting position.
— Ask the child to get on to the floor and then stand up (in order to demonstrate Gower's sign).
— Ask the child to lie down and to sit up without using his arms.

Gait

— *Hemiplegic gait:* The affected leg is rigid with knee extended, hip adducted, ankle plantar flexed and foot inverted (that is, pyramidal pattern). In order to move forwards the foot describes a semicircle and the toe scrapes the floor: this pattern is called circumduction. In hemiplegia the arm will also be in the typical pyramidal pattern with the elbow flexed, wrist flexed and palmar/finger extension.

— *Paraplegic gait/spastic diplegia*: This classically causes the scissoring gait, and the child uses his hips primarily for movement. The knees are partially flexed. This is often called the 'waddling through mud gait'.

— *Waddling gait:* Here the pelvis drops on each side as the foot of the same side leaves the floor. This is caused by weakness of the pelvic girdle muscles.

— *Sensory ataxia (dorsal column loss gait):* This is classically a stepping or stamping gait. There is a wide-based gait and the patient looks intently at the floor since he relies on visual clues as his proprioceptive input has been lost. A cause of this includes Friedreich ataxia.

— *Drop foot gait:* This occurs when there is an inability to dorsiflex the foot. Thus the foot and the leg on the affected side have to be lifted higher in order to avoid hitting the floor. Possible causes include lateral popliteal nerve palsy, poliomyelitis, or peroneal muscular atrophy (Charcot–Marie–Tooth syndrome).

Neurological examination in an infant

Because the infant is still developing motor skills, part of the examination will also look at development.

Inspection
— Undress the infant to the nappy. Look at the posture of the infant. See if he is moving all four limbs. If the baby is crying, is this of normal strength and pitch? Are there any abnormal movements?

— Since it is going to be impossible to assess power formally you must pay attention to movements and in particular look for antigravity movements.

— Look at and feel the fontanelle.

— With a bright object see if the infant can fix and follow.

Tone
— This requires experience but take both of the infant's arms in your hands and push and pull them in all directions in order to get an idea of the tone and power. This is usually strongly resisted by the baby. Then do the same with the legs.

Reflexes
— Don't use a reflex hammer unless the child is over about one year of age. Before this you can use your fingertip to elicit the reflexes. You may perform a few of the other reflexes such as the moro (may persist in cerebral palsy), grasp reflex, rooting reflex and the asymmetrical tonic neck reflex, and placing or stepping reflex all of which usually disappear by 3–6 months. The parachute reflex appears at about 6–8 months. You should be looking for the presence and symmetry of these reflexes.

Developmental screen
— Place the baby in the prone position and observe to see the degree of head lifting and posture of the back.

— Then perform ventral suspension.
— Then pull the baby to sit by pulling the shoulder tips forwards and not from the hands (looking for head lag).
— Examine back (for stigmata of spina bifida).
— Examine the cranial nerves. This has to be done in an opportunistic fashion and you will not be able to do this systematically. For example seeing that the baby has a symmetrical smile and closes both eyes normally and frowns implies that the motor division of the facial nerve is intact. Look for normal eye movements. At the end of the examination you will tell the examiner that you would also like to also examine the gag reflex, corneal reflex and perform fundoscopy for completeness.

Gastroenterology 6

Paediatric gastroenterological problems are common in clinical practice and this is reflected in the large number of questions that relate to it in the examination. I have attempted to include most of the question possibilities that you are likely to encounter as well as useful background information.

GUT EMBRYOPATHOLOGY

There are many paediatric problems that may arise from abnormal embryological development and it is important to be familiar with these. The examination now seems to place a greater emphasis upon the basic science knowledge underlying paediatric conditions.

Oesophageal atresia

At about four weeks of age the foregut is separated into a ventral part called the respiratory primordium and a dorsal portion, the oesophagus by an oesophagotracheal septum. Oesophageal atresia is thought to occur as a result of a posterior deviation of this septum. The most common variety (85% of abnormalities) consists of a blindly ending proximal oesophageal segment with the distal segment usually connected to the trachea by a narrow fistula just above the bifurcation. Other possibilities include no fistulous connection between the oesophagus and trachea (8%) or there may be an H-type fistula where there is a non-obstructed oesophagus and a fistula half way down the trachea (5%).

Intestinal embryology and malrotation

During normal development the primitive intestinal loop herniates into the umbilical cord between the fourth to the fourteenth weeks of fetal life. The apex of this loop is in continuous connection with the yolk sac via the vitelline duct. In about 2% of people a remnant of this duct may persist in the form of a Meckel's diverticulum and may contain ectopic gastric or pancreatic mucosa causing ulceration, haemorrhage or act as an apex of an intussusception. If the vitelline duct remains patent there will be a fistula between the lumen of the ileum and the umbilicus and faecal discharge may be seen at the umbilicus. Vitelline cysts may also be present in the site of the previous vitelline duct. The midgut loop rotates 270° counter clockwise around the superior mesenteric artery. The proximal part of the jejunum is the first part to return into the abdomen and occupies the left side of the abdomen. The colon is the last part to return. The failure of the intestinal loops to return to the abdominal cavity will result in an omphalocoele (exomphalos) covered by amnion or gastroschisis (no covering). See later in this chapter.

Incomplete rotation

This occurs when only 90° of rotation occurs with the colon and caecum returning first to produce a left-sided colon with the small bowel on the right side of the abdomen. The small bowel in this case has a very narrow mesenteric attachment and can be prone to volvulus and subsequent infarction. Sometimes there is reversed rotation of the gut with a 90° clockwise rotation such that the transverse colon passes and lies behind the duodenum and superior mesenteric artery. Arrested caecal descent describes the case where the caecum remains in the subhepatic position and may result in the production of Ladd's bands which are abnormal peritoneal bands that may cause neonatal bowel obstruction involving the second part of the duodenum. There is also a possibility of recurrent volvulus later in life, again caused by a narrow mesenteric attachment (see later).

Intestinal stenosis and atresia

These are the result of interference in the normal process whereby the solid intestinal segment vacuolates and forms a lumen. The commonest site is the duodenum and this produces a distension of the proximal duodenum with a very under-developed distal segment (see later for presentation and radiographic appearances).

Duplication cysts

These may occur anywhere in the gastrointestinal tract but are most commonly seen in the ileum (mesenteric side). They are either double lumen or encysted in nature. The encysted variety may be in continuity with the bowel lumen. The mucosa of these duplications can be of gastric or pancreatic tissue and bacterial overgrowth may result. Obstruction may be seen.

Hindgut abnormalities

The hindgut ends in a membrane called the cloacal membrane which is an endoderm-lined cavity which is in direct connection with the ectoderm outside. This cloaca later divides into an anterior primitive urogenital sinus and a posterior anorectal canal separated by the urorectal septum. At the distal end of the anorectal canal lies the anal membrane. In simple cases the anal canal ends blindly at the anal membrane (which usually breaks down at eight weeks). Deviation of the urorectal septum in a dorsal direction causes anorectal agenesis which can be of two types: in high types the bowel ends above the pelvic floor and in low types below it. High types commonly have fistulas into the vagina, bladder or urethra (usually no visible anus is present at birth and the presence of one not continuous with the bowel would imply rectal atresia which is very rare).

Hirschsprung disease

There is a failure of the autonomic ganglion cells (the submucosal and myenteric plexuses) to reach the hindgut region at about 4–7 weeks of fetal life. This failure results in the area involved being tonically contracted producing obstruction (see later).

NUTRITIONAL STATUS

Methods of assessing nutritional status in children are important. There are several available and they include:

— The simplest and most commonly used in the clinic would involve a detailed history of diet over a typical period of time. This itself may reveal significant nutritional deficiencies.

— Growth charts of height, weight and head circumference (particularly serial measurements) are easy to obtain and very useful.

— Measurements of mid-arm circumference and triceps and subscapular skinfold thickness give an indication of the body build of the child and these values can be compared with standards for age and sex.

— Laboratory investigations can also be used and in particular mineral and electrolyte concentrations can be assayed. Protein malnutrition can be assessed by measuring the plasma proteins such as albumin (half life of about 20 days) and transferrin (half life of about 10 days), as well as determining the ratio of albumin to globulin which may decrease in protein malnutrition.

You should be familiar with the advantages of breast feeding to (a) the baby and (b) the mother. This information is available in most paediatric textbooks.

Nutritional aspects of milk

You should know about the constituents of breast milk. There have been questions asking for approximate values, but even if these are not committed to memory one should be familiar with the main quantitative and qualitative differences between the varieties of milk (see Table 6.1).

Milk constituent summary
The main carbohydrate component in all the types of milk is lactose. It is easily digestible and fermented by the lactobacilli in the gut to produce acidic stools. The main protein in breast milk is whey, which is more digestible than

Table 6.1 Comparison of the constituents of different types of milk

Values per 100ml	Breast milk	Cow's milk	Modified milk
Calories (g)	70	67	65
Protein (g)	1.1	3.3	1.6
Casein: whey ratio	3:7	8:2	4:6
Fat (g)	4.2	3.7	3.3
Sodium (mg)	15	52	21
Potassium (mg)	60	140	70
Phosphorus (mg)	15	98	49
Calcium (mg)	35	120	55

the cow's milk protein casein (which is more likely to curdle). The other proteins in breast milk that are important are the immunoblobulins IgA and IgM, lysozyme, lactoferrin and lactalbumin, which are important in immunological transfer. Lymphocytes and macrophages also add to this protection. Hind milk at the end of a feed contains more fat than foremilk. Breast milk has lower levels of vitamin K (thus haemorrhagic disease of the newborn is more likely) but there are higher levels of vitamins A, C and E compared with cow's milk. Note in Table 6.1 the relatively lower levels of sodium and potassium in breast milk compared to cow's milk: this means that hypernatraemia is less likely to produce a problem in the breastfed baby. Colostrum is the milk that is produced in the first 48 h and is straw coloured with a high protein content and lower fat and carbohydrate content compared to normal milk. The introduction of bottled cow's milk is deferred until the age of one year because of the low iron and vitamin content and the risk of chronic subclinical gastrointestinal bleeding.

The average calorific requirements for a one-month infant are approximately 100 kcal/kg/day. Standard cow's milk formula contains about 100 kcals/100 ml.

Contraindications to breastfeeding

Maternal

— Untreated maternal TB.
— Maternal hepatitis B SAg +ve.
— Maternal drugs such as amiodarone, cytotoxics, indomethacin, lithium, tetracyclines, theophylline, colchicine, senna, carbimazole, chloramphenicol, dapsone, thiouracil and sulphonamides all of which are secreted in significant quantities in breast milk.
— Maternal HIV infection. This is not the case in Third World countries where the risk of death from malnutrition is greater.

Neonatal

— There are various congenital anatomical abnormalities such as cleft lip and palate.
— Inborn errors of metabolism such as phenylketonuria and galactosaemia.

You should be familiar with the malnutrition syndromes and the clinical consequences of mineral and vitamin deficiencies.

BIOCHEMICAL ABNORMALITIES CAUSED BY GASTROENTEROLOGICAL CONDITIONS

These commonly come up in many parts of the examination and you should be familiar with them.

Vomiting

Low sodium, potassium and chloride.

Persistent vomiting or hypertrophic pyloric stenosis

See also later in this chapter. Hypochloraemic or hypokalaemic metabolic alkalosis. The urinary pH, contrary to what would be expected, is usually acidic. This is because the kidney conserves potassium in preference to hydrogen ions.

Remember the other possible causes of a hypokalaemic hypochloraemic metabolic alkalosis that should be considered (this is a common question) and beware: they may have similar clinical presentations. It can be caused by renal and extra-renal chloride loss. The causes are Barrter syndrome, cystic fibrosis, chloridhorrhoea, diuretic or purgative abuse or prolonged vomiting due to any cause. Hyperaldosteronism should also be considered.

Remember that if vomiting is severe there may also be evidence of dehydration with raised urea, hypernatraemia and possibly raised haemglobin. There may also be hypoglycaemia.

Malabsorption syndromes

Malabsorption syndromes can cause low iron, calcium, phosphate, ferritin, albumin, red-cell folate levels and raised ALP and INR levels. Hepatic cholestasis results in reduced fat absorption and of the fat-soluble vitamins A, D, E and K. Thus vitamin D malabsorption can cause rickets and vitamin K malabsorption a raised INR. Reducing substances in the faeces gives an indication of carbohydrate malabsorption. Faecal A1AT collection can assess protein absorption, and elastase in the faeces is a specific marker of pancreatic function.

Abdominal pain and hyponatraemia

This syndrome pattern repeats itself time and time again in questions and you should be familiar with the causes. It is discussed in the section under clinical scenarios later in this chapter.

Diarrhoea

Hypo/hypernatraemia or normal serum sodium. The potassium may be raised initially because of the metabolic acidosis secondary to bicarbonate loss, but if the diarrhoea is persistent it invariably falls. The glucose may initially be raised and this may cause some confusion with diabetes mellitus (DM) in some questions. Testing the stools for reducing substances is useful to determine if there is sucrose/lactose malabsorption (faecal pH may also be low because of bacterial fermentation).

Remember that excessive mucus production by the bowel can produce a normal anion gap metabolic acidosis (like renal tubular acidosis, ingestion of HCL, sometimes in uraemia and in ureteric diversion into the small bowel). The biochemical picture of an extremely low plasma chloride and potassium and high plasma bicarbonate should lead you to suspect congenital chloridorrhoea caused by abnormal active chloride absorption in the ileum. Confirm it by finding very low urinary chloride and plasma levels and excessive faecal chloride levels (usually more than 100 mmol/l with a normal range of approximately 5–15 mmol/l). It presents early and is often associated with hyperbilirubinaemia. There is growth and developmental delay. Treatment consists of potassium chloride (KCL) replacement (this may occur in a data interpretation question).

MALABSORPTION

This is a useful classification.

Malabsorption as a result of mucosal damage

— *Coeliac disease*: (mainly proximal small bowel affected with mucosal damage decreasing in severity towards the ileum as gluten is degraded into smaller and smaller non-toxic fragments).

— *Crohn disease*: which can affect any part of the small bowel but has a propensity for the terminal ileum (Vitamin B12 and bile acids).

— *Intestinal lymphangiectasia*: where the intestinal villi are dilated either congenitally or secondary to obstruction (see later).

— *Abetolipoproteinaemia*: (see later).

Intraluminal causes of malabsorption

— *Intestinal hurry* such as may occur post gastrectomy or ileal resection.

— *Defective secretions into the gut*: (a) cholestasis resulting in decreased intestinal bile salts and thus defective fat absorption including fat soluble vitamins; (b) pancreatic enzymes: cystic fibrosis, chronic pancreatitis and the Diamond–Schwachman syndrome (see chapter 14).

— *Infections*: Giardiasis is the commonest but consider also *Strongyloides* and hook-worm infestation.

— *Bacterial overgrowth*: Typically in blind loops but also in duplication cysts can classically produce fat and vitamin B12 malabsorption.

— *Enzyme deficiencies*: the commonest being the disaccharidase deficiency lactase deficiency, but also others such as congenital lactase deficiency.

GUT DISORDERS AND HAEMATOLOGY

Anaemia

Anaemia can be caused by a wide range of gastrointestinal pathologies.

Blood loss

This causes a typical iron deficiency anaemia pattern (see chapter 8). The following should be considered: reflux oesophagitis, oesophageal varices, peptic ulceration, gastritis, cow's milk protein intolerance, inflammatory bowel disease, haemangioma or telangiectasia (look for telangiectasia elsewhere), Meckel's diverticulum and, chronic NSAID administration (for example for chronic arthritides). Worldwide, the hookworm is the commonest cause. Remember that an acute bleed may not have any effect in haematological indices initially within a few hours.

Reduced red cell production

The other gastrointestinal causes of anaemia are induced by reducing red cell production. The main ones are vitamin B12 and folate deficiencies which cause a megaloblastic anaemia (see chapter 8). The vitamin B12 intrinsic factor complex is absorbed in the terminal ileum.

— *Vitamin B12 deficiency* can be caused by achlorrhydria (possibly as part of pernicious anaemia) where there is reduced intrinsic factor production (derived from parietal cells), fish tapeworm infection, terminal ileal resection or terminal ileal disease such as Crohn disease.

— *Folate deficiency*. Folate is absorbed in the proximal bowel and its absorption will therefore be affected by proximal bowelopathies such as coeliac disease. Chronic diarrhoea states can also produce folate deficiency by a secondary deficiency in the intestinal enzyme necessary to convert dietary folate into the absorbable form.

Causes of an abnormal jejunal biopsy

Having taken a jejunal biopsy in the investigation of malabsorption and obtained a histological report of villous atrophy the differential diagnosis is commonly asked for.

The possibilities are:

— Coeliac disease. For a definite diagnosis an initial biopsy is required followed by a normal one six weeks' later, following a gluten-free diet. A third is sometimes taken following a challenge of gluten (rarely required nowadays). Remember that in children under two years repeat biopsy is more important since transient gluten intolerance is more common. Antibody studies are also useful (see later).

— Temporary gluten intolerance is usually secondary to gastroenteritis.

— Post gastroenteritis.

— Cow's milk/soya milk protein intolerance.

— Giardiasis.

— Severe combined immunodeficiency.

— Post chemotherapy.

— Hypogammaglobulinaemia (although this may be secondary to complicating giardiasis).

— Kwashiorkor in the tropics.

— Tropical sprue, a malabsorption syndrome encountered in the tropics.

Following a jejunal biopsy there are other histological possibilities that may be obtained. In *giardiasis* it is occasionally possible to see organisms. If concerned about a disaccharidase deficiency then various histochemical staining techniques can be carried out to confirm this. In abetolipoproteinaemia (see later for details) characteristic swollen and fat-laden epithelial cells can be found. In intestinal lymphangiectasis dilated mucosal lymphatic vessels may be seen (see later).

Occasionally there is a slide of a jejunal biopsy taken from a child with coeliac disease. These are the characteristic features:

1. Villous atrophy which diminishes in severity the more distal the intestine.

2. Heavy infiltration of the lamina propria with chronic inflammatory cells (lymphocytes and eosinophils).

3. Elongation and deepening of the intestinal crypts.

HEPATOLOGY

Bilirubin metabolism

This is a prime example of a basic science topic that will be popular with examiners; it is extremely important in understanding many clinical conditions in paediatrics.

Post-mature erythrocytes → removed by the reticuloendothelial system → globin broken down to amino acids and iron reutilised → haem → biliverdin (water soluble) → biliverdin reductase (all tissues) → unconjugated bilirubin (water insoluble) → transported to the liver attached to albumin → bilirubin taken up by the hepatocyte membrane and transported to the smooth endoplasmic reticulum (by carriers such as ligandins) → UDP glucoronyl transferase → conjugated with two molecules of glucoronic acid → bilirubin diglucoronide (water soluble) → actively transported into the bile canaliculi → bile in the intestine → in terminal ileum hydrolysed by bacteria to release free bilirubin → reduced to urobilinogen which has three fates: → (1) most of it is oxidised to stercobilin (faecal pigment), (2) some is absorbed by the terminal ileum and transported back to the liver by the enterophepatic circulation, (3) some is reabsorbed by the blood and is excreted in the urine.

You must know the following classification. I have included neonatal and childhood causes of jaundice.

Unconjugated hyperbilirubinaemia

Unconjugated bilirubin is water insoluble and there is thus no bilirubin in the urine (acholuric jaundice). There is however an increased amount of urobilinogen in the urine.

Increased bilirubin production

— Haemolysis for any reason: extracellular (immune, drugs), intracellular (red-cell membrane defects, haemoblobinopathies – after six months of age) and red-cell enzyme defects (G6PD deficiency, pyruvate kinase deficiency).

— Sepsis: congenital or acquired

— Haematoma

— Polycythaemia.

Decreased bilirubin uptake or metabolism
— Gilbert syndrome
— Crigler–Najjar syndrome
— Lucey–Driscoll syndrome
— Hypothyroidism
— Sepsis, acidosis and hypoxia
— Congestive cardiac failure
— Physiological jaundice of the newborn.

Altered enterohepatic circulation
— Breast milk jaundice
— Intestinal obstruction
— Receiving antibiotics.

Conjugated hyperbilirubinaemia

The intrahepatic causes produce a mainly mixed picture (with conjugated and unconjugated hyperbilirubinaemia). The extrahepatic cholestatic causes produce a mainly conjugated hyperbilirubinaemia. Bilirubin will be found in the urine (since conjugated bilirubin is water-soluble). Clinically one would expect dark urine and pale stools and pruritis.

Neonatal hepatitis syndrome
— Congenital infection e.g. rubella, CMV, toxoplasmosis

— Metabolic. A1AT deficiency, cystic fibrosis, CHO metabolism: galactosaemia (test for reducing substances), fructosaemia, glycogen storage disease type IV. Protein metabolism: tyrosinaemia. Lipid metabolism: Wolman disease. Storage diseases: Gaucher disease, Niemann–Pick disease. Copper metabolism: Wilson disease

— Idiopathic giant cell hepatitis.

Abnormalities in excretion of bilirubin by the hepatocyte:
— Dubin–Johnson, Rotor syndrome.

Non-neonatal hepatitis
— *Infection:* This includes the hepatitis viruses A, B, C and Echo, Reo, CMV, EBV, *Leptospirosis*

— *Chemical and drug induced:* carbon tetrachloride, ethylene glycol — including other solvents such as in glue sniffing — alcohol (ethanol and methanol), halothane, isoniazid and rifampicin, paracetamol, methotrexate

— Autoimmune.

Intrahepatic cholestasis
— Alagille syndrome (see chapter 14)
— Byler disease (progressive familial intrahepatic cholestasis — AR)
— Zellweger syndrome (see chapter 14)
— TPN cholestasis (mechanism unclear).

Extrahepatic cholestasis
— Biliary atresia, choledocal cyst (typically a variable jaundice), mass/neoplasia, stone, high intestinal obstruction.

There are a wealth of questions relating to jaundice in the paediatric examination and we will endeavour to cover them now in their various forms through examples. We will refer to the classification above throughout.

The baby who presents with jaundice on the first day of life

A baby who presents with jaundice on the first day of life is always abnormal. You must know that the causes include:

Haemolytic causes
— *Blood group incompatibilities:* rhesus haemolytic disease, ABO incompatibility, and anti-C, E, Kell and Duffy haemolysins.

— *Red cell membrane defects:* hereditary spherocytosis.

— *Red cell enzyme defects:* glucose-6 phosphate dehydrogenase deficiency (commoner in black, oriental and Mediterranean peoples). Remember that haemoglobinopathies (such as sickle cell disease and thalassaemia) will not present in the neonatal period since fetal Hb predominates.

Sepsis
Septicaemia, UTI, congenital TORCH-like syndrome.

— *Investigations* therefore include: full blood count, blood film, blood group of baby and mother and any atypical maternal antibodies, direct Coombs' test, G6PD assay depending on the ethnic group of parents, TORCH screen especially if conjugated hyperbilirubinaemia present. Infection screen (blood culture, urine for MC&S and so on).

The baby referred to hospital with jaundice at three weeks of age

This is another common question. The causes of prolonged neonatal jaundice must be divided up into conjugated and unconjugated hyperbilirubinaemia. Of course a detailed history and clinical examination would be expected.

— *Conjugated hyperbilirubinaemia* causes include the conditions under the titles neonatal hepatitis syndrome, intrahepatic and extrahepatic cholestasis and disorders of bilirubin excretion (in jaundice classification above).

— *Unconjugated hyperbilirubinaemia* causes include hypothroidism, haemolytic anaemia, breast milk jaundice, sepsis, Gilbert syndrome, Crigler–Najjar syndrome, Lucey–Driscoll syndrome and transient familial hyperbilirubinaemia.

— *Investigations:* Initially: FBC, blood group and direct Coombs' test, liver function test including a split bilirubin estimation, U&Es, blood culture, urine for MC&S, urine for reducing substances, TFTs. These will be useful for an initial screen, and if the jaundice turns out to be unconjugated and the other tests are normal (and the baby is clinically well) then a wait and see policy is usually recommended. If the mother is breast feeding then this will be the usual cause.

However if there is a conjugated hyperbilirubinaemia then the necessary biochemical and serological tests must be carried out as soon as possible to exclude the aforementioned causes. Initially liver function tests, bacterial and viral cultures, metabolic screening tests and hepatic ultrasound will be organised. After these have been performed, and if there is still no specific cause found it is imperative to differentiate between biliary atresia and idiopathic neonatal hepatitis, usually with radioisotope studies and possibly a liver biopsy. In extrahepatic biliary atresia (which may also present with deranged clotting, raised transaminases and a raised ALP and GGT) there is delayed excretion of radioisotope into the extrahepatic ducts and intestine. The 99Tc labelled HIDA scan is used with less than 5% excretion of the drug in 72 h. The rose bengal test is an older method. The need for rapid diagnosis is because any delay in the Kasai procedure (see below) beyond about six weeks of age reduces its chances of success. NB: In biliary atresia the onset of jaundice may be delayed for up to four weeks after birth.

— *Kasai procedure:* A hepatic portoenterostomy. This involves forming a connection between the porta hepatis and the bowel lumen. Post-operative complications include: intestinal obstruction, ascending cholangitis (early and late), peristomal breakdown and progressive biliary cirrhosis. Success of the operation is judged by an improvement in biliary flow. Approximately 50% of cases are unsuccessful with ongoing inflammation and biliary cirrhosis. Consider liver transplantation as an alternative option.

A baby found to be jaundiced on the second day of life

Hb	16.2 g/dl
PLT	164
Unconjugated bilirubin	294 µmol/l
Conjugated bilirubin	0 µmol/l
Mother's blood group	O Rh +ve
Baby's blood group	B Rh +ve
DCT	Weakly positive
Blood film	Numerous spherocytes seen

The most likely answer to this question is ABO incompatability. Being blood group O the mother has anti-A and anti-B antibodies and since the baby is blood group B this is a feasible explanation. There is also no Rhesus incompatibility. Not all blood group incompatibilities will result in haemolysis since in most cases the maternal antibodies are IgM and not IgG and therefore will not cross the placenta. ABO incompatibility usually produces a relatively mild jaundice and only very rarely is exchange transfusion required (compared with Rhesus haemolysis — see Table 6.2). Other general features that would make haemolysis more likely is an increased reticulocyte count, reduced serum haptoglobin and a drop in the Hb concentration.

NB. A more detailed account of haemolytic disorders is found in chapter 8.

A child who has a prodromal illness of 1–2 weeks and then presents with jaundice

Unconjugated bilirubin	61 µmol/l
Conjugated bilirubin	42 µmol/l
ALT	1949 IU/l
AST	1041 IU/l
ALP	310 IU/l
GGT	489 IU/l
Urine: Bilirubin	+ve
Urobilinogen	−ve

Table 6.2 Comparison of ABO and Rhesus incompatibility

ABO incompatibility	Direct Coombs weakly +ve	Numerous spherocytes
Rhesus incompatibility	Direct Coombs strongly +ve	No spherocytes

The most likely cause would be an infectious type of hepatitis and the commonest in this country is hepatitis A, although also consider EBV and CMV as possibilities. Hepatitis B and C are blood-borne and therefore these should be considered if the history suggests such.

The hepatitis has produced hepatocellular damage as manifested by the raised AST and ALT. There is also an element of cholestasis as manifested by the raised ALP and GGT levels.

Remember that in the exam you should be able to discuss a full differential diagnosis and list the other questions that you might like to ask in the history in a child who presents with jaundice. These are ethnicity, recent injections or transfusions, contacts with jaundiced individuals, presence of dark urine or pale stools, recent drug therapy, the period from onset of first symptoms to jaundice (hepatitis A: usually 2–6 weeks and hepatitis B: 2–6 months), abdominal pain (hepatitis, stones), recent surgery (halothane toxicity) and family history (e.g. for Gilbert syndrome — unconjugated).

A four-year-old child with recurrent episodes of jaundice since birth with a normal examination

Haematology	normal
Reticulocytes	1.8
Unconjugated bilirubin:	13 µmol/l
Conjugated bilirubin:	67 µmol/l
Urine: Bilirubin	+ve
Urobilinogen	−ve

This clearly demonstrates a conjugated hyperbilirubinaemia. The answer is Rotor syndrome. In paediatrics there are a number of conditions that produce recurring or fluctuating levels of jaundice and they can be classified into two main types:

Haemolytic disorders
Haemolytic disorders are where haemolytic crises tend to occur as a result of endogenous stressors such as infection or exogenous stressors such as drug administration or surgery. Examples of such haemolytic disorders are sickle cell disease and G6PD deficiency.

Inherited disorders of bilirubin uptake, conjugation and excretion
These are Gilbert and Crigler–Najjar syndromes (unconjugated hyperbilirubinaemias), Dubin–Johnson and Rotor syndromes (conjugated hyperbilirubinaemias).

— *Gilbert syndrome*: AD. 1–2% of population, bilirubin usually less than 35 µmol/l. Diagnosis by exclusion of other causes. Biopsy is rarely necessary. Prognosis excellent. Defect-decreased uptake and conjugation of bilirubin.

— *Crigler–Najjar syndrome*: Type I AR Type II AD. Very rare and presents in the neonatal period with high levels of unconjugated hyperbilirubinaemia and can progress to kernicterus. The defect in type I: completely deficient conjugating enzyme resulting in early death (orthotopic liver transplant may be successful). Type II: partial deficiency and may respond to phototherapy and phenobarbitone.

— *Dubin–Johnson syndrome*. AR. Rare. Conjugated hyperbilirubinaemia. Presents usually after puberty. Liver stained black by centrilobular melanin. Late rise in bromosulphthalein (BSP) elimination curve at 90 min but normal at 45 min. Abnormal cholecystogram. Defect: decreased hepatic excretion of bilirubin.

— *Rotor syndrome*. AR. Rare. Conjugated hyperbilirubinaemia. Presents at a younger age. Liver biopsy normal. Raised BSP at 45 min and no secondary rise at 90 min. Normal oral cholecystogram. Defect unknown.

Neonatal hepatitis B immunisation

This is a common question in the exam and relates to the protocol for immunisation of babies born to mothers who are hepatitis B surface antigen positive. It is essential to know the serology of the mother.

We can divide the mother who is hepB SAg +ve into three main types depending on her serology.

1. *High infectivity*: 'e' Ag and no 'e' antibodies. Risk of baby being hepatitis BSAg +ve is 80%.
2. *Intermediate infectivity*: No 'e' markers.
3. *Low infectivity*: 'e' antibodies and no 'e' Ag. Risk of baby being hepatitis BSAg +ve is 10%.

In the first two cases it is recommended that active immunisation and passive immunisation be given into different thighs. In the third case of low infectivity it is recommended to give just the active immunisation. In all cases it is advised that passive or active immunisation take place within the first 12 h of the baby's life. The active vaccine doses are repeated at one and six months and seroconversion tested at one year of life. If negative then a repeated booster of active vaccine is given. A booster is given at five years of age.

The importance of neonatal immunisation is to reduce the risk of cirrhosis and hepatoma in later life.

GASTROENTEROLOGY RADIOLOGY

When looking at an X-ray of the abdomen be sure to have it the right way around. If the gastric bubble still appears to be on the right and liver shadow on the left then this may represent situs inversus. Ask to see a CXR to look for dextrocardia.

Hypertrophic pyloric stenosis

A plain X-ray may show absence of air distal to the pylorus. It is usually demonstrated well on barium meal: a normal gastric outline followed by a narrow, elongated pyloric channel referred to as the 'string sign', delayed gastric emptying and 'mushroom' appearance of the duodenal cap. Ultrasound demonstrates a thickened pylorus and is often diagnostic with a typical history.

Duodenal atresia

Because of the distension of the first part of the duodenum this gives the characteristic appearance of the 'double bubble' with the larger gastric bubble (left) adjacent to a smaller duodenal bubble (right).

Crohn disease and ulcerative colitis

Barium studies are the radiological investigations of choice.

— *Crohn disease*: strictures, 'rose thorn' ulcers, 'cobblestone' mucosal appearance (secondary to mucosal oedema) and skip lesions. Any part of the bowel may be involved but most commonly it involves the small bowel and therefore a barium meal and follow through is the investigation of choice.

— *Ulcerative colitis*: This will only effect the colon in a continuous fashion starting distally. Thus a barium enema will be the investigation of choice. Classic findings are: shortening of the colon and loss of the haustra producing the 'drain-pipe' colon (also backwash ileitis with terminal ileum involvement rarely).

Necrotising enterocolitis

There are four classic features that may be present. (a) Fixed oedematous loops of bowel with thickened wall; (b) Intramural gas-pneumatosis intestinalis; (c) Free air in the peritoneal cavity if there is a perforation present (ask for a lateral film); (d) Gas in the biliary tree.

Intestinal obstruction

Erect and supine films are important. Generally there may be gas-filled distended loops of bowel with multiple horizontal fluid levels. Remember the differences between small and large bowel radiologically. Small bowel have plicae circulares which completely cross the lumen and occupy a central portion of the abdomen and large bowel have haustra that do not completely cross the lumen and occupy the outer portion of the abdomen often with a distended caecum.

Intussusception

Characteristically on a plain film there is a lack of gas in the right iliac fossa and features of small bowel obstruction. Barium enema can be both diagnostic and therapeutic in bringing about reduction. Characteristically shows the 'coiled spring' appearance. As the barium moves proximally a knuckle of obstructing bowel can be seen. Ultrasound shows a mass which is made up of concentric layers.

Hirschsprung disease

Absent gas in the pelvis on a plain abdominal radiograph of the abdomen in the prone position strongly suggests the diagnosis. A barium enema is best done on an unprepared colon (that is, no prior enemas). It may demonstrate the transition zone between ganglionic and aganglionic segments. This gives a characteristic 'ice cream cone' appearance at the transition zone, as the aganglionic section is tonically contracted and the rectal diameter is classically narrower than the sigmoid diameter.

Volvulus

This can cause a 'corkscrew' appearance with other features of intestinal obstruction (see above).

Meconium ileus

There is characteristic bubbling (ground glass appearance) in the meconium plug with the other features of obstruction proximal to it. There may be an associated distal microcolon seen in contrast studies.

GI perforation

This will produce air under the diaphragm if the child is erect and there may be delineation of the falciform ligament.

Paralytic ileus

Gas is distributed diffusely throughout the bowel.

Opacities on the X-ray

This is divided up into the various possibilities.

— *Intestine*: foreign body, meconium peritonitis, TB.
— *Peritoneum*: speckled peritoneal calcification caused by bowel perforation, meconium ileus antenatally.
— *Liver*: gallstones, TB, haemangioma, hydatid cyst/amoebic cyst.
— *Kidney*: renal stones, nephrocalcinosis (remember hyperparathyroidism).
— *Bladder*: stones, foreign body, schistosomiasis.
— *Tumours*: Wilm, neuroblastoma.
— *Abdominal wall*: Post surgery in scar tissue or calcified haematoma.

Microcolon

This is usually a slide of a barium enema with a section of very narrow colon. It is associated with Hirschsprung disease; meconium ileus and a left microcolon which is associated with the infant of a diabetic mother.

Anorectal atresia

Contrast X-rays of a fistula between rectum and bladder/urethra/vagina or of a radio-opaque anal marker failing to reach the air bubble in the rectum.

CLINICAL SCENARIOS

In paediatrics there are a number of diseases that can present with abdominal pain that do not derive from the gastrointestinal system and may therefore produce some confusion. These include: pneumonia (especially right lower lobe), pharyngitis (especially *Streptococcal*), pyelonephritis, renal colic, nephrotic syndrome, pericarditis, haemolytic crisis (such as sickle crisis), migraine (family history or history of recurrent abdominal pain), infectious mononucleosis (hepatic or splenic origin), hypoglycaemia, diabetes mellitus (especially ketoacidosis), hypokalaemia, porphyria and lead poisoning.

Recurrent abdominal pain

This is a common clinical presentation in children. Ninety per cent of cases have no organic cause. A diagnosis of 'the syndrome of abdominal migraine' is made in a child who is thriving, with periumbilical pain (remember the further the pain is from the umbilicus the more likely pathology is present — Appley's law). There may be recurrent nausea and vomiting and a positive family history of migraine or recurrent abdominal pain. The episodes are usually not long or severe and may be triggered by certain situations. Irritable bowel syndrome is being increasingly diagnosed and is suggested by a history of recurrent abdominal pain, bloating, alternating diarrhoea and constipation often in children who are described as 'worriers'. Minimal investigations might include FBC, ESR, AXR and urine for MC&S.

Abdominal pain with hyponatraemia

There are many questions that present a case of a child with abdominal pain and a biochemistry picture of hyponatraemia. You must know the differential diagnosis, which, includes the following possibilities:

— *Nephrotic syndrome*: here the abdominal pain results from splanchnic ischaemia (as a result of vascular volume depletion) and the hyponatraemia from dilution.

— *IDDM*: especially ketoacidosis. Look for other clues in the biochemistry picture.

— *Addison disease*: there may be other signs of hypotension and shock. The potassium will usually be raised.

— *Acute intermittent porphyria*: abdominal pain is common during attacks and hyponatraemia occurs secondary to SIADH caused by hypothalamic involvement. There may be dark urine, neurological features and skin pigmentation without blistering in sun exposed areas.

— *Gastrointestinal cause*: for the abdominal pain and hyponatraemia. Hyponatraemia secondary to diarrhoea and vomiting.

Abdominal pain with neurological features

Another useful pattern to be familiar with in the examination and in clinical practice is the combination of abdominal pain and neurological features. Here the differential diagnosis includes.

— *Lead poisoning* (an exam favourite). This produces abdominal features (abdominal pain, vomiting and constipation) as well as neurological features such as signs caused by raised intracranial pressure, seizures, sixth nerve palsy, ataxia and peripheral neuropathy (mainly motor). Neurological features result from cerebral oedema, vasculitis and increased capillary permeability. In addition there may also be a microcytic hypochromic anaemia, haemolytic anaemia and basophilic stippling. Fanconi syndrome may occur and lead lines may be seen radiologically (growth arrest lines at the metaphysis of long bones). Test the urine for Fanconi type picture (glycosuria, phosphaturia and so on). There is an increased urinary coproporphrin, increased delta aminolaevulinic acid and normal porphobilinogen. Note that sometimes there is a clue in the question: for example, if the child lives in an old house (walls often painted with lead-containing paint).

— *Acute intermittent porphyria* (dealt with in chapter 10). During attacks this can produce abdominal pain, vomiting, constipation and dark urine. Neurological features may include personality changes, and varying neurological problems ranging from mild peripheral neuropathy to quadriplegia and respiratory failure (caused by neuronal damage and demyelination). In order to differentiate it from lead poisoning (during attacks) there is an increased urinary delta aminolaevulinic acid and raised urinary porphobilinogen.

— *Sickle cell crisis* may well have combined abdominal pain and neurological features (usually with a preceding characteristic history in an appropriate racial setting).

— *Hypoglycaemia*.

— *Wilson disease* (see later).

Abetolipoproteinaemia

Think of the rare AR disorder of abetolipoproteinaemia in a child who presents with diarrhoea or steatorrhoea and progressive neurological features with a progressive ataxia, neuromuscular degeneration and retinitis pigmentosa (neurological features seen after the age of approximately 10 years old). A blood film may show acanthocytosis (erythrocytes with spiny projections from surface – seen also post splenectomy). Typically there is no post-prandial lipaemia. Retinitis pigmentosa and acanthocytosis are thought to be secondary to vitamin E deficiency. It is caused by defect in apoprotein B production by the intestine which leads to defective LDL, VLDL and chylomicron synthesis and thus failure of lipids transportation from the intestine or liver (including malabsorption of fat and fat-soluble vitamins A, D, E and K). Other features include very low levels of cholesterol and triglycerides and the consequences of A, E and K deficiency. Treat with medium-chain triglycerides and fat-soluble vitamins.

Pus collection

With any clinical history where there is a swinging temperature with an abdominal mass you must think of a pus collection which may be in the liver, gall bladder, bowel, kidney or tumour. Remember that the kidney may be obstructed and therefore give rise to a culture negative urine specimen despite the presence of an abscess in the kidney. Perform an ultrasound scan (consider IVU or DMSA scan if considering renal origin).

Tuberculosis

If the history is one of several weeks to months of general malaise, anorexia, weight loss and any GI symptoms then always consider tuberculosis in the differential diagnosis especially if the patient is Asian or immunocompromised. In addition there may be an abdominal mass, hepatosplenomegaly and ascites.

Discharge from the umbilicus

This may be seen in a number of conditions. You should be aware of the different possibilities. These include: (a) umbilical sepsis; (b) patent urachus – urine discharge from bladder; (c) patent vitello-intestinal duct — faecal discharge; (d) umbilical granuloma (see embryology notes earlier in chapter).

Omphalocoele or gastroschisis

You may be shown a slide of an omphalocoele or gastroschisis. In an omphalocoele abdominal contents are herniated into a sac comprising amnion and peritoneum (as a result of deficiency of the umbilical ring). The umbilical cord is attached to the vertex of the sac (exomphalos minor contains gut and exomphalos major — larger defect — contains gut and liver). It is associated with Beckwith–Wiedemann syndrome, cardiac defects (for example tetralogy of Fallot), imperforate anus and trisomies 13 and 18. In gastroschisis the small bowel herniates through a defect which is found to the right of the umbilical cord because of a defect in the anterior abdominal wall. There is no peritoneal covering. The exposed bowel is at risk of infarction.

Complications of both include heavy losses of protein and fluid as well as heat loss and infection. Initially occlusive film is placed over the hernial sac and free drainage of gastric contents is performed in order to prevent gut distension. Intravenous fluids and plasma are given, monitoring haemodynamic status and urine output.

A closure is then performed (usually in two stages). Complications of returning the bowel into the abdomen include bowel infarction and occlusion of the inferior vena cava.

Hereditary spherocytosis

In a Caucasian child who presents with a Coombs' negative haemolytic anaemia and splenomegaly then consider hereditary spherocytosis (AD). In about 20% of cases of hereditary spherocytosis splenomegaly will be absent. There may be a history of neonatal jaundice in about half the cases. Diagnosis is usually made on blood film. Remember that the red-cell fragility test is not reliable until about six months of age. These patients may come to clinicians in aplastic crisis (like sicklers) if infected with the human parvovirus type B19 (see chapter 8).

In some questions use is made of the connection of a child who has a haemolytic disorder (for instance, hereditary spherocytosis) and develops recurrent abdominal pain. In addition to haemolytic crises (especially sicklers) think of the formation of pigment gallstones producing biliary colic, acute and chronic cholecystitis and perform an ultrasound scan to confirm.

Anaemia and abdominal pain

In a child presenting with anaemia and abdominal pain you must not forget the potential sites of bleeding in the gastrointestinal tract. These may present as haematemesis, malaena, frank blood PR or in occult loss so that the symptoms and signs of anaemia predominate. Know your lists of causes of GI bleeding, many of which lead to painless loss of blood: oesophagitis, swallowed maternal blood at birth or through cracked nipples (these last two a cause of rectal bleeding in neonates), Mallory–Weiss tear/syndrome, gastritis, peptic ulcer, Meckel's diverticulum (diagnose with a technetium isotope scan which is taken up by gastric mucosa), inflammatory bowel disease, foreign body, haemangioma, bacterial gastroenteritis (especially *Salmonella*, EHEC, *E. coli*, *Campylobacter*, *Shigella* and *Yersinia*), intussusception, NEC (in neonates), volvulus, polyps, cow's milk protein intolerance, vasculitis e.g. HSP, anal fissure, sexual abuse and coagulopathies.

GOR

In a baby who presents with persistent vomiting you should know the differential diagnosis which is available in most paediatric texts. Don't forget the huge range of possibilities ranging from raised intracranial pressure through to a metabolic disorder. Your investigations will be directed from the history and examination. For example a common cause of persisting vomiting in a three-month-old baby who may have an element of failure to thrive is gastro-oesophageal reflux (GOR). Remember another common presentation of GOR which is coughing and possibly apnoea especially shortly after feeds. Your investigations of choice will therefore be a pH probe study and barium swallow. However a baby who is vomiting and has a head circumference increasing disproportionately to the rest of the body will need a cranial scan etc. Thus your history and examination will direct your evaluation.

Bruising around labia majora and anus

A not uncommon finding of bruising around the labia majora and anus, including excoriation and erythema, does not necessarily cause concern about sexual abuse (although this should always be considered in such cases). This is especially so when there is no involvement of the labia minora or the vaginal orifice itself. The leading diagnosis would indicate that some sort of irritation such as allergy to washing detergent, for example, or threadworms — (*Enterobius vermicularis* — nocturnal itching prominent) is causing the problem. You would carry out a detailed history and examination and test for threadworms with the sellotape test (where eggs can be identified microscopically). Although as paediatricians you should have a high index of suspicion of abuse this question is really seeing whether you have a sensible and discriminatory approach to your patients.

Necrotising enterocolitis

A question dealing with a premature baby who develops abdominal distension, bile-stained vomiting or bloody stools should immediately suggest to you the possibility of necrotising enterocolitis. However in the exam the presentation may not be so obvious. There may be non-specific signs such as vomiting, hypotension, thrombocytopenia, temperature instability, apnoeas and lethargy. The babies have almost always been fed. There may also be an antenatal doppler report of reversed end-diastolic flow (associated with NEC). Know your investigation and management.

Crohn disease

A teenage child who presents with an insidious onset of weight loss, abdominal pain, unexplained fever and possibly diarrhoea should alert you to the possibility of Crohn disease, which is on the increase in children. Indeed the failure to thrive may well precede any gastrointestinal symptoms. There may be a right iliac fossa mass. It may present as an acute ileitis resembling acute appendicitis. Anal lesions (skin tags, fissures and fistulas) are common. In the exam, questions will of course make use of the huge range of extraintestinal features common to the condition: delayed puberty, short stature (the last two are a common accompaniment to most chronic inflammatory conditions), clubbing, arthritis — 20% have joint involvement at presentation and it is usually mild, assymetrical and migrating, resolving without deformity, usually involving lower limb joints. Arthritis may precede GI symptoms. In addition apthous ulcers, angular cheilitis, erythema nodosum, uveitis, episcleritis, conjunctivitis and also occasionally concurrent liver involvement (chronic active hepatitis, gallstones and biliary cirrhosis) may occur. Ulcerative colitis (UC) shares many non-GI manifestations with Crohn and clinically can be difficult to distinguish from it. However rectal bleeding (often bloody diarrhoea), mucus passed rectally and abdominal pain (lower abdomen) are usually commoner features in UC. A formed stool implies rectal disease and diarrhoea implies more extensive disease. Investigation of choice for UC is colonoscopy and biopsy and barium follow through for Crohn.

Aphthous ulcers

A question may present a child with recurrent aphthous ulcers (or aphthous stomatitis). Most are idiopathic but may be associated with Crohn disease, ulcerative colitis and occasionally in coeliac disease, Behçet disease and neutropenia. Behçet disease has three main features consisting of recurrent painful oral and genital ulceration (scrotum, penis and labia) often the presenting feature, ocular inflammatory disease (pain, iritis, posterior uveitis) and neurological involvement including aseptic meningoencephalitis, pseudotumour cerebri and severe brainstem and cord lesions. Gastrointestinal symptoms may also occur and are varied. Lesions resembling erythema nodosum may occur. A medium–large sized joint arthritis may be seen. A migratory vasculitis (thrombophlebitis) may occur. Males are twice as commonly affected as females. HLA B-5 associated. The pathergy test involves a sterile subcutaneous puncture (for example a blood test), which in Behçet may give rise to a bullous/pustular reaction within a couple of days. It usually has a benign relapsing and remitting course.

'Toddler's diarrhoea'

A child who is thriving and well nourished but presents to the clinician with chronic diarrhoea with no obvious cause given in the question leads one to consider 'toddler's diarrhoea' as the diagnosis. Key points in the history that you should look for are the typical age that is, 6–24 months; parents often report seeing particles of undigested food in the stools; and the absence of failure to thrive. Management is reassurance and it usually resolves spontaneously at 2–3 years (obviously in the clinic additional investigations such as a stool sample would be also carried out).

Pseudomembranous colitis

This is a potential case in the exam. It is caused by an alteration in the normal balance in gut flora by antibiotic therapy with resulting overgrowth of *Clostridium difficile* (it is the A and B toxins of *Cl. difficile* that are pathogenic). Children present with varying degrees of symptoms ranging from mild watery diarrhoea with crampy abdominal pain to severe watery/bloody diarrhoea with a high fever, raised white cell count and even toxic megacolon and perforation. It is most commonly associated with the use of clindamycin, ampicillin, penicillins and cephalosporins.

Symptoms may begin during the course of antibiotic treatment or up to six weeks following the course. Sigmoidoscopy reveals the characteristic yellow necrotic areas on the mucosal surface. Stool culture for *Cl. difficile* or assays for its toxin can be carried out. It is less reliable for infants and neonates many of whom commonly carry both the organism and the toxin in their bowel. Treatment consists of oral vancomycin and metronidazole.

Bezoars

You may come across bezoars in the exam. They are collections of indigestible swallowed material in the gut, most often seen in the stomach. They may be made up of undigested milk proteins or hair collections (seen in trichillomania, often in adolescent girls and possibly psychiatric disturbance). The importance of bezoars is that they may result in obstruction. Keep them in your differential diagnosis of obstruction. Treatment often ends up being surgical.

Parotitis

Occasionally there are questions about parotitis in children. The commonest cause is mumps which has a 2–3-week incubation period. Check the MMR immunisation status. It most commonly affects the parotid glands but submandibular glands may also be affected. Acute suppurative parotitis is most commonly caused by *Staph. aureus*, and *Strep. pyogenes* and occurs in debilitated patients who are dehydrated. Acute sialadenitis (more commonly affecting the submandibular gland in about 80% of cases) is caused by a duct calculus. Increasingly, recurrent parotitis is being seen in HIV infection. Recurrent acute inflammation may be seen in children without stones or strictures and usually improves with time (recurrent parotitis of childhood). It produces a painful parotid gland (unilateral or bilateral) with erythema around Stensen's duct (or occassionally pus discharging from the duct). Chronic parotitis may be a result of salivary duct dilatation (sialectasis) resulting in recurrent infection. Sjogren syndrome is an autoimmune disorder that principally affects the salivary and lacrimal glands causing dry eyes and dry mouth. One-third of patients have chronically enlarged slightly tender parotid glands. Investigations for parotitis would include X-ray for stones, MC&S of the expressed pus from Stenson's duct, sialograms of the glands and possibly an HIV test.

Pelvic appendix abscess

A question that you should recognise is the child who may have symptoms of appendicitis that may settle and then recur with the patient in urinary retention (usually with a palpable bladder). The cause is a pelvic appendix abscess which often causes urinary retention.

CF with malaena or haematemesis

A case may describe a child with cystic fibrosis who presents to the casualty department with malaena or haematemesis. The causes of such a gastrointestinal haemorrhage include: (a) portal hypertension having given rise to oesophageal varices with their subsequent rupture; (b) reduced fat-soluble vitamin absorption and thus reduced vitamin K absorption with consequent deficiency of clotting factor synthesis; (c) liver involvement in cystic fibrosis may affect clotting factor synthesis; (d) in a child it may sometimes be difficult to distinguish between haematemesis and haemoptysis; (e) hypersplenism secondary to portal hypertension causing thrombocytopenia.

Coeliac disease

Failure to thrive after onset of weaning (thin, muscle wasting especially buttock wasting, hypotonic and pale), diarrhoea (soft, pale and sticky) and abdominal bloating should alert you to the possibility of coeliac disease. Oedema, rickets, iron deficiency anaemia may also occur and the children are often depressed and irritable.

Onset is usually by two years of age and symptoms usually start at the introduction of cereals at 5–6 months of age. You may be shown a growth chart of a child where the weight begins falling and crossing centiles from the age of gluten introduction. Vomiting is more common the earlier the onset of the disease. It is associated with HLA-B8. Late complications include gastrointestinal lymphoma (heralded by a worsening in clinical state), myopathies, neuropathies, hyposplenism and later in life gastric and oesophageal carcinoma. Don't forget the association with dermatitis herpetiformis.

A typical slide question might show a miserable child with wasted buttocks and a bloated abdomen. An important differential diagnosis is *Giardiasis* which can present with bloating, flatulence, diarrhoea, abdominal pain and malabsorption with steatorrhea and failure to thrive. It is investigated by repeat stool microscopy (since *Giardia* is excreted in intervals), looking for cysts or trophozoites or duodenal aspiration. Treatment is with metronidazole which is sometimes given empirically on suspicion only. Initial investigations in coeliac disease would include antibodies (IgA antigliadin, antiendomyseal and antireticulin antibodies — remember however that 3% of coeliacs have IgA deficiency), jejunal biopsy (see before), examination of jejunal mucosa and jejunal aspirate for *Giardia*.

Other differentials include cow's milk protein intolerance which causes vomiting, diarrhoea occasionally with blood, failure to thrive, rash, wheeze and eczema. Treatment of coeliac disease is with a gluten free diet (no wheat, barley or rye but maize and rice products may be eaten).

Mediterranean fever

Recurrent episodes of fever with abdominal pain in a child of Mediterranean origin (Sephardic Jews, Turks and Arabs for example) should lead you to suspect familial Mediterranean fever. It is a disorder of polymorphonuclear cells. Attacks usually start between five and 15 years but this is not always the case. Attacks consisting of fevers (over 38.5°) with serositis (mainly abdominal pain with tenderness, but also pleuritic pain, large joint arthritis and pericarditis rarely) occur approximately monthly for a few days, but the frequency decreases with age. Skin lesions such as erysipelas may occur. A family history may be present in half the cases. The question may have presented a child with a recurrent acute abdomen having been operated on several times with no pathological finding. WCC and ESR are raised during attacks but normal in between. Genetic testing for the commonest mutations can be carried out. Treatment is with colchicine. A serious complication is amyloidosis (mainly vascular involvement).

Abdominal tumours

Know about the commoner abdominal tumours in infancy which include nephroblastoma (can have haematuria and rarely cause tricuspid regurgitation because of invasion of IVC), hepatoblastoma which is associated with an increased platelet count and increased alphafetoprotein (the first two tumours are associated with Beckwith–Wiedemann syndrome) and neuroblastoma. All these can present with an abdominal mass. An IVP of a nephroblastoma reveals a filling defect which distorts the calyceal system, displaces the kidney and does not cross the midline. The IVP in neuroblastoma may cause displacement of the kidney with little distortion of the calyceal system since it is extrarenal (usually adrenal gland). CT scan will also differentiate the two since one is extrarenal and the other intrarenal (see chapter 4 for more details).

Acute pancreatitis

This is rare in children but may turn up in a question. Symptoms include severe abdominal pain radiating to the back with shock and tachycardia. The main causes in children include trauma, drugs, viral illness, hyperlipidaemia, CF and hyperparathroidism. Look for a raised amylase in the biochemistry.

Hirschsprung disease

This can present in a number of ways. Most commonly it is seen in males (M:F ratio 4:1): (a) delay in passing meconium in first 24 h (90%); (b) intermittent bowel obstruction or chronic constipation; (c) failure to thrive; (d) a severe enterocolitis (commoner in neonates) may perforate the bowel (and may occur even post repair). Most cases (90–95%) of Hirschsprung present in the first year of life (90% of these in the first month) but may present later. There can be short segment or more extensive involvement. The anal canal and rectum are usually free of faeces and the examiner may feel a tight grip on the examining finger (see earlier notes on radiology). A rectal biopsy under sigmoidoscopy may identify absence of ganglion cells, and staining for acetylcholinesterase reveals abnormally prominent nerve fibres (a possible slide question). Also perform manometric studies on the anus. The internal anal sphincter is always involved and extends proximally a variable distance.

Treatment of neonatal Hirschsprung consists of producing a defunctioning colostomy, removing the aganglionic segment and then pull through repair at a later age. Another anatomical abnormality that may be associated with constipation includes an anteriorly located anus where the anal canal and external sphincter are anteriorly placed. In anterior ectopic anus the external sphincter is in the normal position but the anal canal and internal sphincter are anterior (this can be felt as a shelf projection on PR examination). Anal fissures may also cause constipation as a result of pain and inhibition behaviour. Remember that any cause of chronic constipation may cause soiling. Fluid faeces pass around the hard impacted faecal mass since the distended rectum fails to control the bowel motion.

Recurrent episodes of vomiting

These can be bile-stained and occur with abdominal pain, both of which may resolve spontaneously and can be caused by recurrent volvulus which is most commonly a result of malrotation. Can also be because of duplication cysts or Ladd's bands (see notes on malrotation earlier in chapter).

Protein-losing enteropathy

In a question that presents a child with chronic diarrhoea and a low protein count one has to consider a protein-losing enteropathy.

1. Exudation from ulcerated mucosa, for example intestinal TB.
2. Defective lymphatic drainage, for example intestinal lymphangiectasia.
   NB Look also for low Ig levels and very low lymphocyte count with a normal remainder of the WCC.
3. Others include coeliac disease, food allergy and CF.

Coma and hepatic dysfunction

A pattern that comes up in questions and you should be familiar with is the child who presents with (1) coma or near coma; and (2) hepatic dysfunction. Apart from hepatic failure and concurrent encephalopathy be familiar with the other causes.

The list includes *Reye syndrome*: suspect this in any question where a child develops an acute onset of encephalopathy associated with hepatic dysfunction. Peaks at 5–6 years of age. Usually a biphasic illness with a viral URTI followed about 5–6 days later by intractable vomiting. This is associated with confusion, agitation and a deepening level of unconsciousness (the result of raised intracranial pressure). There is no jaundice, no fever and the liver may be enlarged. Investigations: bili — normal, NH_3 — raised, PT time — increased, hypoglycaemia in approximately 15%. Unknown aetiology but associated with *Influenzae* A, B, *Varicella* and the administration of aspirin in children under 12 years. Histology — a possible slide question — shows fatty accumulation with no necrosis or inflammation and swollen mitochondria in the liver and other tissues. Treatment is supportive including treatment of hepatic failure and fluid restriction. Other differential diagnoses to exclude are as follows: (a) fatty acid oxidation, amino acid and mitochondrial electron transfer defects; (b) urea cycle defects (more likely in infants); (c) salicylate and carbon tetrachloride poisoning; (d) sepsis and (e) hypothermia.

Wilson disease

A rare syndrome but very common exam topic is Wilson disease and answering the related questions requires recognising the classic presentation patterns. These include: (a) presentation usually after the age of eight or nine years of age; (b) chronic liver disease (which may present with hepatosplenomegaly, cirrhosis, jaundice, hepatitis and/or fulminant hepatic failure). Liver disease may be absent at disease presentation; (c) neurological features may be the first presentation and include intellectual impairment/behavioural change (manifest often in questions as reduced school performance) and extrapyramidal movement disorder (tremor, rigidity); (d) haemolytic anaemia; (e) Fanconi syndrome; (f) cataract (sunflower type).

You may be asked for your investigations to confirm. These are: low serum caeruloplasmin (also seen in nephrotic syndrome, malabsorption and protein-losing enteropathy), high urinary copper excretion increasing with penicillamine challenge, slit-lamp examination of the eyes for detection of Kayser–Fleischer rings (dull green/gold coloured granular deposit at the limbus of the cornea — almost pathognomonic). A raised copper level in a liver biopsy specimen. Also screen siblings (AR). Treat with D-penicillamine. Pathology: failure of liver to excrete copper into bile so that accumulation causes suppressed caeruloplasmin levels and excess copper spills out of the liver into the circulation and deposits in various tissues causing the above pathology.

Alpha–1 antitrypsin deficiency

Hepatomegaly and a prolonged neonatal conjugated hyperbilirubinaemia is a common exam pattern and you should know the differential diagnosis given earlier in the chapter. A rare condition but relatively common in the exam is alpha-1 antitrypsin deficiency. It is important to know the different ways in which it can present. The commonest is in adults with premature emphysema and bronchitis (not seen before the first decade). Less commonly it presents in infancy with neonatal cholestasis (a cause of prolonged neonatal jaundice), hepatomegaly, cirrhosis and liver failure and there is a longer term risk of hepatic carcinoma. Eighty-five per cent are asymptomatic.

In the question you are usually directed to it being the most likely diagnosis after other metabolic screens are negative, radioisotope labelling tests are normal and an ultrasound scan for a choledocal cyst (which presents with variable jaundice) is negative. Since A1AT enzyme is an acute phase reactant its level may be artificially raised to normal levels in inflammatory disorders. Therefore Pi (protease inhibitor) typing is performed. Genes express co-dominant inheritance. Infants with the ZZ phenotype are at risk of the neonatal hepatitis and later in life of lung disease. The MM-phenotype is normal and the heterogeneous MZ-phenotype may or may not have hepatic disease. Treatment is a liver transplant which converts the recipient to the Pi phenotype of the donor.

Primary haemochromatosis

This is an autosomal recessive inherited disorder in which there is excessive iron absorption from the gut. This excessive iron may be deposited in the pancreas (leading to diabetes), heart (leading to cardiomyopathy), synovial membranes (leading to arthropathy and chondrocalcinosis), testicles (leading to feminisation in males) and the liver leading to hepatomegaly, cirrhosis, liver failure (and a long-term risk of hepatocellular carcinoma). The children gradually develop skin pigmentation (secondary to melanin deposition – sometimes referred to as 'bronzed diabetes'). The serum iron is raised and there is an almost totally saturated serum iron-binding capacity. The serum ferritin may be raised. Liver biopsy shows perilobular fibrosis with excessive iron deposition. Treatment is with repeated venesection. A secondary form of haemochromatosis is seen in children needing repeated blood transfusions for example in beta thalassaemia major (see chapter 8).

Chronic active hepatitis

In a girl (usually over 6–7 years of age) who presents with an insidious onset of jaundice, general malaise (including weight loss and anorexia) and hepatosplenomegaly consider chronic active hepatitis which is usually autoimmune. Test for nuclear autoantibodies, smooth muscle antibodies, antiliver microsomal antibodies. Treatment with steroids +/– azothioprine. F:M 3:1 ratio. Prognosis: post therapy 70% are normal at five years and the remaining 30% develop cirrhosis and liver failure. Pathology demonstrates piecemeal necrosis.

ABDOMINAL CLINICAL EXAMINATION

This is a commonly assessed system in the short cases and you should have a good, reproducible and effective system. For the sake of simplicity this clinical section also incorporates the examination of the renal system (as it does clinically) in order to save on repetition in the renal chapter. As in other systems (if you are given a choice) I advise you to examine the system fully before presenting your findings to the examiner rather than presenting as you examine. It appears more professional and you are less likely to make blunders.

First, introduce yourself to the patient/parent. Then expose the abdomen from the nipples to the knees keeping the child's pants on and generally maintaining the dignity of the patient with a blanket (if available).

General inspection

Observe the child from the end of the bed. Look for whether thriving or not, dysmorphic features, race (for example, Afro-Caribbean for sicklers, Asian for thalassaemia) and presence of a nasogastric tube. Telangiectasia, spider naevi (in region drained by superior vena cava that is, above the nipple line).

More than three spider naevi are significant (chronic liver disease, ataxia telangiectasia or hereditary telangiectasia).

In order to impress your examiners look also for complications of GI diseases such as erythema nodosum, arthritis, iritis or complications of treatment such as the cushingoid features of steroid use for example IBD; gum hypertrophy seen in cyclosporin use: for example, post-renal transplant (also seen in phenytoin use and M4, M5, AML).

Abdominal inspection

Inspect the abdomen fully including the flanks for scars (don't forget renal angle and liver biopsy scars), distension (the Fs), caput medusae, umbilical hernia (Afro-Caribbean, Down, hypothyroidism, mucopolysaccharidoses and prematurity).

— Take both hands and inspect both palmar aspects and the nails. Look particularly for palmar erythema, anaemia (nailbed and palmar creases), clubbing (know the causes) and koilonychia (iron deficiency).

— Look at the eyes. Inspect the sclera for jaundice and the conjunctivae for anaemia. Although uncommon clinically, look for Kayser–Fleischer rings seen in Wilson disease (not uncommon in exam short cases).

— Inspect the mouth. Perioral pigmentation in Peutz–Jaegers syndrome. Look for aphthous ulcers. Ask the patient to stick his tongue out. Macroglossia is associated with hypothroidism, Beckwith–Wiedemann syndrome and the mucopolysaccharidoses. In Down the tongue protrudes secondary to hypotonia but is not enlarged. Look at the dentition.

— Ask the patient to sit forwards and with both hands gently palpate the cervical lymph nodes from behind.

— Having inspected the abdomen fully before (after general inspection) you now palpate the abdomen. It is absolutely essential that you look at the child's face during palpation since any discomfort elicited will usually be obvious and you can adjust your palpation accordingly (a scream from the child in pain as a result of your examination does not impress the examiner and could fail you). In addition it also shows that you are a sensitive doctor. The examiners will be looking for this caring and gentle approach throughout the clinical examination. In fact this may be a good time to interact and distract the child (obviously depending on the age — for example, 'So let's see if I can feel what you had for breakfast'). Don't forget that the examiner is looking for a general rapport with children and will be awarding marks for it, since after all it is a paediatric examination.

— Bend down or kneel to the level of the abdomen and with the flat palmar aspect of your hand superficially palpate the four quadrants in turn. Then repeat this with deeper palpation (being sensitive to signs of guarding which are most unlikely in the short cases). Children will sometimes tense their abdominal muscles making palpation difficult. Try flexing both knees in order to loosen the abdominal muscles. Any masses should be delineated and measured approximately.

— You must now palpate for organomegaly. First palpate the liver starting from the right iliac fossa and work your way up. Try and synchronise the palpation with the child taking a breath in, and try and feel the liver edge flick across your fingertips. In younger children a liver edge that is soft can usually be felt up to 1–2 finger breadths below the right costal margin and is normal.

Then palpate for a spleen again from the right iliac fossa and again synchronising with deep inspiration. In order to facilitate feeling for an enlarged spleen turn the child over on to their right side and palpate again with the child taking a deep breath (your free hand should be on the left side of the rib cage in order to stabilise it). It may be just palpable in an infant however a palpable spleen in an older child is never normal (since it must be three times its normal size in order to be felt on palpation).

Now palpate for the kidneys. This is always done bimanually with the left hand over the loin posteriorly and the right hand palpating deeply anteriorly. Perform one side and then the other. In infants the kidneys are often felt normally and this is sometimes facilitated by flexing the hips.

— Percuss the child's abdomen over the main quadrants and over the liver and spleen. Remember to percuss out the upper border of the liver in suspected hepatomegaly since hyperinflated lungs may push the liver down causing this apparent hepatomegaly. (Some children might be scared so it is always worthwhile warning them before that 'I am going to make you sound like a drum').

— Now you must auscultate the abdomen listening for bowel sounds and bruits especially over the aorta, renal arteries and liver and any masses that you may have palpated. You can use this time to start putting your findings together in your mind.

— If the abdomen is distended or there are signs of chronic liver disease then you should test for ascites. This is done in two ways. (1) Shifting dullness. Starting from the umbilicus percuss towards the flanks and mark the skin over which dullness was first heard. Then turn the child on to that side and again percuss as before and see if the dullness has moved significantly towards the midline (implying the presence of fluid in the peritoneal cavity). (2) Fluid thrill (positive only if there is a large amount of ascitic fluid). Place one hand on one side of the abdomen and then flick the skin of the contralateral side to see if there is transmission in the form of a thrill. However since it will also be transmitted by the subcutaneous fat politely ask the examiner's assistance (or child if old and co-operative enough) to place a hand vertically in the midline pressing gently on the skin.

— It is now essential as part of your paediatric abdominal examination that you sit the child forwards to inspect the back for scars and signs of spina bifida/occulta (which may be responsible for an enlarged bladder or faecal soiling etc.).

— You must then turn to the examiner and say that ideally you would also like to examine the genitalia, the anal area and look for herniae and perform a rectal examination to complete the abdominal examination as well as plotting the height and weight on a centile chart. The examiner will usually say 'No, that's fine'.

Presenting to the examiners

By this time you should hopefully have some sort of idea as to what you think the pathology is. Now comes the all-important presenting to the examiners. Remember to keep your hands still and look at the examiner and not the patient.

Say 'On abdominal examination …'. First mention a general observation: for example 'Charlie looked well/thriving/ thin/obese'.

Then mention the following whether they are present or not (since they are important to the differential diagnosis): Presence or absence of jaundice, anaemia and clubbing. Also mention any other findings such as scars, spider naevi or umbilical hernia if present.

Now you can mention the findings on the examination of the abdomen itself blending the results of palpation, percussion and auscultation: this makes you sound confident and coherent. A model example would be: 'The abdomen was generally soft and non-tender apart from a smooth mass that could be palpated 5 cm below the right costal margin which moved with respiration, could not be got above and was dull to percussion with no abnormal associated sounds'.

Finally formulate a diagnosis if you can: 'These findings are consistent with hepatomegaly'. In the short cases this is probably as far as you can go not having done a complete examination. However you will probably be quizzed as to the possible causes of hepatomegaly in the child.

USEFUL CLINICAL HINTS IN THE EXAMINATION OF THE ABDOMEN

Differentiating an enlarged left kidney from an enlarged spleen

You must know the differences:

1. It is usually possible to be able to get a hand above a kidney, however this is not possible with an enlarged spleen.

2. The spleen usually enlarges along a direction that approximates to the line made by the ninth rib (diagonally from the left costal margin to the right iliac fossa).

3. The kidneys can be ballotted bimanually but this is not possible with a spleen.

4. In the case of an enlarged spleen it is usually possible to palpate the splenic notch on its leading border (however the notch may be absent in the younger child).

5. There is usually dullness to percussion over an enlarged spleen but this is not so in the case of an enlarged kidney which is retroperitoneal and therefore has resonant bowel over it.

Know the following patterns of clinical signs indicating disease

Chronic liver disease

Jaundice, palmar erythema, clubbing, leukonychia, spider naevi, foetor hepaticus from breath, hepatomegaly, splenomegaly (secondary to possible portal hypertension), ascites, caput medusae (secondary to portal hypertension) and peripheral oedema.

In addition if you have picked up on these signs, go a step further and look for a cause, for example. Kayser–Fleischer rings in Wilson disease, or clinical lung disease in cystic fibrosis.

Chronic renal failure

Pallor, sometimes uraemic colour to skin (lemon tinge), pulmonary and peripheral oedema, pleural effusions, pericarditis, scars relating to renal surgery, peritoneal dialysis scars, AV vascular access sites. **NB** Any evidence of renal disease should instinctively lead you to take the blood pressure (and test the urine if provided).

Causes of hepatomegaly and splenomegaly

If predominantly hepatomegaly or splenomegaly, indicated as H or S respectively in brackets after the condition. If no S or H then hepatosplenomegaly is seen.

Haemolytic

Sickle cell disease (S) felt before splenic infarction (which occurs at 2–4 years of age), thalassaemia, hereditary spherocytosis (S).

Infections

— *Bacterial*: bacterial septicaemia, brucellosis, tuberculosis. SBE (S).
— *Viral*: hepatitis A, B, EBV, CMV.
— *Protozoal*: toxoplasmosis, malaria (S).
— *Parasitic*: hydatid disease, schistosomiasis.

Metabolic

— *Storage disorders* Mucopolysaccharidoses, lipidoses, glycogen storage disorders (H).
— *Others* Wilson disease, galactosaemia (H), alpha-1 antitrypsin deficiency (H), cystic fibrosis, Reyesyndrome (H).

Congestive cardiac failure
Neoplastic causes

Hepatic tumours primary and secondary (H), leukaemias, lymphoma, neuroblastoma.

Gastrointestinal
Chronic hepatitis (H), biliary atresia (H), inflammatory bowel disease, portal hypertension (usually S but depends on cause) prehepatic, hepatic and posthepatic.

Chronic diseases
SLE, JCA.

Causes of enlarged kidneys

Unilateral enlargement
Hydronephrosis, kidney with cyst or cysts, tumour e.g. Wilm tumour, renal vein thrombosis.

Bilateral enlargement
Hydronephrosis for example posterior urethral valves, stones, ureterocoeles, polycystic kidneys, tumour such as Wilm tumour (remember that 5–10% are bilateral), also infiltration secondary to leukaemia and lymphoma.

Other masses in the abdomen
These may include: faecal impaction (sometimes indentable), transplanted kidney (with overlying scar in the lower abdomen), palpable bladder (examine back for spina bifida), right iliac fossa mass in Crohn disease and tumours.

ABDOMINAL SCARS

You should have a basic knowledge of the common scars that you may encounter in the examination.

— A common scar is the so-called gridiron scar over the RIF which runs parallel and above to the inguinal ligament and is the result of a previous appendicectomy.

— A laparotomy scar usually takes the form of a midline, right or left paramedian scar and implies exploratory or major abdominal surgery e.g. bowel resection in Crohn disease.

— A so-called Kocher incision in the region of the liver implies hepatic surgery e.g Kasai procedure for biliary atresia (see notes earlier in chapter). Smaller scars may be found in the region of the liver and may be the result of liver biopsies for the investigation of liver disease.

— A scar in the lower abdomen may be the result of a transplant and you should be able to feel a kidney beneath it. Renal biopsy scars are small and located on the back over the loins.

— Small scars on the lateral aspects of the sides of the abdomen (usually on a line between umbilicus and anterior superior iliac spine) may be the result of previous peritoneal dialysis. In cases of suspected chronic renal disease look for arteriovenous fistulae (usually on the arms and they should have an associated thrill and bruit if functional).

— Colostomies are usually flush with skin surface and are usually in the region of the left iliac fossa. Ileostomies usually protrude slightly from the skin's surface and are located in the right iliac fossa (performed usually in the treatment of IBD and proximal colonic obstruction). Both types can be temporary or permanent. Examine the surrounding skin for excoriation and the scar itself for dehiscence or herniation.

Endocrinology

THYROID DISORDERS

Thyroid physiology

The thyroid gland begins embryologically as an out-pouching from the floor of the pharynx and migrates caudally to its final position in the lower neck anterior to the trachea. This is the pathway of the thyroglossal duct from the foramen caecum of the tongue (junction of anterior two-thirds and posterior one-third of the tongue) down in front of the hyoid bone to the thyroid gland. Remnants of the thyroglossal duct may present in the form of a cyst, sinus or fistula (mostly in the midline and move with swallowing). Iodide ingested in the food is actively concentrated in the thyroid gland. Peroxidase converts it into iodine which is then incorporated into tyrosine residues in thyroglobulin using peroxidase. The tyrosine residues are either iodinated at either one or both ends (producing monoiodothyronine — MIT — or diiodothyronine — DIT). Coupling then occurs and MIT may combine with DIT to form triiodothyronine (T3) or two DITs can combine to form tetraiodothyronine (T4). The thyroglobulin is then secreted into the colloid for storage and under the influence of TSH endocytosis of thyroglobulin together with hydrolysis liberates free T3 and T4. All T4 is produced from the thyroid gland but 85% of T3 (considered the active hormone) is derived from peripheral conversion of T4 (by the enzyme 5' monodeiodinase). The hormones are bound to thyroxine binding globulin (TBG) and albumin and it is the free component which is biologically active.

A negative feedback loop exists between TRH (hypothalamus), TSH (anterior pituitary) and thyroid hormones. The thyroid hormones control the basal metabolic rate, affect growth, mental development, sexual maturation and increase the sensitivity of beta-receptors to catecholamines.

— *Changes occurring at birth*: At birth there is an outpouring of TSH from the pituitary gland resulting in very high levels of TSH which usually fall to adult levels by the end of the first week (and this is followed by parallel changes in T3 and T4 levels).

Congenital hypothyroidism

This is a common slide question and you should be able to recognise it (it may sometimes be difficult to distinguish from a Down baby on a picture slide). It is most commonly caused by agenesis or dysgenesis although there may also be ectopic thyroid tissue present (the majority of cases are sporadic). In agenesis there will obviously be no goitre. In the minority of cases (about 5%) there is a dyshormonogenesis, and a goitre will be present, the commonest being Pendred syndrome which is associated with sensorineural deafness (often euthyroid). Other causes include pituitary failure and maternal ingestion of goitrogens during pregnancy.

Clinical features include coarse facial features, dry skin, prolonged jaundice, large fontanelles, posterior fontanelle (>1 cm), cutis marmorata, bradycardia, hypothermia, hoarse cry, cold extremities, hypotonia, lethargy and poor feeding, constipation, umbilical hernia, macroglossia and oedema. The brain is extremely sensitive to the presence of thyroid hormones from the end of pregnancy until the first few weeks of life and if left untreated may result in irreversible mental retardation.

Screening involves testing for serum TSH levels at seven days of life (following the postnatal TSH surge). The TSH levels will be very high (> 20 μmol/l most >50 μmol/l) but be aware that this method will not pick up hypothyroidism caused by a low TSH (pituitary failure). You should also be alerted to the possibility of a more generalised hypopituitary problem if in addition there is hypoglycaemia, small phallus or midline defects (see later in this chapter).

Juvenile hypothyroidism

A question may describe a child who may be short for his age, suffers from constipation, has recently become less sociable, and recently gained weight; his school performance is deteriorating and he is intolerant of cold. There may also be a presenting goitre. These features should point you in the direction of juvenile hypothyroidism. They have typical facies with pale dry skin and periorbital puffiness. They may be short. Typically there is no effect on intellect (compared with congenital hypothyroidism). Causes include: Hashimoto thyroiditis (more common in girls who may have initial thyrotoxicosis or be euthyroid or hypothyroid at presentation). Hashimoto may be associated with Down, Turner and Klinefelter syndromes as well as SLE and other autoimmune disorders. Hashimoto is the commonest cause of hypothyroidism in children. A goitre may be present initially with no clinical features of disturbed thyroid function at first. Antithyroglobulin and antimicrosomal antibodies are found. Bone age is delayed. Other causes of juvenile hypothyroidism include ingestion of goitrogens, iodine deficiency, hypothalamic/pituitary disorder (secondary hypothyroidism — TSH low) and post thyroidectomy. Treatment is with thyroxine.

Hyperthyroidism

This is described as primary with decreased TSH and secondary with increased TSH (pituitary). It may present with weight loss, increased growth rate, nervousness and irritability, fatigue, increased sweating, diarrhoea, increased appetite, dislike of hot weather, palpitations, tachycardia, fine tremor, hyperreflexia, proximal myopathy, goitre, thyroid bruit and lid lag (caused by sympathetic overactivity). It is most commonly a result of Graves disease and this is caused by thyroid stimulating immunoglobulins (TSIs) directed against the TSH receptor. Females are more commonly affected (F:M 5:1). Additional features of Graves disease include pretibial myxoedema and Graves ophthalmology (chemosis, diplopia and exophthalmos). Other causes of thyrotoxicosis include a toxic adenoma, subacute thyroiditis (often painful goitre) and initially in Hashimoto thyroiditis. Treatment may require carbimazole (or second line propylthiouracil); propranolol is used especially for thyroid storm. Thyroidectomy and radioactive iodine in older patients.

Neonatal hyperthyroidism

You should be aware of the rare case of neonatal hyperthyroidism caused by the transplacental transfer of thyroid stimulating immunoglobulins. It occurs in 1–2% of cases of maternal Graves disease. Remember that since the condition is caused by immunoglobulins and not thyroid hormone transfer the mother may not be clinically thyrotoxic around the time of birth. The baby presents within the first week with irritability, diarrhoea, temperature instability, tachycardia (sometimes supraventricular tachycardia), diarrhoea and weight loss; there may be features of heart failure. The disease is transient and disappears with the disappearance of the antibodies, usually within 2–3 weeks.

— *Thyroid storm* may occur if thyrotoxicosis is undetected and left untreated and it presents with fever, tachycardia, irritability, sweating and diarrhoea. Treat with i.v. carbimazole, i.v. beta-blockers and rehydration.

Goitre

A goitre may be classified as (a) toxic goitre: Graves disease, toxic adenoma, subacute thyroiditis, toxic multinodular goitre; (b) non-toxic goitre: Hashimoto thyroiditis, simple goitre of iodine deficiency (especially at puberty where there are increased requirements), ingestion of goitrogens, inborn errors of metabolism caused by dyshormonogenesis, or euthyroid goitre, a simple colloid goitre, common in the second decade, that may resolve spontaneously in later life or become a multinodular goitre.

Investigations of thyroid function

— *TSH:* Normal range 0.4–4.0 µmol/l. Raised in primary hypothyroidism and low in secondary hypothyroidism. Low in thyroid hyperthyroidism and raised in pituitary hyperthyroidism.

— *Total T3 and T4:* This gives measurements of thyroid hormones bound to binding proteins and thus are unreliable since they can be increased by for example oestrogen treatment and decreased by protein-losing states such as nephrotic syndrome.

Table 7.1 Examples of typical results obtained in a TRH stimulation test

Time after TRH injection	0	20	60
TSH (hypothyroid)	4.7	24	59
TSH (hyperthyroid)	0.8	1.2	0.7
TSH (hypothalamic)	1.3	4.1	6.7

— *Serum free T3:* Rises early in thyrotoxicosis (cf. T4) and so is more important in detecting thyrotoxicosis.

— *Serum T4* falls earlier than T3 in hypothyroidism and is thus more important in detecting hypothyroidism.

— *TRH test:* This may be a data interpretation question and you will be expected to recognise the main graphical types. This test is used if the patient is suspected of having thyroid disease but the TFTs are equivocal. It involves the measurement of TSH levels before, 20 min and 60 min post-TRH administration. In normal individuals the TSH levels rise by 20 min (by 1–20 µmol/l) and fall to normal levels by 60 min. In primary hypothyroidism there is an exaggerated response, with very high levels of TSH continuing to rise even after 60 min. In hyperthyroidism there is a flat response (because of inhibition by thyroxine) and in hypothalamic disease there is a delayed response. See Table 7.1.

— *Autoantibody screen — Graves:* thyroid stimulating immunoglobulin (TSI), thyroid growth immunoglobulin (effects size of goitre), thyroid ophthalmological immunoglobulin (causes eye signs) Hashimoto thyroiditis: antimicrosomal and antithyroglobulin antibodies.

— *Bone age:* delayed in hypothyroidism.

— *Ultrasound:* If nodules are felt consider ultrasound.

— *Thyroid scan:* detects uptake of pertechnetate (hot areas). Useful to identify ectopic thyroid tissue.

ADRENAL DISORDERS

Adrenal physiology

The adrenal gland has two main regions: (a) the adrenal cortex; and (b) the adrenal medulla. The adrenal cortex in fetal life produces cortisol and dehydroepiandrosterone (DHEA). After birth the cortex has differentiated into the zona glomerulosa (outermost), zona fasciculata (middle) and reticularis (innermost). Their function is in the production of (a) glucocorticoids; (b) mineralocorticoids; and (c) androgens.

The zona glomerulosa produces mineralocorticoids (aldosterone). Its production and release is under the control of renin (released from the kidney in response to reduced renal perfusion). Renin results in the conversion of angiotensinogen to angiotensin I which as a result of the action of angiotensin converting enzyme (ACE) in high concentration in the lungs, causes the conversion of angiotensin I to angiotensin II. Angiotensin II improves the renal perfusion by (a) increasing the production of aldosterone; (b) directly causing vasoconstriction; and (c) stimulating thirst. Aldosterone acts on the distal convoluted tubule to cause sodium and water reabsorption (in exchange for potassium or hydrogen ions).

The zona fasciculata and reticularis produce glucocorticoids and androgens respectively. The release of these hormones (especially cortisol) is under a negative feedback controlled by ACTH released from the anterior pituitary gland (which itself is controlled by CRH release from the hypothalamus). Cortisol has a diurnal variation with highest levels at 9 a.m. and lowest levels at midnight.

Congenital adrenal hyperplasia

A common question relates to congenital adrenal hyperplasia. See Fig. 7.1.

The commonest enzyme abnormality is the 21 hydroxylase deficiency (accounting for 95% of cases) in which progesterone and 17 OH progesterone fail to be converted to deoxycorticosterone and deoxycortisol respectively resulting in failure of production of aldosterone and cortisol with excessive androgen production. The reduced cortisol production results in increased ACTH secretion which causes adrenal hyperplasia and excess precursor production as well as testosterone hyperproduction. The second commonest enzyme deficiency is that of 11 B-hydroxylase deficiency which prevents deoxycorticosterone and deoxycortisol being converted to aldosterone and cortisol respectively. The clinical presentation of this condition is usually in the neonatal period. Common presentations include:

a. Genital hypertrophy in the male and in the female with hypertrophy of the clitoris and labia, and labial fusion (which may present in more severe cases with ambiguous genitalia). The genitalia may display pigmentation after several weeks because of increased ACTH secretion.

b. Salt-losing crisis presentation in about 70% of the 21 hydroxylase deficiency variety (which may occur from about day 3–4 up to about three weeks).

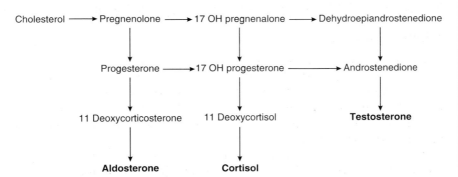

Fig. 7.1 A simplified biochemical pathway demonstrating the main causes of congenital adrenal hyperplasia.

It presents with hypotension, features of dehydration, vomiting, shock and collapse. An early sign is an increase in serum potassium even before clinical signs become evident. Remember that the biochemical pattern of a low sodium and high potassium may occur with acute renal failure as well as aldosterone deficiency and diabetic ketocidosis (however in the latter acidosis is present and the potassium is often normal — despite total body potassium being depleted).

c. Hypoglycaemia

The 11 B-hydroxylase deficiency presents less commonly with salt-losing crisis and hypotension (in fact hypertension is more common) since the build up of 11 deoxycorticosterone appears to protect against hypotension as well as causing hypokalaemia (since it has some mineralocorticoid activity). Partial defects exist where there may be no symptoms until puberty when females may present with amenorrhoea and hirsutism and males with precocious puberty. Delayed clinical presentation also includes excessive growth, but because of premature epiphyseal closure the final height is lower than expected.

— *Investigations*: (here we will discuss the two commoner varieties). Raised 17 OH progesterone levels in 21 OH deficiency and raised 11 deoxycortisol in 11 B hydroxylase deficiency. Urine chromatography may also be used to look for raised urinary 17 ketosteroids (androgen metabolites) and decreased 17 hydroxycorticosteroids (cortisol metabolites). Biochemical abnormalities will depend on the enzyme defect and in 21 OH deficiency if of the salt losing type: low sodium, low glucose, high potassium, metabolic acidosis and high urea and haematocrit. In the 11 B hydroxylase deficiency there may be hypokalaemia. In addition you may want to perform other tests to exclude other causes of ambiguous genitalia (see later).

— *Treatment* acutely involves resuscitation with i.v. fluids such as normal saline, glucose and intravenous hydrocortisone. In the long term one should use regular treatment with hydrocortisone and a salt-retaining mineralocorticoid such as fludrocortisone in order to prevent continued ACTH induced hyperplasia whilst also allowing adequate replacement. Monitor treatment with serum or salivary 17 OH progesterone levels. Further treatment involves assessment of the genitalia and the possible need in girls for surgical correction.

You should be aware that the salt-losing crisis may sometimes be mistaken for a urinary tract infection or hypertrophic pyloric stenosis (however the biochemistry may help you differentiate the conditions).

Adrenal insufficiency

This is not common in childhood but be aware of its mode of presentation, which may be acute or chronic.

Acute forms
Congenital adrenal hyperplasia/hypoplasia, following severe hypotension, trauma or sepsis, or chronic steroid administration followed by sudden

withdrawal (or failure to increase dosage with periods of stress such as trauma or surgery), Waterhouse–Friederichsen syndrome (bilateral adrenal haemorrhage secondary to septicaemia most commonly resulting from meningococcaemia).

Chronic forms
Addison disease, tuberculosis (may be noticed as adrenal calcification on X-ray). Remember pituitary/hypothalamic causes of adrenal insufficiency (referred to as secondary) as a result of lack of ACTH (through surgery, trauma, irradiation or tumour).

Clinical features
In the acute onset look for a precipitating cause with compounding hypotension, salt loss and collapse. Abdominal pain (epigastric), vomiting, hypoglycaemia with metabolic acidosis, hyponatraemia and raised potassium.

In the chronic form there is a slow onset of generalised fatigue and weakness, anorexia, nausea, vomiting, abdominal pain, diarrhoea, postural hypotension and pigmentation of palmar creases and buccal mucosa (if ACTH is high, this is not found in secondary causes of adrenal insufficiency).

Investigations include biochemistry: there will be low sodium, high potassium and low blood glucose.

There may be a normocytic normochromic anaemia: primary disease — high ACTH; secondary disease — low ACTH. The short synacthen (an ACTH analogue) test will help in diagnosing adrenal insufficiency but the long synacthen test differentiates primary (adrenal) and secondary (hypothalamic/pituitary causes). In the short synacthen test a dose of synacthen is given intramuscularly and in adrenal insufficiency there is no increase in cortisol over 30 min. In the long synacthen test a depot intramuscular injection is given daily for three days and cortisol measurements are made subsequently. In Addison disease there will be no increase in cortisol but in secondary disorders there will be a slow rise (as the essentially functional but hypotrophic glands are 'kick started' into action). Remember that Addison disease is associated with other autoimmune diseases, thus an autoantibody screen may also be useful.

Pseudohypoaldosteronism is caused by renal unresponsiveness to aldosterone resulting in very high levels of renin, aldosterone and consequently hypertension (because of angiotensin II) with hyponatraemia and increased levels of potassium. It may be mistaken for CAH but there is no virilisation.

Cushing syndrome

Causes
The causes of Cushing syndrome are: (a) An ACTH-secreting tumour of the pituitary (Cushing disease); (b) adrenal adenoma/carcinoma secreting cortisol (low ACTH); (c) ectopic ACTH production from for example Wilm tumour; (d) rarely hyperplasia; (e) exogenous steroids (the commonest cause). The zona reticularis is mainly involved.

Clinical features

Thinning of the skin with purple striae, easy bruising, pigmentation if ACTH excess, centripetal obesity (moon face, buffalo hump, protuberant abdomen), limb muscle wasting (leading to proximal myopathy), hypertension secondary to sodium retention (cortisol has some mineralocorticoid activity and thus also hypokalaemia and metabolic alkalosis), osteoporosis and peptic ulcer. Androgens may lead to hirsutism and acne (especially in adrenal adenoma/carcinoma) and psychiatric disturbance.

Investigations

(a) Usually cortisol is highest at 9 a.m. and lowest at midnight. In Cushing syndrome this diurnal rhythm is lost; (b) 24 h urinary cortisol levels are high; (c) dexamethasone is a synthetic glucocorticoid which in normal individuals binds to cortisol receptors in the pituitary gland and causes a decrease in ACTH secretion reducing cortisol production (sometimes measured as urinary 17 OH corticosteroids) by the adrenal glands. The overnight (low dose dexamethasone suppression test) will distinguish between Cushing syndrome and stress, obesity and depression. In the latter three (which can sometimes mimic Cushing) the serum cortisol will become lowered by the dexamethasone (but not in Cushing). In the high dose dexamethasone suppression test cortisol is suppressed in Cushing disease but not in adrenal or ectopic causes of Cushing syndrome; (d) biochemically there may be a high sodium and low potassium and plasma glucose may also be high; (e) in the insulin stress test (see later) the cortisol should rise to more than double the normal baseline in normal individuals – this normal rise does not however occur in Cushing. Treatment depends on the cause and tumours may require surgery (such as adrenelectomy or transphenoidal microadenectomy).

DIABETES MELLITUS

Diabetes questions come up regularly but there appears to be a familiar repertoire of topics relating to it.

Basic physiology

Insulin is an anabolic hormone whose main action is on muscle and adipose tissue where it causes uptake of glucose and promotes its storage as glycogen. It also causes uptake of amino acids, stimulates protein production and promotes fat synthesis. When insulin is lacking these processes go into reverse with hyperglycaemia causing an osmotic diuresis and consequently dehydration, break down of muscle to amino acids (muscle wasting), breakdown of fat to glycerol and fatty acids and ketogenesis (lipolysis with B-oxidation resulting in ketone production via acetyl coenzyme A) with consequent metabolic acidosis. Anti-insulin hormones include glucagon, adrenaline, cortisol and growth hormone.

Examples of question topics relating to diabetes

Hyperglycaemia

The finding of hyperglycaemia on blood testing (often following a prompt from finding glycosuria on dipstick). Glycosuria with a normal blood glucose indicates a problem with proximal tubular reabsorption (but is also seen in some individuals, about 1% of the population, who have a reduced renal threshold for glucose and is called renal glycosuria).

Hyperglycaemia has many causes including: (a) pancreatic disease: cystic fibrosis, haemachromatosis, pancreatectomy, chronic pancreatitis; (b) endocrine disease: Cushing syndrome, growth hormone secreting tumour, thyrotoxicosis, phaeocromocytoma; (c) drugs: steroids, thiazide diuretics; (d) inherited disorders such as Friedreich ataxia. Other causes include: infections (especially associated with high fever), stress, intracranial tumours/infections and following seizures. Hyperglycaemia is accompanied by polyuria (secondary to an osmotic diuresis).

The clinical history of a few weeks of increased thirst, polyuria, weight loss and lethargy in addition to excluding features of the above causes of hyperglycaemia will help you make your diagnosis of DM. Remember that infection may accompany the presentation of diabetes (leading to pruritis vulvae or balanitis). You may be given data relating to a high plasma osmolality with normal sodium, potassium and urea and thus the remaining osmotically active particle contributing to the hyperosmolality must be glucose (see chapter 10).

The Smogyi effect

This is a fairly common question which relates to the child who appears to be a well controlled diabetic (the question may give you clues to this such as a normal glycosylated haemoglobin, no glycosuria in clinic visits, a reliable child and well informed and sensible parents). There is, however, early morning glycosuria and ketonuria. On closer investigation there appears to be an adequate dosage of insulin for their age/weight. This may have prompted an increase in insulin dose administration without improvement in glycosuria or ketonuria. The likely cause is the Smogyi effect which describes the phenomenon where the child experiences night-time hypoglycaemia (although this may also occur during the day as well). This may manifest as nightmares, tremor and rarely fits though usually no manifestations are present but it sets in motion compensatory hormonal mechanisms which lead to rebound hyperglycaemia with the resulting glycosuria and ketonuria. It can be investigated by a 24 h urine collection (ideally every 4 h) which shows excess glucose in the urine during the night time compared with day time or preferably overnight blood glucose sampling.

The Smogyi effect is more common when fast acting insulins are used. Treatment involves carefully reducing the dose of insulin or using a longer acting insulin. Other causes of finding early morning glycosuria are: (1) non-compliance with insulin regime; (2) dawn phenomenon (hyperglycaemia resulting from growth hormone secretion (which peaks at about 4–5 a.m.); (3) inadequate insulin administration — here there is no nocturnal hypoglycaemia and this can be improved by increasing the insulin dose.

Children with poor diabetic control

Be aware of the clinical features of diabetic dwarfism (Mauriac syndrome) which results from very poor diabetic control over a long period. These children are characteristically short with delayed bone age, obese (although weight is low on centile charts because of short stature) and delayed sexual maturation. They characteristically have hepatomegaly. Biochemical features of hyperglycaemia, ketosis and hypertriglyceridaemia may also be seen. Co-existing disease which can produce short stature and obesity must also be considered such as Cushing syndrome (including steroid treatment for any medical condition) and hypothyroidism although the presence of hepatomegaly will help distinguish these causes. Moderately poor control may result in some weight loss and these children tend to be slim.

Infants of diabetic mothers

Infants of diabetic mothers present with a number of problems with which you should be familiar. Essentially maternal hyperglycaemia causes fetal hyperglycaemia via placental diffusion which in turn results in fetal hyperinsulinism, which being anabolic causes macrosomia with visceromegaly (including placenta and cord) with characteristic facies and head comparatively smaller than the rest of the body. These effects have the possible consequences of obstructed labour, birth injuries and birth asphyxia. Poorly controlled diabetes causes placental vascular disease and may conversely result in an IUGR baby. Another characteristic feature is the presence of hairy ears (a possible slide). Neonatal hypoglycaemia as a result of excess insulin in the blood may occur and is usually transient lasting a few hours or may be more troublesome (treat with early feeds, possible i.v. dextrose and regular frequent blood glucose testing). Hypocalcaemia may also occur. These babies may have respiratory distress resulting from respiratory distress syndrome, persistent fetal circulation, polycythaemia or as a result of transient tachypnoea of the newborn (as a consequence of the increased caesarian section rate). Polycythaemia results in poorly compliant lungs, increased levels of jaundice, increased risk of vascular thrombosis and necrotising enterocolitis (NEC).

There is an increased incidence of congenital heart disease with a transient hypertrophic obstructive cardiomyopathy with echo showing asymmetrical septal hypertrophy and thickening of the left ventricular wall. Other types of CHD are also more common. Sacral agenesis occurs more commonly. Microcolon most commonly affecting the descending and sigmoid sections is diagnosed by barium enema and often resolves spontaneously, but a colostomy may be required (microcolon is also seen in CF and meconium ileus). A possible slide of an infant of a diabetic mother (IDM) will show a typical macrosomic baby with an i.v. infusion (dextrose), plethoric facies and possible forceps marks on the face.

Diabetic ketoacidosis
A common question relates to the child who presents with abdominal pain and hyponatraemia. The differential diagnosis includes diabetic ketoacidosis (see chapter 6).

Consider diabetic ketoacidosis in any metabolic acidosis with an increased anion gap. About 25% of all childhood cases of diabetes present with diabetic ketocidosis. The child may typically be severely dehydrated, with Kussmaul breathing (secondary to the metabolic acidosis), vomiting, abdominal pain (may mimic acute abdomen), confusion and coma may occur. Infection may be present secondary to the ketocidosis or as a causative factor leading to insulin resistance. Diagnosis is confirmed by finding hyperglycaemia with ketosis and a metabolic acidosis (with a raised anion gap and increased measured osmolality). Hyponatraemia is common (as a result of water moving into the extracellular fluid from the cells). Serum potassium may be normal or increased (despite total body potassium stores being depleted). Remember that children are very sensitive to too rapid replacement of fluids as this may result in cerebral oedema.

Polyuria and polydipsia
When given a history of polyuria and polydipsia your differential diagnosis should include: IDDM, diabetes insipidus, renal tubular acidosis (secondary to hypokalaemia), any cause of hypokalaemia, chronic renal failure, relief of prolonged obstruction of the urinary tract and psychogenic polydipsia.

Common slide questions
Common slides on the diabetic child include: *diabetic scleradactyly* — shown by the failure to be able to place the palmar aspects of both hands flat against each other because of thickening of the skin around the joints of the fingers ('prayer sign'). *Necrobiosis lipoidica diabeticorum* — seen as waxy yellow raised skin lesions with erythematous and atrophic areas in the centre most commonly occurring over the shins. *Lipoatrophy/hypertrophy* may be seen over injection sites and the importance of these is to advise the patient to stop using these injection sites because of unpredictable absorption from them.

Impaired glucose tolerance
You should know a list of syndromes and conditions associated with impaired glucose tolerance: Friedreich ataxia, cystic fibrosis, Duchenne muscular dystrophy, Cushing syndrome, ataxia telangiectasia, Prader–Willi syndrome, Down syndrome, Turner syndrome.

HYPOGLYCAEMIA

A low blood glucose can be caused by deficiencies of substrates for glycogenolysis or gluconeogenesis or enzymatic abnormalities in these pathways, or disturbances in the insulin/anti-insulin hormone system. The symptoms of hypoglycaemia are divided into two types:

a) *Neuroglycopenic symptoms*: Headache, irritability, confusion, seizures, coma. Jitteriness, apnoea and hypotonia in the neonatal period.

b) *Adrenergic features*: tremor, tachycardia, sweating, hunger, pallor, visual changes.

The causes of hypoglycaemia are also divided into two types: (1) ketotic; (2) non-ketotic.

Ketotic causes

Here there is reduced glucose production and a corresponding low insulin level. It is ketotic because insulin is lacking and thus lipolysis results in ketone body formation.

— *Low substrate levels*: malnutrition (including poor feeding after birth), birth asphyxia, prematurity, IUGR, malabsorption, infection. These causes are the commonest immediately after birth and are usually transient and resolve after appropriate treatment.

— *Liver disease* such as Reye syndrome.

— *Enzymatic defects in gluconeogenesis and glycogenolysis:* Von Gierke disease (GSD type 1), galactosaemia (latter two are associated with hepatomegaly).

— *Reduced levels of circulating anti-insulin:* adrenaline, growth hormone, cortisol, glucagon and hypopituitarism.

— *Ingestion of drugs*: such as alcohol and salicylates (alcohol inhibits gluconeogenesis but plasma glucose can usually be maintained from glycogen breakdown).

Non-ketotic causes

Here there is an excess of insulin (inappropriate because of low blood glucose): non-ketotic since insulin promotes fat synthesis and no ketone bodies will be formed.

— Too much insulin administration in diabetics: including missed meals and excessive exercise.

— Infant born to a diabetic mother.

— Nesidioblastosis (thought to be caused by B-cell hyperplasia in the pancreas and curative treatment may involve removal of part or whole of the pancreas).

— Islet cell adenoma.

— Rhesus isoimmunisation.

— Beckwith–Wiedemann syndrome.

— Islet cell insulinoma.

— Münchausen by proxy (maternal exogenous administration).

— Fatty acid oxidation defects, carnitine deficiency.

In the first year of life after birth transient forms are commoner and are usually ketotic in nature but sustained forms tend to be non-ketotic in nature. From one year of age ketotic forms occur more commonly.

The commonest cause of hypoglycaemia between the ages of one and seven years is ketotic hypoglycaemia (accelerated starvation). It usually begins after the first year and clinically presents after a period of prolonged fasting (typically more than 7–8 h) and/or in combination with a concurrent illness (typically viral). M:F ratio 2:1.

Reactive hypoglycaemia (post-prandial hypoglycaemia) occurs soon after eating a meal with blood glucose levels less than 3 mmol/l. It is seen in up to 25% of healthy individuals and improves spontaneously.

Clues in the examination must be sought in order to determine a possible cause. Look for the features of Beckwith–Wiedemann syndrome (macrosomia or macroglossia for instance). Look for hepatomegaly found in glycogen storage disease. Look for evidence of hypopituitarism (most commonly secondary to a craniopharyngioma or idiopathic) associated with short stature (height usually less than the third centile), delayed sexual characteristics, immature round facies often with midline defects such as cleft palate or optic hypoplasia.

Blood should be taken for hormonal assay (insulin, cortisol, growth hormone, glucagon), fatty acid metabolism indicators (ketones, free fatty acids), gluconeogenic pathways (lactate, pyruvate and alanine). Urine during hypoglycaemia should be tested for ketones. Urine should also be sent for a drug and toxicology screen in selected cases.

Measurement of insulin levels during a period of hypoglycaemia is important in the diagnosis of an insulinoma. Firstly the presence of a fasting glucose together with a normal or high insulin level is suspicious (that is, the insulin/glucose ratio is high). Then perform the insulin suppression test where insulin is infused into a patient. Normally because of the hypoglycaemia produced the insulin level falls, but this is not the case in an insulinoma. However insulin levels cannot be measured since we will not be able to distinguish between the endogenous and exogenous sources. Thus C-peptide is measured which is secreted from the B cells of the pancreas in equimolar amounts to insulin. A plasma C-peptide concentration in excess of 1.2 μg is indicative of an insulinoma. Measurement of C-peptide will also distinguish nesidioblastosis from Münchausen by proxy.

ABNORMALITIES OF GROWTH

Growth abnormalities are common accompaniments to many paediatric problems. You should be able to discuss the causes, recognise the commoner clinical scenarios and be able to investigate appropriately.

Background information

As a general rule growth is critically dependent on different factors at different ages:

— *Infancy:* Nutrition.
— *Childhood:* Growth hormone.
— *Puberty:* Growth hormone and sex steroids.

The average rate of growth during childhood is between 5–7 cm per year (increasing to 7–12 cm/year around puberty). Growth can be monitored using standard growth charts or growth velocity charts. Growth velocity charts will usually detect a slowing down in growth before it will be appreciated on a normal growth chart.

The mid-parental centile gives an expected range for the child's height given the parental heights.

— *For a boy:* The mid-parental height is determined by taking the mother's height + 13 cm and marking it on the height axis and then taking the father's height and marking it on the height axis. The mid-point between these heights is the mid-parental height and 10 cm on either side of this point equivalates to the third and 97th percentiles.

— *For a girl:* Take the father's height –13 cm and mark it on the height axis and then take the mother's height and mark it on the height axis. The mid-point between these two measurements is the mid-parental height and the third and 97th centiles lie 10 cm on either side of this point.

Skeletal maturation appears to be more closely related to physical development than to chronological age.

Causes of growth abnormality

Normal variants

— Familial short stature: here the parents are short. There is no delay in bone age and children continue to grow along their centiles.

— Constitutional short stature: M > F. Children are born with a normal weight and length and then during the first few years of life the rate of growth begins to fall. This is however temporary and height eventually returns to normal. There is a delayed bone age but serial bone ages will show advancement in parallel with the child's age. Children usually reach a normal adult height eventually, although growth may occur well into late teens after having no obvious growth spurt at the time of expected puberty. The bone age is usually 1–4 years behind the chronological age but is appropriate for the height. Puberty is often delayed. Often a positive family history of a similar tempo of growth in one of the parents is available. Ask about the age at onset of menarche in the mother since there is often a family history of constitutional delayed puberty. The diagnosis is only made when other diseases have been excluded.

Nutritional disorders

These may be a result of reduced intake or malabsorption.

Chronic disease

Many chronic diseases will result in poor growth. These include renal failure, renal tubular acidosis, congestive cardiac failure and chronic severe asthma. Bone age will be delayed and if the underlying disease is left untreated then there will be a progressive deviation from the chronological age.

Endocrinopathies

Rare but treatable. Unlikely if growth rate is more than 5 cm/year in childhood.

— Hypothyroidism and growth hormone deficiency (these two produce a delay in bone age). Growth hormone deficiency children are short (a deviation from the normal growth rate occurs after the age of about six months) with a doll-like face and may present with hypoglycaemia early in life. Provocation tests are required to confirm GH deficiency such as after 20 min exercise, or insulin, glucagon, clonidine and arginine tests. See insulin stress test below.

— Cushing syndrome and precocious puberty both cause an advancement in bone age. They result in an initial increased growth velocity but a final reduced height as a result of premature fusion of the epiphyses.

— Hypopituitarism presents as short stature, round face, saddle nose, short neck, small larynx with a high pitched voice, small hands and feet, delayed sexual development, microphallus and fine scalp hair and loss of body hair (including axillary and pubic cf. anorexia), pallor (as a result of loss of melanocyte-stimulating hormone (MSH) activity of ACTH) and hypoglycaemia. The causes are idiopathic or secondary to trauma, radiation, syndromes associated with midline defects, tumours (such as a craniopharyngioma caused by an expanding remnant of Rathke's pouch), infections and bleeds.

— Remember that tumours in the piuitary gland cause in addition other endocrinological disorders (either hypo- or hypersecretion depending on the nature of the tumour), diabetes insipidus (posterior pituitary involvement) as well as visual field defects (classically a bilateral hemianopia) and hydrocephalus as a result of obstruction to the third ventricle.

— Psychosocial deprivation is known to cause reduced secretion of growth hormone.

Other causes

a. Dysmorphic children with syndromes such as Turner (perform a chromosome analysis in a girl if suspicious of Turner syndrome), Noonan, Aarsog, Prader–Willi, Russell–Silver and Down syndrome. Some questions may give you some measurements of the trunk and limbs (normal ratio is 1:1). Remember that achondroplasia gives rise to a normal sized trunk and short limbs and spondyloepiphyseal dysplasia gives rise to a short trunk and normal limbs (spinal irradiation may also cause a shortened trunk).

b. Non-dysmorphic children born IUGR or prematurely.

Table 7.2 A typical set of results obtained following an insulin tolerance test

Minutes after insulin injection	0	15	30	45	60
Glucose concentration	5.1	1.9	4.5	10.2	9.7
GH	2.2	5.9	4.3	3.7	2.5
Cortisol	516	931	886	611	498

Example: In this patient there is both growth hormone deficiency and Cushing disease (see earlier explanation for the reasons).

The insulin stress test

The insulin stress test is a common data interpretation question. This test is also used for assessment of cortisol and prolactin secretion in addition to growth hormone secretion. It is only carried out in specialised centres. Insulin is injected and GH measured at 15, 30, 45, 60 and 120 min, with hypoglycaemic symptoms and signs occurring at 15–30 min. There should be a reduction in basal glucose values by more than 50% or < 2.2 mmol/l. If peak GH levels are less < 7 mU/l then this suggests GH deficiency and levels in excess of of 15 mU/l exclude the diagnosis. In normal subjects cortisol levels should double the basal level (see Table 7.2). Examples of other pituitary function tests include the LHRH and TRH tests.

The pituitary gland

Secretion of hormones from the pituitary gland.

— *Anterior pituitary gland*
   Chromophobe cells: non-secretory.
   Acidophil cells: GH, prolactin.
   Basophil cells: FSH, ACTH, LH, TSH.
— *Posterior pituitary gland*
   Oxytocin, ADH.

Bone age (see also chapter 11):

— *Cortisol*: Cortisol excess: delayed. Cortisol deficiency: normal.
— *Thyroxine*: Thyroxine excess: slightly advanced. Thyroxine deficiency: delayed.
— *Growth hormone*: Growth hormone excess: normal. Growth hormone deficiency: delayed.
— *Androgens*: Androgen excess: considerably advanced. Androgen deficiency: normal.

PUBERTY

Puberty is the consequence of the interaction of the hypothalamic/pituitary/gonadal feedback loop. Hypothalamic Gn-RH results in pituitary release of LH and FSH (pituitary gonadotrophins) which in turn cause gonadal hormonal release. Puberty coincides with an increase in the concentration of circulating gonadal hormones (testosterone in boys and oestradiol in girls). The oestrogen is mainly responsible for breast enlargement, the red vaginal mucosa turning to pink, increased prominence of the labia minora in girls and increase in penis size in boys. Pituitary gonadotrophins are mainly responsible for increase in testicular size. Adrenal androgens are mainly responsible for pubic hair and virilisation (facial hair, acne, deepening voice and increased muscle mass).

The order of pubertal changes in boys is as follows: testicular enlargement (size may be determined using a Prader orchidometer) with reddening and rugosity of scrotal skin → pubic hair → penile enlargement → axillary hair. The order in girls is as follows: breast enlargement → pubic hair → axillary hair → menarche. In boys and girls the growth spurt occurs during puberty.

Tanner staging is expected knowledge in the clinical examination. It involves the assessment of genital development in boys, breast development in girls and pubic hair growth in both sexes. All scales are from I–V.

Precocious puberty (sexual precocity)

Defined as the development of secondary sexual characteristics before eight years of age in a girl and nine years in a boy. It is much commoner in girls compared to boys (F:M = 5:1). Eighty per cent of cases are not related to pathological causes in girls, whereas 80% have pathological causes in boys.

Classification
— *True*: Puberty is synchronous: that is, it occurs in an orderly fashion as described above (suggesting an intact hypothalamic/pituitary axis) — sometimes referred to as intracranial.

  — Idiopathic.
  — Secondary to trauma, tumours, haemorrhage, hydrocephalus, neurofibromatosis, primary hypothyroidism (the only cause of precocious puberty with short stature and delayed bone age).

— *False (Pseudopuberty)*: Puberty is not synchronous and is pituitary independent. Sometimes called extracranial.

  — *Adrenal*: Cushing syndrome, congenital adrenal hyperplasia and tumours.
  — *Gonadal*: Ovarian cyst/tumour (for example, granulosa cell). Testicular tumour (such as Leydig cell tumour). Albright–McCune syndrome = café au lait spots, polyostotic fibrous dysplasia (with irregular borders – 'Coast of Maine') and precocious puberty caused by primary ovarian cysts secreting oestradiol (also associated with Cushing and hypothyroidism).
  — *Ectopic*: gonadotrophin secreting tumour: for example, hepatoblastoma, dysgerminoma. Exogenous hormone administration (such as ingestion of birth control pills).

Questions may ask you to distinguish the two forms. Remember that in true precocious puberty FSH and LH levels are high (you should also perform oestradiol and testosterone levels in an initial evaluation and adrenal hormones such as cortisol and 17-OH progesterone might also be taken). In pseudopuberty FSH and LH levels are low.

A Gn-Rh stimulation test with basal and peak LH, FSH and sex steroids distinguishes true precocious puberty (resembling an adult response) from pseudopuberty (prepubertal response with low FSH and LH levels). In boys with true precocious puberty the testes are almost always large but in pseudopuberty the testes are small (< 2 ml). Other useful tests may include skull X-ray/MRI, pelvic ultrasound scan and bone age. Isolated premature thelarche (isolated premature breast enlargement) caused by ovarian cysts is common and there are no other signs of puberty or advanced growth (however these patients require careful follow up). Pubertal gynaecomastia is common in boys passing through puberty, and usually coincides with Tanner stages III and IV. It is caused by an increase in the oestrogen/androgen ratio seen at this time and is sometimes tender. A full history and examination usually excludes other causes. It usually resolves spontaneously. Additional causes of gynaecomastia include: pituitary tumour, testicular/hepatic oestrogen secreting tumour, hyper/hypothyroidism, liver disease, Klinefelter syndrome, testicular failure (if oestrogens > androgens), feminising tumours and drugs: oestrogens, phenothiazines, spironolactone, digoxin. Localised causes include: haemangioma, carcinoma, lipomas and abscesses.

You may be shown a slide of swollen breasts in a newborn baby. This is referred to as neonatal mastitis or neonatal breast engorgement rather than gynaecomastia. It is common and is a result of the effect of maternal oestrogen on the breast tissue (occasionally 'witches' milk' may be seen from the nipples). Rarely it may be complicated by abscess formation when antibiotics become appropriate.

Premature adrenarche (isolated pubic hair development) is also common but again follow up is essential. Beware if in addition there is clitoromegaly and other signs of masculinisation where you should consider the possibility of an androgen-secreting tumour.

Management of precocious puberty involves understanding the causes and investigating appropriately children in which pathology is suspected. In the majority (especially in girls) little more than reassurance is required and investigation only in cases in which there are other suspicious features or for example you suspect Klinefelter syndrome (perform a karyotype). Bone age will be advanced in many of the forms of precocious puberty especially if there is adrenal involvement. The longer the exposure to sex steroids and the higher their concentration the more advanced will be the bone age. The most important long-term complication caused by precocious puberty (other than any underlying pathology) is accelerated growth that occurs initially, eventually leading to premature fusion of the epiphyses and a short adult height.

DELAYED PUBERTY

This is defined as the absence of signs of puberty by 14 years in a boy and 13 years in a girl.

Causes

— *Constitutional:* often goes along with growth delay (see earlier).

— *Hypogonadotrophic hypogonadism:* decreased FSH and LH. Defective hypothalamus/pituitary. Isolated gonadotrophin deficiency which may be idiopathic or associated with a syndrome, for example Kallman syndrome (associated with anosmia, microphallus, cryptorchidism and renal defects), Prader–Willi syndrome. Hypothalamic/pituitary damage: trauma, infection, irradiation, tumours, congenital malformations, surgery. Here other hormones will usually be affected in addition to gonadotrophin release. Others: chronic disease, hypothyroidism, Cushing disease, diabetes, anorexia and in athletes.

— *Hypergonadotrophic hypogonadism:* Increased FSH, LH. Defective gonads. In females this may be the result of primary ovarian failure, such as occurs in Turner syndrome. Also consider chemotherapy and post irradiation. In males this may be caused by primary testicular failure such as cryptorchidism or Klinefelter syndrome. Also consider testicular feminisation, chemotherapy and post irradiation.

Investigations for delayed puberty include the following (most are similar to tests for short stature): bone age, FSH, LH, TFTs, testosterone, oestradiol, Gn-RH stimulation test, HCG stimulation test (HCG is injected and testosterone release is measured from the testes), visual field analysis, skull X-ray (looking at the pituitary fossa, clinoid processes and for calcification) and cranial MRI (if hypogonadotrophic hypogonadism is suspected).

AMBIGUOUS GENITALIA

This topic can cause confusion. Differentiation starts at six weeks and is complete by the end of the first trimester. See Fig. 7.2.

Classification of ambiguous genitalia

Female pseudohermaphrodite

Genetically female (XX) and normal internal ducts but there is masculinisation of the external genitalia. From Fig. 7.2 we can see that this may arise from inappropriate androgen stimulation. Maternal causes include: androgen exposure in first trimester, or from an androgen secreting tumour. Fetal causes include congenital adrenal hyperplasia.

Male pseudohermaphrodite

Here the baby is genetically a male (XY) with testis, but with ambiguous genitalia. This may be due to an inborn error of metabolism of testosterone biosynthesis, defective 5-alpha reductase deficiency (AR) and the testicular feminisation syndrome in which there is complete or incomplete deficiency of androgen receptors (that is, end organ resistance). In addition there can be abnormal testicular development with defects such as Leydig cell hypoplasia.

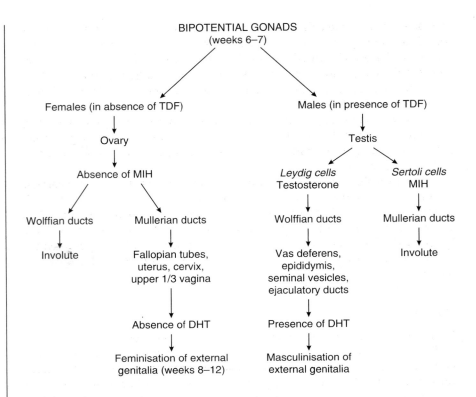

Fig. 7.2 A simplification of the events that lead to sexual differentiation.

TDF=Testes determining factor. MIH=Mullerian inhibitory factor. DHT=diydrotestosterone (testosterone is converted to DHT in target tissue by 5-alpha reductase)

There may be a structural defect such as severe hypospadias unrelated to androgen production.

True hermaphrodism
This is in practice extremely rare and occurs when both testicular and ovarian tissue is present and there is frequently ambiguous genitalia. They may be genotypically 46XX (most commonly), 46XY or mosaicism.

History and examination

The history should exclude maternal androgen ingestion or previous neonatal death, for example CAH or familial genetic disorders. Examination should involve palpation of the gonads (a male pseudohermaphrodite may occasionally be confused with a female with bilateral inguinal herniae). Blood pressure should be taken and you should look for pigmentation (ACTH induced in CAH). If the gonads are palpated then the baby is definitely male. An ultrasound should then be performed to look for a uterus. If present then this may be the result of abnormal testis such as Sertoli cell hypoplasia, or a true hermaphrodite. If not present then the causes are for a male pseudohermaphrodite listed above. If gonads are not palpable the baby may be genetically male or female. In this case the ultrasound looking for a uterus will differentiate between a male and female pseudohermaphrodite.

Apart from obvious parental distress caused by the ambiguous genitalia, of prime importance to the paediatrician is to exclude and treat the potentially life-threatening complications of a possible congenital adrenal hyperplasia and salt-losing crisis.

A common slide and grey case question in the examination is to recognise ambiguous genitalia. Subsequent questions ask for your list of investigations. These are pelvic ultrasound, karyotype and measurement of 17-OH steroids as the three main expected answers. In addition tests may include HCG (to see if HCG stimulates testosterone release from Leydig cells on the testis) and androgen binding sites on genital skin fibroblasts (for testicular feminisation).

Management

Viva or grey cases may ask you to discuss the management.

First discuss the way that your investigations have narrowed your differential diagnosis down (slides often ask for three investigations of choice: ultrasound of pelvis for uterus, karyotype and 17 OH progesterone). This may involve resuscitation of a shocked infant with a salt-losing crisis, continual psychological support to the parents and advising against naming of child until all investigations and appropriate consultations have taken place. In addition to having determined the genetic sex, decisions have to be made as to what sex to rear the baby. These are joint decisions with surgeons, endocrinologists, paediatricians and the parents. It is surgically easier to reconstruct female genitalia compared to male genitalia, and so many genetic males are reared as females. If CAH is diagnosed hormone replacement is necessary. Psychological support is necessary for parents in addition to support groups; genetic counselling if there is a genetic cause.

Causes of micropenis

— Idiopathic
— Hypopituitarism with growth hormone or gonadotrophin deficiency
— Hypothalamic disorders such as Kallman syndrome
— Testicular feminisation syndrome
— Other syndromes: Prader–Willi, Noonan, Down, and Smith–Lemli–Opitz syndrome.

Causes of macropenis

— Congenital adrenal hyperplasia (look for scrotal pigmentation)
— Precocious puberty.

DISORDERS OF ADH METABOLISM

Syndrome of inappropriate ADH secretion (SIADH)

This is a common question and should always be considered in a child who presents with, hyponatraemia (possibly with clinical sequelae such as seizures) and an inappropriately concentrated urine. ADH is secreted from the posterior pituitary gland in response to hyperosmolality or hypovolaemia. In SIADH there is an inappropriate secretion of ADH (in the absence of the usual physiological stimuli mentioned above) that occurs in a number of conditions.

Causes include:

(a) Intracranial causes such as head injury, meningitis/encephalitis, space occupying lesions, tumour, abscess, haematoma; (b) pulmonary causes: IPPV, pneumonia, asthma attack; (c) ectopic hormone production: rare in children, usually tumours in older patients; (d) drugs: carbamazepine, chlorpropamide, cyclophosphamide, vincristine, morphine, rifampicin. Some children receive therapeutic DDAVP (for example, in nocturnal enuresis) and this can cause an SIADH picture. Features include:

— A low plasma osmolality with a low volume of inappropriately hypertonic urine.

— A hyponatraemia caused by both dilution and natriuresis.

— A high urinary sodium excretion > 20 mmol/l. This is secondary to release of natriuretic peptides because of volume receptor stimulation (for example antinatriuretic peptide (ANP) from the atria), and secondly because of fluid overload there is no renin drive and consequently no aldosterone production leading to urinary sodium loss.

— An increase in total body water without the presence of oedema caused by sodium loss. Water is distributed equally between the intracellular and extracellular compartments.

— Renal function including GFR is unaffected.

— In order to make the diagnosis it is important to exclude hypovolaemia (clinically as perfusion, pulse, b.p. as well as Hb and urea in investigations) in the child. The child must have normal adrenal and renal function. Finally the child must not have received loop diuretics recently.

Thus in questions look for (a) the plasma osmolality and (b) the urinary osmolality: typically inappropriately high relative to the plasma osmolality.

Under normal circumstances the urinary osmolality should be less than 130 mOsmol/kg in the presence of hyponatraemia. In SIADH the urinary osmolality is typically higher.

Treatment involves fluid restriction to two-thirds maintenance. The plasma sodium and osmolality should be measured regularly, as well as frequent weighing. If hyponatraemia is causing complications such as seizures then a quicker return of plasma sodium to normal is required and can be achieved using intravenous administration of hypertonic saline (3%) and concurrent frusemide administration if there is also an element of fluid overload. Sometimes an ADH antagonist such as domeclocycline may be used.

Diabetes insipidus (DI)

This is a common condition in examinations and should be thought of in a child who presents with polyuria, polydipsia, frequency, nocturia and nocturnal enuresis. If drinking is continued and there are no additional fluid losses that cannot be kept up with such as fever or diarrhoea, then dehydration will not result. However this balance is not always seen in practice (that is, drinking is not always kept up) and dehydration will develop. Clinical features of dehydration — including fever (especially in infants), constipation, vomiting and cerebral venous thrombosis — may occur with ironically good urine output. Blood tests may reveal hypernatraemia with increased urea as well as a raised haemoglobin and haematocrit. Usually a data question presents a patient with a high sodium, high urea and an unexpectedly low urinary osmolality.

Diabetes insipidus refers to two conditions.

— *Central DI:* here there is a deficiency of ADH secretion from the posterior pituitary gland (idiopathic or secondary to hypothalamic disease e.g. craniopharyngioma), post-head trauma, meningoencephalitis. Don't forget histiocytosis X or familial causes — AD.

— *Nephrogenic DI:* there is an insensitivity to ADH of the collecting ducts in the kidney. It may be acquired e.g. hypokalaemia, hypercalcaemia, sickle cell disease and lithium intake. It may occur following prolonged polyuria for any reason (because of a reduction in medullary interstitium tonicity) such as occurs in obstructive nephropathy, interstitial nephritis and Fanconi syndrome.

Differential diagnosis of polyuria and polydipsia

This is a common grey case scenario and, includes:

— Diabetes mellitis
— Diabetes insipidus (central and nephrogenic and their causes)
— Chronic renal failure (can usually be excluded if there is a normal urea and creatinine) and following relief of a chronic obstructive nephropathy
— Psychogenic polydipsia.

The water deprivation test

This is a useful test to distinguish between diabetes insipidus and psychogenic polydipsia. You may be asked to interpret such a test in a data question. Here the aim is to demonstrate an inappropriately dilute urine in the presence of a concentrated serum. It is potentially a very dangerous procedure and meticulous care should be taken to measuring clinical parameters hourly (such as weight, pulse, b.p and urine output). The test is carried out until there is a 3% loss in weight. At the start of the test the patient voids urine; this is discarded and then the fast begins. After the test the urine and plasma osmolalities are measured.

In the normal patient following water deprivation the urine osmolality is usually > 800 mOsmol/kg — however in a normal patient in which there has been prolonged polyuria, the urinary osmolality may be as low as 600 mOsmol/kg such as following chronic psychogenic polydipsia. In diabetes insipidus the urine osmolality is usually < 200 mOsmol/kg. A urinary concentration > 200 mOsmol/kg makes DI very unlikely (or may be possible in a partial defect). DDAVP may be given at the end of the test and will cause concentration of the urine in cranial DI and produce no change in nephrogenic DI. In practice a concentrated urine > 800 mOsmol/kg in the presence of a normal serum osmolality < 290 mOsmol/kg excludes DI.

ANOREXIA NERVOSA

Because of the vast array of clinical presentations of anorexia, it comes up in the examination not infrequently. It is about 10 times more common in females, with an average age of onset during adolescence (males mean age: 12 years; females: 16 years). Psychologically there is a disturbed sense of body image with a morbid fear of obesity, and relentless pursuit of low body weight. Physically there is a body weight more than 25% below the standard weight and there is often amenorrhoea. Additional features are as follows: evidence of vomiting, excessive exercising or laxative abuse; uncontrollable bingeing (bulimia) followed by remorse and efforts to vomit or lose the weight in other ways.

Know about other features that can sometimes cause diagnostic confusion: constipation (very common), hypotension (often postural), bradycardia, hypothermia, sensitivity to cold, amenorrhoea (may precede weight loss in 25% of cases), hypoglycaemia, alopecia (sparing axillary and pubic hair cf. hypopituitarism), lanugo hair on the trunk and extremities, ankle oedema, leucopenia, vomiting and purgation may cause hypokalaemia, alkalosis, cardiac arrhythmias, dental erosions and knuckle calluses (Russell sign) and tooth decay (as a result of self-induced vomiting).

Hormonal changes in anorexia

— *Decreased:* LSH, FSH, testosterone, oestrodiol, T3 and T4.
— *Increased:* prolactin, growth hormone and cortisol.
— *Differential diagnosis* includes: thyrotoxicosis (especially in a slide of a face), diabetes mellitus, neoplasia, malabsorption, inflammatory bowel disease and hypopituitarism.

One third recover fully, one third partially recover and in one third it remains a severe chronic disease. Poor prognosis is associated with male sex, later age of onset, bulimia, purgation, unstable family relationships and the greater the weight loss.

OBESITY

When faced with an obese child you must always have a list of secondary causes to exclude.

— *Endocrine problems:* Cushing, hypothyroidism, Mauriac syndrome, polycystic ovarian disease.
— *Syndromes:* Prader–Willi, Laurence–Moon–Biedl.
— *Hypothalamic disorders* e.g post infection or trauma.

In babies macrosomia may be caused by Beckwith–Wiedemann, Sotos syndrome (also macrocephaly, large hands and feet) and having diabetic mothers.

Polycystic ovarian disease

Polycystic ovarian disease or (Stein–Leventhal syndrome) presents with obesity, hirsutism (sometimes with acne) and irregular periods (also primary or secondary amenorrhoea) usually from puberty and the symptoms deteriorate with time. Numerous ovarian cysts are seen on ultrasound. Androgen levels are elevated (SHBG low) and there is a raised LH:FSH ratio with a normal or low FSH (that is, LH is high). Infertility is a common problem later on, and treatment with clomiphene or wedge resection of the ovary can be effective.

CALCIUM METABOLISM

Calcium physiology

In plasma 50% of calcium is in the free ionised state, 45% is albumin bound and about 5% is complexed with citrate and phosphate. It is the free ionised calcium that is biologically active. Distribution between these various forms is affected by: (a) pH — increased acidity displaces calcium from albumin increasing ionised calcium; (b) increased serum albumin increases serum total calcium; (c) precipitation in diseases e.g. pancreatitis can lower serum calcium; and (d) alterations in bone turnover. Laboratories measure total calcium. Corrected calcium may be useful to see if the apparent hypercalcaemia might be caused by increased albumin concentration (or vice versa). It can be calculated as follows.

1. If the albumin level is more than 40 g/l: e.g 45 then (45 – 40) multiplied by *0.02* = 0.1 which is then subtracted from the total calcium concentration.

2. If the albumin concentration is less than 40 g/l e.g. 35 then (40 – 35) multiplied by *0.02* = 0.1 which is then added to the calcium concentration.

Calcium concentration in the blood is mainly controlled by two hormones namely vitamin D and parathyroid hormone (PTH). Increased ionised calcium concentration inhibits PTH release whilst low serum calcium concentrations have the reverse effect. Calcitonin is released from the C cells in the thyroid gland in response to hypercalcaemia but physiologically has little effect.

Vitamin D
Its main effect is an increase in calcium and increase in phosphate. Cholecalciferol (vitamin D3) is derived from the diet or from the UV light

conversion of 7 dehydrocholesterol. This is hydroxylated in the liver to 25-OH cholecalciferol (by the 25 hydroxylase enzyme) which is then hydroxylated in the kidneys (by 1-alpha hydroxylase enzyme) to 1,25 dihydroxycholecalciferol (the biologically active form).

— *Gut effect:* increases calcium and phosphate reabsorption.
— *Bone effect:* stimulates osteoclast resorption.

Parathyroid hormone

Its main effect is an increase in calcium and decrease in phosphate levels.

— *Bone effect:* rapid release from bone, increased osteoclast resorption (longer effect).
— *Renal effect:* increased calcium reabsorption, decreased phosphate reabsorption, stimulation of the 1-alpha hydroxylase enzyme.

Hypercalcaemia

Causes

Primary hyperparathyroidism (85% adenoma, 15% hyperplasia), hyperalbuminaemia (however if corrected as above calcium will be in the normal range), chronic renal failure with tertiary hyperparathyroidism, milk-alkali syndrome, vitamin D excess, thiazide diuretics, sarcoidosis, tuberculosis, neonatal hypercalcaemia (secondary to maternal hypoparathyroidism), thyrotoxicosis, Addison disease, factitious (with venous stasis on blood taking).

Symptoms

Anorexia, nausea, vomiting, abdominal pain, constipation, rarely peptic ulceration and pancreatitis, polyuria, polydipsia (acquired nephrogenic diabetes insipidus), muscle weakness, depression and poor concentration. Hyperparathyroidism is more likely to present with renal stones (nephrocalcinosis), peptic ulceration, pancreatitis and chondrocalcinosis as compared to hypercalcaemia from other causes.

Hypocalcaemia

Causes

Hypoalbuminaemia (if corrected however calcium will be in normal range), chronic renal failure, acute pancreatitis, prematurity, vitamin D deficiency, hypomagnesaemia (Mg needed for PTH activity), hypoparathyroidism (usually autoimmune but also parathyroid agenesis in Di George syndrome and as a complication of thyroidectomy) and pseudohypoparathyroidism (hereditary end organ resistance to PTH: affecting males more commonly, PTH levels are very high, and they have a characteristic phenotype with short stature, moon face, mental retardation, calcified basal ganglia and short fourth metacarpal bone). In hypoparathyroidism if i.v. PTH is infused there will be an increase in urinary cyclic AMP but there is no response in pseudohypoparathyroidism. In pseudopseudohypoparathyroidism there is a similar phenotype to pseudohypoparathyroidism but they have normal biochemistry.

Symptoms
Muscle weakness, tetany and cramps (Kvostek sign — carpopedal spasm; Tinnel sign — tap over parotid gland causes facial muscle twitching). Remember that tetany can also occur with a normal calcium under conditions of alkalosis (because of decreased biologically active ionised calcium), stridor, parasthesiae and numbness, cataracts, short stature and behavioural changes.

PHAEOCHROMOCYTOMA

Phaeochromocytomas may come up in a grey case. They are catecholamine secreting tumours of neuroectodermal tissue. Ten per cent are bilateral, 10% malignant and 10% extra-adrenal. Ten per cent are associated with other syndromes, for instance neurofibromatosis or type II MEN. The adrenal tumours mainly secrete adrenaline and extra-adrenal tumours mainly secrete noradrenaline. Clinical features include: hypertension (50% sustained, 50% intermittent), weight loss, headaches, chest pain, attacks of sweating, flushing, tachycardia and palpitations, polyuria and nocturia, and glycosuria with impaired glucose tolerance. In addition anxiety, nausea and behavioural changes may occur. In chronic situations a blunting of the normal sympathetic response may be seen with postural hypotension. Paroxysms usually last 15–45 min.

Investigations: 24 h urinary analysis for catecholamine byproducts (metanephrines — VMA vanilmandelic acid; HMMA—hydroxymethoxymandelic acid). False positives are seen in stress, illness, caffeine, bananas and vanilla consumption, beta-blockers and others. Plasma catecholamines, CT scan and MIBG scan. Beta-blockers may result in a paradoxical rise in blood pressure. Surgery cures in 75% of cases and is carried out with alpha- and beta-blockade.

Neuroblastomas may also secrete catecholamine but to a much lesser extent.

THE CARCINOID SYNDROME

A rare syndrome which is caused by a tumour of the argentaffin cells in the ileum, appendix or bronchi. Ileal carcinoids readily metastasise while the others rarely metastasise. The tumour produces 5HT but this will be metabolised by the liver (in the case of a gastrointestinal carcinoid) unless hepatic metastases are present in which case 5HT enters the systemic circulation. Extraintestinal carcinoids secrete 5HT directly into the systemic circulation. Typical attacks include paroxysms of facial flushing, bronchoconstriction causing dyspnoea, fever, nausea, vomiting, abdominal colic and watery diarrhoea. In addition features of the primary tumour itself may be present, such as gastrointestinal obstruction. Chronic carcinoid syndrome may result in pulmonary stenosis and tricuspid regurgitation (right side of heart).

Investigate with 24 h urinary collection for 5 hydroxyindole acetic acid (5HIAA).

MULTIPLE ENDOCRINE NEOPLASIA (MEN)

These are familial disorders inherited in an autosomal dominant fashion. They describe tumours which may be benign or malignant, or hyperplasia developing in more than one endocrine gland. It is important to recognise these rare syndromes since the presence of one endocrinopathy might lead you to look for other features common to the MEN syndromes especially if there is a family history. They are listed in decreasing order of occurrence.

Type 1

— Parathyroid adenoma/hyperplasia
— Anterior pituitary adenomas e.g. prolactinomas, GH secreting tumours
— Pancreatic islet cell secreting tumours e.g. secreting insulin, glucagon, gastrinoma, VIP
— Adrenal cortical non-functioning adenoma
— Thyroid follicular cell adenoma.

Type 2(a)

— Thyroid medullary cell carcinoma (secreting calcitonin)
— Adrenal medulla phaeochromocytoma
— Parathyroid hyperplasia or adenoma.

Type 2(b)

As for type 2(a) plus marfanoid appearance, perioral mucosal adenomas and visceal ganglioneuromas.

CLINICAL EXAMINATION

The only endocrine abnormality that you are likely to be asked to assess in the clinical examination is the thyroid status of the child.

— Firstly observe the child. See if there is anything immediately obvious (for example, is he thin, proptosis). You may ask the child to look at the ceiling to make a goitre more obvious. Are there any scars present from previous thyroid surgery?

— Take the child's hands and feel them. In hyperthyroidism they will be warm and sweaty whereas in hypothyroidism they will be cold and dry. Ask the child to hold his hands out in front of him (dorsal sides upwards) with outstreched arms and fingers widely spaced. Now place a piece of paper on the hands to demonstrate the fine tremor of hyperthyroidism.

— Now take the pulse feeling for the tachycardia (and frequent ectopic beats) of hyperthyroidism or the bradycardia of hypothyroidism.

— Look at the eyes for proptosis and test for lid lag. This is done by asking the child to look at your finger as you raise it above his field of vision and then gradually lower your finger watching for lid lag: that is, the upper eye lid coming down after the eyeballs do.

— Now examine the neck from behind feeling for a goitre. Ask the child to swallow and feel for any movement in any masses felt (indicative of thyroidal origin). Ask the child to stick his tongue out. Any movement of a structure on protruding the tongue could be caused by a remnant in the thyroglossal tract e.g. thyroglossal cyst. Percuss over the upper sternum if a large goitre is present to check for retrosternal extension.

— Auscultate the thyroid gland for bruits (if a goitre is present).

— Examine all the lymph nodes in the cervical region.

— Look at the legs for necrobiosis and pretibial myxoedema.

— Now examine the reflexes which are increased in hyperthyroidism and sluggish in hypothyroidism. Get the child to kneel on a chair and test the ankle reflexes. In hypothyroidism there will be a slow relaxation phase of the ankle jerks.

— Ask the child to speak to hear the hoarse voice of hypothyroidism.

— Finally offer to plot the child's height and weight on growth charts.

THE DIABETIC PATIENT

Have a list of things that you would look for routinely in a diabetic child.

— You should first of all carry out a general observation looking for obesity, thinness, well looking or not well looking.

— You should examine injection sites making sure that there is no lipoatrophy or lipohypertrophy. Look also for the presence of skin prick test sites (indicating that the child has been checking his blood glucose).

— Get the child to perform the 'prayer sign' with his hands to demonstrate diabetic sclerodactyly (see earlier in chapter).

— Offer to examine the blood pressure and perform a fundoscopy despite the fact that such end organ damage is extremely unlikely in the childhood population.

— Finally offer to plot the height and weight on a growth chart and test the urine with a dipstick test and test for microalbuminuria.

Haematology

Haematology is a frequent topic for questions in the MRCPCH examination.

ANAEMIA

It is important that you have a thorough understanding of the pathophysiology and classification of anaemia since this will give you a framework for discussing many other haematological disorders.

Physiology

Haemoglobin production in the fetus usually starts by the third week of gestation, primarily in the yolk sac. By month 3–4 of fetal life the liver and spleen take over erythropoiesis and finally by month 6–7 the bone marrow becomes the principal production site of blood. At birth haematopoiesis occurs in all the bones but this gradually reduces during childhood so that the central bones are mainly involved as the child ages (vertebrae, ribs, sternum and pelvis) and the long bones play less of a role in blood production.

The normal values for haemoglobin concentration change during the first year of life and it is important to be aware of these changes since it can avoid misdiagnosis and unnecessary investigation in some cases (see Table 8.1). Newborn babies are relatively polycythaemic; the haemoglobin concentration falls to its lowest levels by 2–3 months (physiological anaemia) and then

Table 8.1 Variation in haematological indices during the first year of life

	Haemoglobin values (mean) g/dl	MCV (mean) fl	White cell count ($\times 10$ to power 9/L)*
Term newborn	19	108	5–25
2 months old	11	100	6–15
1 year	12	86	6–15

*Neutrophils (N) predominate at birth compared to lymphocytes (L) (60%: 30% N:L) but this ratio is reversed by six months of age and this is maintained for the first 4–5 years but is reversed yet again by puberty (55%: 40% N:L).

slowly rises again. Low haemoglobin concentrations at six months may be caused by iron and folate deficiency especially in premature babies.

In the fetus haemoglobin is in the form of fetal haemoglobin (HbF, consisting of two alpha chains and two gamma chains) but towards the end of gestation the fetus begins to produce beta globin chains as well so that by birth the baby has 20% HbA (adult haemoglobin — two alpha chains and two beta chains) and 80% fetal haemoglobin. Fetal haemoglobin has an oxygen dissociation curve to the left: that is, it has a very high affinity for oxygen but is less good at giving it up. This was ideally suited to intrauterine life. The average child has haemoglobin that is made up of 95% HbA (adult haemoglobin) and the remainder HbF 0.5–2% and HbA2 2–3% (two alpha chains and two lambda chains). The rapid increase in PaO_2 at birth causes a reduction in the production of erythropoietin which results in greatly reduced red cell production for several weeks. This results in a decrease in haemoglobin concentration by about two months of age (physiological anaemia) and this value is usually not less than 10 g/dl in healthy children, and usually well tolerated by the infants; this fall in haemoglobin is however more dramatic and occurs earlier in premature babies. This reduction in haemoglobin is partly compensated for by the increase in HbA which has an oxygen dissociation curve to the right and thus gives up oxygen more readily. The reduction in Hb results in increased erythropoietin production as a result of reduced tissue oxygenation (negative feedback loop) so that haemoglobin levels begin to rise again with an appropriate reticulocytosis (not to be confused with haemolysis). The normal blood volume in a child is 85 ml/kg.

Lifecycle of red cell
Bone marrow pronormoblast → normoblast → reticulocyte (one day in bone marrow and then released into peripheral blood with a survival of one day in the peripheral blood) → mature red cell.

Reticulocytes
These are an important indicator of (a) bone marrow response to anaemia (increased in haemolysis and decreased in haematinic or aplastic anaemia); and (b) successful response to treatment. A reticulocytosis gives the blood film increased staining called polychromasia. The presence of reticulocytopenia in the presence of anaemia implies: (a) that there is an abnormality at the level of the bone marrow; (b) the picture seen is so shortly after the episode causing the anaemia that the bone marrow has not had time to respond, for example a large haemorrhage or (c) that the reticulocytes are being destroyed, possibly by an immune mediated mechanism.

Reticulocytosis is seen in:

— Haemolytic anaemia
— Acute severe bleeding
— Beginning of a remission in aplasia
— Response to treatment in haematinic deficiency.

Classification of anaemias
It is important to have a system in your mind.

Decreased production
— Reduced haematinics (iron, folate and B12)
— Infiltration
— Aplasia
— Chronic disease.

Increased loss
— Haemorrhage
— Haemolysis:

  a. Intrinsic (membrane defects, haemoglobinopathies, red cell enzyme defects).
  b. Extrinsic (microangiopathic haemolysis, immunological).

Another way of classifying anaemias is to distinguish between microcytic, normocytic and macrocytic causes of anaemia.

1. *Microcytic:* Iron deficiency, beta thalassaemia trait, sideroblastic anaemia, chronic disease (usually normocytic) and lead poisoning.

2. *Normocytic:* Bleeding (acutely), chronic disease, haemolysis.

3. *Macrocytic:* Megaloblastic anaemia (B12, folate), liver disease, myelodysplasia, hypothyroidism, aplastic anaemia, reticulocytosis, chronic alcohol ingestion, newborn and pregnancy.

Blood-film abnormalities

You will face questions that will ask you to interpret blood indices or films and you should be familiar with the commoner blood-film abnormalities.

Target cells
These contain excess membrane or insufficient haemoglobin and are recognised as 'target-like' with red peripheries, central pallor and with a dot of haemoglobin at the centre.

— Post splenectomy
— Haemoglobinopathies (sickle cell, thalassaemia disease plus trait)
— Severe iron deficiency
— Obstructive jaundice.

Anisocytosis
Variation in size of erythrocytes.

— Iron deficiency anaemia
— Beta thalassaemia
— Megaloblastic anaemia.

Howell–Jolly bodies
Dense nuclear round remnants found within erythrocytes. Remnants of DNA and RNA.

- Beta thalassaemia
- Post splenectomy
- Megaloblastic anaemia
- Sometimes found in premature infants.

Poikilocytosis
Variation in shape of erythrocytes.

- Severe iron deficiency
- Beta thalassaemia
- Tear drop poikilocytosis (seen in myeloproliferative disease/other bone marrow infiltrative conditions).

Heinz bodies
Denatured haemoglobin/haemoglobin remnant — stained by supravital staining — seen as a dark dot in erythrocyte.

- Red cell enzyme defects (e.g. G6PD deficiency, pyruvate kinase dficiency)
- Drugs and chemicals causing haemolytic anaemia.

Left shift and leukaemoid reactions
Less mature white cells released prematurely from the bone marrow. Careful examination may be needed to distinguish from leukaemia. Also refers to increased neutrophil/lymphocyte ratio.

- Sepsis (caused by increased demand on neutrophils; less mature cells are released prematurely). Tuberculosis, syphilis, toxoplasmosis
- Down syndrome.

Rouleaux formation
Erythrocytes stacked in rows one on another.

- Inflammation
- Malignancy.

Spherocytes
Seen as spherical cells with no central pallor; give rise to a low MCV.

- Hereditary spherocytosis
- Immune haemolytic anaemia
- Severe burns
- Post transfusion.

Dimorphic blood film
The presence of two differently sized populations of red cells, with increased RDW.

- Sideroblastic anaemia (bone marrow cells unable to utilise iron to form haemoglobin characterised by ring sideroblasts in bone marrow: caused by inherited and acquired causes such as lead poisoning, anti-TB drugs)

— Combination of iron deficiency with a B12/folate deficiency
— Iron deficiency anaemia (with microcytosis) and having received a blood transfusion.

Basophilic stippling
Seen as numerous small dots in the red cell due to alpha chain clumping.

— Lead poisoning
— Beta thalassaemia.

Post splenectomy features
— Howell–Jolly bodies (spleen usually involved in removal of excess cell remnants)
— Acanthocytes (red cells with spiny projections protruding from the surface also seen in abetolipoproteinaemia)
— Target cells
— Schistocytes (portions of disrupted cells).

Leucoerythroblastic picture
Increase in numbers of primitive cells in the blood film, for example nucleated red cells (normoblasts), myeloblasts.

— Malignant infiltration of the bone marrow
— Mycobacterium e.g. TB infection
— Marble bone disease (osteopetrosis)
— Myelomatosis
— Myelofibrosis.

COMMON EXAMINATION HAEMATOLOGICAL DISEASES AND THEIR CORRESPONDING BLOOD FILMS

The blood film may be given to you in the form of a slide or described to you in a data or grey case question.

Hereditary spherocytosis

The main feature is of spherocytes which compared to normal red cells are spherical instead of biconcave, and thus lack their characteristic central pallor. Reticulocytosis is often prominent. Do not forget that if a splenectomy has been performed then features of post splenectomy may also be present (see above).

Beta thalassaemia major

Microcytic hypochromic anaemia (pale sparse small red cells on blood film), marked anisocytosis (variation in size of the red cells), poikilocytosis (variation in shape), basophilic stippling (clumped together alpha chains), target cells and red cell fragments. As a result of bone marrow stimulation there may also be increased nucleated red cells, white cells and platelets; however white cells and platelets may be reduced if there is concurrent splenomegaly causing hypersplenism.

Sickle cell disease

The characteristic feature is of sickling of the red cells. In addition there may be hypochromic, microcytic cells, numerous target cells, polychromasia and numerous nucleated red cells. The presence of Howell–Jolly bodies will indicate splenic function in the child (most children are functionally asplenic by one year of age as a result of repeated splenic infarction).

Malaria

A common slide question is the erythrocyte with a ring form within it. In *Plasmodium falciparum* there are thin small rings, in *P. ovale* there are larger coarse rings each with a single chromatin dot, and in *P. vivax* there is a large ring form with a single chromatin dot.

Iron deficiency anaemia

Hypochromic microcytic anaemia (hypochromia describes when the peripheral pink haemoglobin rim of the red cell is less than two-thirds of the diameter of the entire red cell). Anisocytosis, poikilocytosis, target cells and cigar cells/pencil cells may also be seen. Differential diagnosis of the microcytic hypochromic anaemia includes beta thalassaemia trait, chronic inflammation and sideroblastic anaemia. Lead poisoning also gives rise to a microcytic hypochromic anaemia but one would also expect basophilic stippling in addition.

Megaloblastic anaemia

The red cells are large (macrocytic) with anisocytosis. Neutrophils are larger than normal and have characteristic hypersegmented nucleus (neutrophils usually have up to five lobes in the nucleus but in megaloblastic anaemia this number is greater). This is sometimes called right shift and is also seen in uraemia and hepatic disease. Leucopenia and thrombocytopenia simply reflect ineffective erythropoiesis. The bone marrow is hypercellular with megaloblasts with nuclear/cytoplasmic dissociation.

Lead poisoning

— Microcytic hypochromic anaemia
— Basophilic stippling
— Evidence of haemolytic anaemia.

Infectious mononucleosis

This is characterised by a lymphocytosis and the presence of atypical lymphocytes which are typically amoeboid in appearance, have a large nucleus and abundant cytoplasm.

Haemolytic uraemic syndrome

This is an example of a microangiopathic haemolytic anaemia and the blood film can be identified by hypochromia, fragmented red cells, Burr cells (schistocytes) and a significant paucity in platelets. It is caused by excessive shearing of the red cells. Microangiopathic haemolytic anaemia may also occur in children with prosthetic valves, disseminated intravascular coagulation, thrombotic thrombocytopenic purpura, haemangiomas and in some malignancies.

HAEMOLYSIS

Haemolytic disorders are divided up into those which produce extravascular haemolysis (the majority) where red cells are removed mainly by the spleen leading to splenomegaly if haemolysis is chronic. Intravascular haemolysis occurs when red cells are rapidly lysed within the vasculature with some haemoglobin being lost in the urine as haemoglobinuria.

The consequences of haemolysis

Anaemia (normocytic, normochromic), unconjugated hyperbilirubinaemia, increased urinary urobilinogen, haemoglobinuria (in intravascular haemolysis), decreased serum haptoglobin since it binds to released haemoglobin (**NB** haptoglobin is absent in newborns and may be congenitally absent). Reticulocytosis, polychromasia, fragmented red cells and spherocytes (if hereditary spherocytosis or autoimmune). No urinary bilirubin (acholuric jaundice). Bone marrow erythroid hyperplasia, extramedullary haematopoiesis. 51 chromium labelled red cells can be used to look at red cell survival which is reduced in haemolysis.

Common haemolytic questions

1. A three-year-old Caucasian child is noted to be pale and slightly jaundiced. She has recently had a viral URTI and just has a residual cough. On examination she is noted to have an enlarged spleen and is otherwise well.

Hb	9.8 g/dl
WCC	6.9
Platelets	129
Unconjugated bilirubin	72 µmol/l
DCT	negative
Blood film	numerous spherocytes
Reticulocytes	++

This story is typical of hereditary spherocytosis. It has a mainly AD inheritance but is sporadic in 20% of cases. It is caused by a mutation in the spectrin protein (which is a membrane skeletal protein) leading to membrane fragility and the red cells are removed by the spleen. Symptoms may include those caused by anaemia and intermittent jaundice which may be precipitated by viral illnesses. Chronic haemolysis may result in gallstones. Sudden reduction in Hb concentration may be the result of abrupt haemolysis or infection with human parvovirus infection causing aplastic anaemia (which may also occur in sickle cell disease). **NB** Hereditary spherocytosis is difficult to diagnose during an aplastic crisis. It may present in the neonatal period with jaundice on the first day of life (50% of cases). Because of the presence of spherocytes both in hereditary spherocytosis and ABO incompatibility the two may be difficult to distinguish from each other as a cause of neonatal jaundice. Splenomegaly is common (80% of cases).

Investigations include: FBC (anaemia with reduced MCV), blood film, red cell fragility test (increased red cell lysis in hypotonic solutions compared to normal red cells). There is an increased red cell distribution width (RDW). Treatment consists of splenectomy (to reduce haemolysis and possibility of traumatic rupture) in many cases unless haemolysis is mild or the spleen is only mildly enlarged. This is delayed until after five years of age because of the risk of overwhelming sepsis. In view of this the following precautions are taken prior to splenectomy: Pneumovax, hib vaccine and prophylactic penicillin.

2. A seven-year-old child presents with lethargy and is described by the parents as being paler than usual. The child had had a bad flu two months ago which was slow to resolve and the symptoms of tiredness had really started since then. On examination the sclera are slightly yellow and a mild degree of splenomegaly was found. Blood results were as follows:

Hb	5.4 g/dl (normocytic, normochromic)
WCC	7
Platelets	208
Unconjugated bilirubin	61 µmol/l
DCT	positive (anti-IgG)
Blood film	anisocytosis, polychromasia, reticulocytosis, spherocytosis

The picture here describes an autoimmune haemolytic anaemia. The normochromic normocytic anaemia with a positive Coombs with IgG coating the red cells and spherocytosis make the likely diagnosis a warm antibody autoimmune haemolytic anaemia (IgG antibodies agglutinate red cells preferentially at warm temperatures > 37°C). This form is mainly idiopathic (60%) and associated with thrombocytopenia (not in this case) in 20% of cases (Evan syndrome). The remaining 40% of cases are the result of an underlying disorder such as an autoimmune disorder e.g. rheumatoid arthritis, SLE, lymphoma or other malignancy and drugs (methyldopa, penicillin). Red cells are coated by IgG immunoglobulins giving a positive DAT. Treatment consists of steroids which reduces the interaction between macrophages and coated red cells. If no improvement consider immunosuppressives such as azathioprine. If the condition becomes chronic consider splenectomy which has a success rate of about 60–70%. Blood transfusion should be avoided.

Cold antibody AIHA produces IgM autoantibodies which agglutinate red cells preferentially at lower temperatures (< 37°C). In children it usually follows infections such as mycoplasma and infectious mononucleosis but is also seen in SLE and some lymphomas. DAT IgM is positive (with IgM often directed against the I antigen of erythrocytes) and anti-C3d is positive (detects complement components). Haemolysis tends to be milder than warm AIHA. Treatment involves avoidance of the cold, immunosuppressives, warmed blood transfusion; splenectomy is of no use.

You may be given a question with the rare condition of paroxysmal cold haemoglobinuria. It is classically associated with congenital or acquired syphilis but more commonly follows viral illnesses such as chickenpox, mumps and especially gastroenteritis. Here haemoglobinuria occurs after exposure to the cold. The IgG binds to red cells in the cooler parts of the body (with specificity for the P antigen) and then when it reaches the warmer parts there is complement mediated haemolysis. Investigation involves use of the Donath–Landsteiner biphasic lysis test. Treatment involves avoidance of the cold and possibly immunosuppressive agents.

Other causes of haemoglobinuria include the causes of intravascular haemolysis (especially if acute) such as microangiopathic haemolytic anaemias, for example HUS and paroxysmal nocturnal haemoglobinuria (an acquired sensitivity of a clone of red cells to lysis by complement) and infections such as malaria (blackwater fever).

3. A five-year-old Greek boy is seen in the A&E department of his local hospital feeling generally unwell. According to his mother, he has been passing dark urine for the last couple of days. On routine questioning of the mother about the possibility of ingesting any medications she replied that there was a small possibility. She had come into his room a couple of days ago and removed a container of tablets from him. He had removed the container from the suitcase that they were in the process of unpacking (they had just returned from their holiday in Kenya), but she was sure that there were no tablets missing.

Hb	6.7 g/dl
WCC	15.0
Platelets	239
Reticulocytes	9%
Blood film:	Fragmented red blood cells, Heinz bodies, bite cells (bite cells are cells that look as if a bite has been taken out of them, possibly because of Heinz body removal by the spleen: also called blister cells).

The diagnosis is glucose-6-phospate dehydrogenase deficiency (G6PD deficiency). The child had swallowed several primaquine tablets. It is the commonest red cell enzyme deficiency. It is inherited in a sex-linked fashion with males affected. Female carriers may exhibit some milder features (as in Duchenne muscular dystrophy as a result of random lyonisation). It may be precipitated by oxidative stress, stress of any sort or infection. It is common in

American blacks (10%), and Mediterranean peoples (such as Italians, Arabs and Greeks) as well as in South-East Asians. It affects the hexose monophosphate pathway (within which G6PD holds a vital role) which produces reducing power for the red cell in the form of NADPH (which maintains glutathione in a reduced state). Reduced glutathione is important in combating oxidative stress to the red cell. Absence of reduced glutathione will result in cross-linking of spectrin (leading to red cell rigidity) and haemoglobin oxidation to methaemoglobin with Heinz body precipitation in the cell. Both of these effects will result in haemolysis.

Normal enzyme variants are G6PD type B (found in most whites and 70% of American blacks) and type A+, another normal variant (found in approximately 10–20% of American blacks). Abnormal variants include variant A– seen in Afro-Caribbeans which becomes more unstable and degrades as the cell ages (thus reticulocytes have adequate levels, and so a haemolytic crisis is usually self-limiting resolving when a new population of red cells are formed). This form tends to be very sensitive to oxidative stress and precipitated by drugs such as sulphonamides and primaquine. G6PD-Caucasian/Mediterranean variants are seen in Mediterranean peoples who tend to be particularly sensitive to fava beans. They tend to suffer from chronic haemolysis and acute life threatening haemolytic crises. G6PD-Canton variants are especially prone to haemolysis in the neonatal period. There is of course overlap between all the groups. G6PD appears to protect against malaria. Intravascular haemolysis is common during haemolytic crises causing haemoglobinuria and jaundice. The blood film is as above.

Diagnosis is made by family history, history of oxidative stress and by performing an assay for G6PD enzyme. Remember to repeat this test if it is normal during a crisis since rapid production of reticulocytes (with normal enzyme levels) and loss of the mature enzyme deficient cells may sometimes give false negative results.

Treatment is supportive with treatment of infection, removal of offending drugs and blood transfusion. Splenectomy is usually of no use. In cases of chronic haemolysis folic acid and vitamin E are sometimes given.

Pyruvate kinase deficiency is the second commonest enzyme disorder (glycolytic pathway) inherited in AR fashion. It is also exacerbated by stress or infection.

ABO AND RHESUS HAEMOLYTIC DISEASE IN THE NEWBORN

Many questions relate to ABO and Rhesus haemolytic disease (see Table 8.2)

The Kleihauer test is an acid elution test on maternal blood and relies on the fact that HbF in the fetal cells is acid resistant (compared with maternal cells) so that fetal cells remain pink and maternal cells become colourless. The percentage of the fetal red cells in the maternal blood is then calculated and is a measure of extent of fetomaternal haemorrhage. This test is used by obstetricians to determine the dose of anti-D prophylaxis (given to Rhesus –ve women) to prevent rhesus haemolytic disease in subsequent pregnancies.

Table 8.2 Comparison of ABO and Rhesus incompatibility

	ABO incompatibility	Rhesus incompatibility
Genes found on	Chromosome 9	Chromosome 1
Phenotypes	O (46%), A (42%), B (9%), AB(3%)	CDE/cde. Rhesus relates to D/d. Rhesus +ve (83%), Rhesus –ve (17%)
Naturally occurring antibodies in serum	Present. A = Anti-B, B = Anti-A, O = Anti-A,B, AB = nil	None present
Haemolysis possible	Possible in the first pregnancy (only if anti-A or anti-B antibodies are IgG class; approximately 10% of women).	After the first pregnancy
Direct Coombs' test	Usually negative or weakly positive	Strongly positive
Blood film	Numerous microspherocytes, reticulocytosis	No spherocytes, reticulocytosis
Haemolysis severity	Mild, only very rarely requiring exchange transfusion	Usually more severe than ABO incompatibility

HAEMOGLOBIN ELECTROPHORESIS

Many questions relate to haemoglobin electrophoresis. It is important that you know some of the uses and are able to interpret results from them. This is the single most important investigation in the diagnosis of haemoglobinopathies. The questions may give you percentages or give you a diagram of a haemoglobin electrophoresis. This is usually in the form of a copied diagram or a picture of the actual electrophoresis. Either way the bands are labelled with the haemoglobin type and the width of the band corresponds to the proportion of the haemoglobin type that makes up the haemoglobin being tested.

Normal child: HbA   92%
HbA2   2–3.5%
HbF   0.5%

At birth: HbA 20%, HbF 80%. Charts are available to determine the normal ranges of different Hb types at different ages. The following are examples of average results seen in children.

Sickle cell disease

1. Sickle cell disease: Note no HbA and high proportion of HbF.

    HbS   90%
    HbF   10%
    HbA2   2%
    HbA   0%

2. Sickle cell trait: Note no HbF.

HbS	40–45%
HBA	50–55%
HbA2	2%
HbF	0%

3. Sickle cell B⁺ thalassaemia: This and B° thalassaemia have many clinical features in common with sickle cell disease but is generally less severe.

HbS	65%
HbA	15%
HbF	10%
HbA2	3%

4. Sickle cell B° thalassaemia: Note no HbA cf. sickle cell B⁺ thalassaemia.

HbS	75%
HbF	15%
HbA2	3%
HbA	0%

5. Sickle SC disease: Symptoms similar to sickle cell disease but less severe.

HbS	50%
HbC	50%

NB The following may come in useful in some questions. In sickle cell disease the MCV is normal so that if there is a question that has a high proportion of HbS with a microcytic anaemia consider a Hb sickle/thalassaemia variant (above).

Thalassaemia

1. Beta thalassaemia major (note very high levels of HbF)

   Hb F up to 90% (usually around 75%)
   HbA2 increased but variable between 3.5–8.0%
   HbA absent

2. Beta thalassaemia minor (note raised HbA2)

HbA2	usually 4–7%
HbF	variably increased (1–3%) but not as high as beta thalassaemia major
HbA	rest

Alpha thalassaemia

The alpha chain is encoded by four genes on chromosome 16. Clinical consequences arise with deletion of these genes.

1 gene deletion: Silent carrier.
2 gene deletions: Alpha thalassaemia trait. Hypochromic microcytic anaemia.

3 gene deletions: HbH disease. Anaemia (variable), splenomegaly.
4 gene deletions: No alpha chain synthesis. Four gamma chains are produced leading to Hb Barts and this is commoner in South-East Asia and a common cause of stillbirth.

Electrophoresis will show varying degrees of HbH and Hb Barts in type 3, and in type 4 gene deletion mainly Hb Barts.

If a child is being investigated for a microcytic anaemia and iron studies and Hb electrophoresis are normal but you still think there is a likelihood of a haemoglobinopathy, then consider alpha thalassaemia. It is diagnosed by specific genetic tests.

HPFH (hereditary persistence of fetal haemoglobin) is associated with a normal prognosis.

IRON DEFICIENCY ANAEMIA

Many questions are centred around iron deficiency anaemia. In a child who has an anaemia with a low MCV it is important to distinguish between iron deficiency anaemia and other microcytic causes such as thalassaemia, chronic disease and lead poisoning. This is done with iron studies (see Table 8.3), Hb electrophoresis, possibly ESR and lead studies depending on clinical suspicion. The blood film is described above and examination of the bone marrow would show erythroid hyperplasia and a lack of stainable iron. Iron deficiency anaemia is common towards the end of the first year of life because of increased demands of the body and maternal stores running out. It is commoner in bottle-fed babies rather than breast-fed because of reduced absorbable iron. It may also be caused by prolonged breastfeeding without introduction of sufficient solids. Doorstep cow's milk given before the age of one year can cause GI bleeding. Iron stores at birth last for 5–6 months by which time solids have usually been introduced. Poor diet is the commonest cause of iron deficiency and presents most commonly towards the end of the first year (earlier in premature babies). Premature and low weight infants should receive iron supplements for at least the first year.

Remember the slide of koilonychia (spoon-shaped nails) associated with iron deficiency anaemia. In case histories also remember that iron deficiency is associated with pica and brittle hair. Iron in the body is stored mainly in the form of ferritin (soluble) and is found chiefly in the bone marrow. It is in equilibrium with the cell ferritin so that serum ferritin gives an indication of the

Table 8.3 Differentiating the causes of a microcytic anaemia based on iron studies

	Serum Fe	TIBC	% Saturation	Ferritin
Iron deficiency	Low	High	Approx. 10%	Low
Chronic disease (Hb rarely less than 9 g/dl)	Low	Low	Normal	Normal or increased
Beta thalassaemia trait/disease	Normal or increased	Normal	Normal	Normal
Sideroblastic anaemia	Increased	Increased	Approx. 100%	Increased

total body stores. Plasma iron is attached to a plasma protein called transferrin which is the main transport protein for iron. Synthesis of transferrin by the liver is inversely proportional to the body's iron stores and is therefore increased in iron deficiency. TIBC (total iron binding capacity) is a functional measurement of serum transferrin concentration and is approximately 33%, that is, one-third saturated. Remember that plasma ferritin is an acute phase reactant and may be raised even in the absence of body iron stores.

Sometimes questions will ask you to differentiate between iron deficiency and beta thalassaemia trait based only on a full blood count. (a) Look at the MCV which in the beta thalassaemia trait is usually disproportionately low (usually between 50 and 60) compared to the mild anaemia that one sees (severe anaemia could be a result of beta thalassaemia major but would usually have been indicated to you in the history). On the contrary however the lower the MCV in iron deficiency usually the more severe the anaemia. Other useful indicators are (b) that the red cell count is usually raised in beta thalassaemia trait but reduced in iron deficiency. (c) The RDW (red cell distribution width) is very high in iron deficiency anaemia (> 14) but normal in beta thalassaemia trait (this does not always occur in clinical practice). In practice Hb electrophoresis and iron studies (as above) would be performed for confirmation.

Differences between the dietary, haematinic anaemias are commonly referred to in examinations (see Table 8.4).

Table 8.4 Comparison of haematinic causes of anaemia

	Iron deficiency anaemia	B12 deficiency anaemia	Folate deficiency anaemia
Physiology	H+ in stomach causes $Fe^{3+} \rightarrow Fe^{2+}$ which can then be absorbed in the duodenum and jejunum. Iron absorption increased by iron deficiency, vitamin C and reduced by phytates.	Vitamin B12 (hydroxycobalamin) combines with intrinsic factor in the stomach which is produced by parietal cells. It is carried to the terminal ileum where it is absorbed.	Folate from the diet is absorbed unchanged in the duodenum and jejunum.
Sources	Red meat, egg yolk, green vegetables. Requirements 1–2 mg/kg/day.	Animal origin foods e.g fish, meat, eggs and milk. Requirements 1–3 µg/day. Stores last 3–4 years.	Most foods esp. liver and spinach. Requirements 100 µg/day. Body stores last 3–4 months.
Causes of deficiency	(1) Haemorrhage esp. GI bleeds e.g. peptic ulcer, ulcerative colitis, Meckel's diverticulum, hookworm; (2) Inadequate intake in premature infants,	(1) Inadequate intake e.g. vegans. (2) Malabsorption: post gastrectomy, pernicious anaemia, Crohn disease, ileal resection, fish	(1) Reduced intake rare in children. (2) Increased utilisation e.g chronic haemolytic anaemia, pregnancy (3) Antifolate drugs

Table 8.4 *Continued*

	Iron deficiency anaemia	B12 deficiency anaemia	Folate deficiency anaemia
	presents between 6–12 months because of increased needs. Esp. Asian families, late weaning from breast milk, bottle-fed babies; (3) Malabsorption e.g. achlorhydria, post gastrectomy, coeliac disease.	tapeworm, intestinal blind loops (B12 and fat malabsorption).	e.g. phenytoin, antimetabolite cytotoxics e.g. methotrexate.
Clinical signs	Features of anaemia + koilonychia, glossitis, brittle hair and pica.	Features of anaemia + glossitis, jaundice because of ineffective erythropoiesis, bleeding tendency because of reduced platelet production, increased infections, reduced white cell production. Neurological sequelae.*	Features of B12 deficiency anaemia without the neurological features.
Investigations	Microcytic hypochromic anaemia, Fe studies (see above). Blood film (see above). Hb of < 10 g/dl after six months of age. Bone marrow, erythroid hyperplasia and reduced stainable iron.	Macrocytic anaemia, hypersegmented neutrophils, leucopenia and thrombocytopenia, Howell–Jolly bodies. Bone marrow hyperplastic, megaloblasts with nuclear/cytoplasmic dissociation (nucleus more primitive cf. cytoplasm). B12 tests.**	As for B12 deficiency. Serum and red cell folate.
Treatment	Treat underlying cause. Oral/i.m. iron and rarely transfusion. Continue treatment for three months after stabilisation of Hb to replenish stores.	Treat underlying cause. i.m. hydroxycobalamin injections if intrinsic factor (IF) a problem or malabsorption. Otherwise oral B12.	Treat underlying cause and give folate supplements.

*Neurological features of B12 deficiency include peripheral neuropathy, optic atrophy, mental retardation and subacute combined degeneration of the spinal cord (with co-existing degeneration of the dorsal columns and pyramidal tracts).
**In B12 deficiency there is a reduced serum B12 level and red cell folate is normal or reduced since folate entry into the red cell is dependent on vitamin B12. Serum folate is thus normal or increased (since not entering the red cell). In folate deficiency, serum and red cell folate levels are reduced and serum B12 levels are normal.

The Schilling test

An important test of vitamin B12 handling is the Schilling test and you may be asked to interpret some results. The test is carried out as follows: firstly, storage sites are saturated with vitamin B12 following an i.m. injection (this is so that any extra B12 entering the body will be excreted in the urine). The child then takes oral radiolabelled hydroxycobalamin. Because of the saturated storage body sites of B12 normally a proportion of ingested radiolabelled B12 will pass into the urine and thus the urine is collected for 24 h (expected amounts are between 10–30%). A reduction in expected excretion indicates reduced absorption of vitamin B12. This test is called Schilling 1. The next test (called Schilling 2) involves giving radiolabelled vitamin B12 this time with intrinsic factor to see if urinary excretion increases. If it does then there is an abnormality with intrinsic factor production. If there is no increase with added intrinsic factor then there is a problem at the level of the terminal ileum.

CLOTTING DISORDERS

These are common in data interpretation questions and in order to answer them you should have a basic understanding of the following principles (see Fig. 8.1).

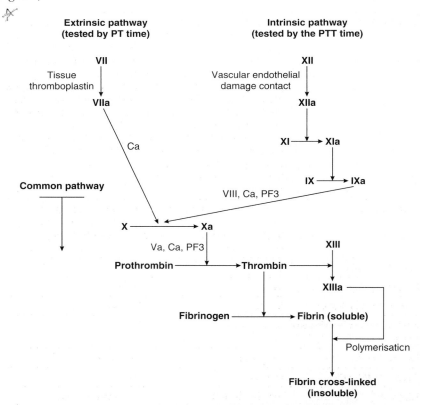

Fig. 8.1 A simplified clotting pathway. NB PT time and PTT times reach adult levels at one week and 2–10 months respectively.

You shoiuld be able to distinguish haemophilia A and von Willebrand disease. See Table 8.5.

Table 8.5 A comparison between Haemophilia A and von Willebrand disease

	Haemophilia A	von Willebrand disease
Pathophysiology	Congenital deficiency of Factor VIII resulting in interference in intrinsic pathway	Deficiency or abnormality in Factor VIII: VWF results in Factor VIII deficiency and decreased platelet adhesion
Inheritance	X-linked recessive. Affects males but random lyonisation may result in heterozygote female carriers having reduced Factor VIII levels and symptomatic under extreme haemostatic demands. High mutation rate (one-third spontaneous mutation rate).	The VIII: VWF gene is found on chromosome 12. Inheritance in the majority of cases is autosomal dominant although autosomal recessive forms exist.
Clinical features	Depends on Factor VIII levels: (a) < 1% — severe (50% of cases) Spontaneous haemorrhage into muscle, joint, GIT, soft tissue from early life. (b) 1–5% — moderate. Usually bleeding problems after trauma. (c) > 5% — mild. Only minor symptoms e.g. prolonged bleeding post surgery or bleeding after severe trauma.	Clinical features mainly reflect the platelet function abnormality (easy bruising, purpura, mucous membrane bleeding, menorrhagia and epistaxis). Reduced Factor VIII levels may give rise to similar features of haemophilia A but are usually much milder.
Investigations	Involves (a) coagulation tests (b) factor assays (c) diagnosis of carriers and DNA probes.	Involves (a) coagulation tests (b) factor assays (c) ristocetin assay
Platelet count	Normal	Normal
Bleeding time	Normal	Increased
Prothrombin time	Normal	Normal
Partial thromboplastin time	Increased	Increased
Factor VIII:C	Decreased	Decreased
Factor VIII:VWF	Normal	Decreased
Ristocetin co-factor assay	Induces platelet aggregation	Ristocetin (a platelet aggregator) will not

Table 8.5 Continued

	Haemophilia A	von Willebrand disease
		induce platelet aggregation in the absence of VWF
Treatment	1) Treat bleeds with i.v. Factor VIII concentrate (half life 12 hours). 2) DDAVP for minor bleeds or to increase Factor VIII levels before surgery. 3) Register with haemophiliac centre for support	Treatment is usually the same as for mild haemophilia with DDAVP before surgery and treatment of bleeding episodes with Factor VIII concentrates.

To understand the pathophysiology you must know that the stable Factor VIII consists of two components (Factor VIII: C and Factor VIII: VWF,). In haemophilia A no Factor VIII: C is produced but Factor VIII: VWF (stable on its own) is. In von Willebrand disease Factor VIII: C is produced but there is failure to produce Factor VIII: VWF. Factor VIII: C is unstable in the absence of Factor VIII: VWF and is destroyed leading to features of VWF deficiency (defective platelet function) and features of Factor VIII: C deficiency (similar to but milder than haemophilia A — see Fig. 8.2).

Complications of haemophilia treatment

1. About 10% of treated patients develop Factor VIII: C antibodies which is usually treated using high levels of the factor or alternative clotting factor intermediates (activated prothrombin complex) which may bypass the inhibitor or porcine Factor VIII.
2. Allergic reactions.
3. Risk of acquiring bloodborne disease e.g. hepatitis B,C.

Acquired coagulation defects

You should be able to compare the features of acquired coagulation defects (see Table 8.6).

Causes of DIC include sepsis, malignancy, trauma, burns, hypovolaemic shock and neonatal asphyxia.

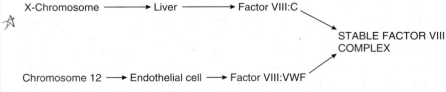

Fig. 8.2 The formation of stable Factor VIII complex.

Table 8.6 Comparison of acquired coagulation disorders

	Vitamin K deficiency	Liver disease	Disseminated intravascular coagulation (DIC)
Bleeding time	Normal	Normal or increased*	Increased
Prothrombin time	Increased	Increased	Increased
Partial thromboplastin time	Increased	Increased	Increased
Thrombin clotting time	Normal	Normal	Increased**
Factor assays	Decreased Factors II, VII, IX, X (normal Factor V)	Decreased Factors II, VII, IX, X (also low Factor V)	All clotting factors decreased. Increased FDPs.

*Because of functional abnormalities of platelets in liver failure as well as possible associated hypersplenism leading to thrombocytopenia.
**Thrombin time is sometimes included in some questions. It is essentially a measure of active fibrinogen. It is increased in patients receiving heparin, in hypofibrinogenaemia and in the presence of inhibitors of the formation of the fibrin polymer such as FDPs in DIC. Protamine corrects the thrombin time in all the cases except hypofibrinogenaemia. The reptilase test is a direct test for hypofibrinogenaemia.

Products
— Fresh frozen plasma is the result of freezing one unit of blood at −30°C to supply approximately 200 ml of fluid with all the clotting factors.
— Cryoprecipitate contains Factor VIII: C, Factor VIII: VWF and fibrinogen.

HAEMATOLOGY AND RADIOLOGY

There are several slides that you may be expected to recognise that relate to haematological problems:

— *Lead poisoning* has some characteristic features. You may be shown linear densities in the metaphysis of bones (similar to growth arrest lines), or split sutures seen on a SXR caused by raised intracranial pressure. In addition you may be shown a slide of an abdominal X-ray in a child with symptoms and signs of lead poisoning. Look for radio-opaque material in the intestine because of accidental ingestion.

— *Beta thalassaemia major* is a common slide. Compensatory bone marrow expansion occurs secondary to haemolysis and produces the characteristic 'thalassaemic facies' with frontal bossing and maxillary prominence. Radiologically this can be seen typically in the skull bones with widening of the cortex giving rise to the 'hair on end' appearance (also called 'sun-ray' appearance). Instead of appearing bilaterally concave, phalanges may appear rectangular or bilaterally convex. AXR may show hepatosplenomegaly.

— *Sickle cell disease*. There may be a slide of a hand of a child with dactylitis showing considerable soft tissue swelling. A CXR may be shown with basal infiltrates, consolidation, areas of collapse and atelectasis in a child who is described as being febrile with breathlessness or chest pain. These features indicate acute chest syndrome. You may be shown a hip with avascular necrosis of the femoral head related to sickle cell disease.

— *Radial aplasia*. See chapter 11.

— *Haemophilia*. Look for evidence of arthritis if shown a knee of a child with haemophilia. The most obvious feature of arthritis is the loss of joint space but in addition look for osteophytes, subchondral bone sclerosis and cyst formation. A psoas muscle bleed can be massive and may be seen on a plain AXR but should be accurately assessed with CT scan.

HAEMATOLOGICAL CLINICAL SCENARIOS

There are a number of haematological conditions that have structural skeletal defects associated with them.

Diamond–Blackfan syndrome

This is an example of pure red cell aplasia. Ninety percent present before the age of one year, mostly before the age of six months. Physical abnormalities can be found in about 30%. These include short stature, web neck, cleft lip and a triphalangeal thumb (instead of the usual diphalangeal thumb). The anaemia is normocytic and normochromic and notably has a low reticulocyte count. The red cells have certain fetal characteristics that persist, which include occasional increased MCV, elevated HbF and the presence of I antigen. Bone marrow reveals a selective absence of red cell precursors such as normoblasts. Treatment is with steroids with an initial response of 75% and this response may continue or be of limited duration in which case regular red cell transfusions are required. There is a possibility of bone marrow transplant in some. A similar condition called transient erythroblastopenia of infancy (TEC) must be distinguished from the above. It is self limiting and presents slightly later. There are no fetal characteristics of the red cells. The children are phenotypically normal. It may be preceeded by a viral illness such as human parvovirus infection.

Fanconi anaemia

This is a form of aplastic anaemia that presents at around five years of age. It is inherited as autosomal recessive with an M:F ratio of 2:1. These children can be recognised by shortness, microcephaly, horseshoe kidney, absent/abnormal thumbs, absent radii (radial aplasia) and sometimes hyperpigmentation. Cytogenetic problems are common such as chromosome breaks/gaps. There is an increased risk of AML. Reticulocyte count is low and thrombocytopenia may present before full pancytopenia. HbF is increased. It may be diagnosed by performing a white cell chromosome fragility test and looking for characteristic cytogenetic abnormalities. Compared to other aplastic anaemias there is a more favourable response to androgens and high dose steroids. However, treat it like any other aplastic anaemia.

TAR syndrome

This is inherited in an autosomal recessive fashion. The syndrome consists of thrombocytopenia and bilateral radial aplasia (TAR). Radial aplasia is a common slide and you should recognise it immediately. It consists of shortening of the forearm and marked deviation of the wrist in a radial direction. Causes include TAR syndrome, VATER syndrome, Fanconi anaemia and the Holt–Oram syndrome.

Risks of treating thalassaemia major

Treatment of thalassaemia major aims to allow normal growth and development while at the same time inhibiting extramedullary haemopoiesis, marrow hyperplasia and preventing bony abnormalities. Be aware, however, of the risk of overtransfusion and iron overload. Beta thalassaemia major patients often require regular transfusions approximately every 2–4 weeks to keep the haemoglobin above 10 g/dl. This has problems of iron overload, atypical antibody formation leading to difficult cross-matching and increased risk of infection. In cases of increased transfusion requirements or hypersplenism, splenectomy may be of help. In order to prevent iron overload these patients require iron chelation therapy (using subcutaneous overnight pumps of desferrioxamine which may cause local and systemic allergic reactions as well as reversible cataract of the lens) with regular measurement of serum ferritin (which should always be below 1000 μg/ml). One should also perform regular assessment of end organ damage by iron (for example liver function tests). Folate supplements should be given. Treatment using bone marrow transplantation (which has a high incidence of graft vs. host disease) and gene therapy using modified retrovirus vectors to introduce complete globin genes into the bone marrow are being investigated.

Iron overload

Any haematological condition requiring regular transfusions runs the risk of iron overload. Features of iron overload syndrome (haemosiderosis) are damage to the liver (leading to hepatomegaly, cirrhosis and possible hepatoma and hepatic failure), pancreas (leading to diabetes mellitis), heart (leading to arrhythmias and heart failure), skin pigmentation, delayed puberty, and *Yersinia* gastrointestinal infection (*Yersinia* utilises iron for growth) which can present with abdominal pain, sometimes with severe diarrhoea, and is treated with ciprofloxacin.

Sickle cell disease

Sickle cell disease is a common question. The molecular defect is substitution of valine for glutamic acid at position 6 on the B globin chain. Twenty-five per cent of black Africans are carriers of the gene. Remember other variants that are inherited in a co-dominant way such as beta thalassaemia, sickle cell beta thalassaemia with a variable presentation and sickle cell-HbC disease which has an increased incidence of thrombosis as one of its features.

The pathology occurs when the HBS molecules are deoxygenated or become acidotic. The molecules polymerise. This causes the red cell to become sickle shaped which results in (a) reduced life span of the red cell leading to haemolysis; and (b) impaired circulation through small vessels leading to vascular occlusion. Known precipitating factors include: hypoxia, acidosis, dehydration, cold and infection. Because of the presence of HbF (which has anti-sickling effects) the condition does not usually present before six months of age.

Heterozygotes are usually asymptomatic except when exposed to hypoxia e.g. under anaesthesia or when flying. Haematuria and concentrating problems may occur.

You may be presented in a question with any of the large spectrum of presentations.

a. Chronic haemolytic anaemia with varying degrees of anaemia (usually between 5–10 g/dl), unconjugated jaundice and — like all chronic haemolytic disorders — there is expansion of the bone marrow cavity leading to sickle facies with maxillary hyperplasia;

b. Hand and foot syndrome: seen primarily in toddlers with recurrent pain and swelling often with fever;

c. Bone pain;

d. Chest pain often pleuritic in nature;

e. Priapism;

f. Renal papillary necrosis often with haematuria which may lead to loss of renal concentrating ability (leading to polyuria and enuresis) and long term renal failure;

g. Abdominal pain may be the result of infarction of organs such as the spleen or liver (and may present as an acute abdomen) but also may be a sign of the presence of pigment gallstones.

h. Infection which is the leading cause of mortality is often caused by encapsulated organisms such as pneumococcus;

i. Osteomyelitis — often with unusual organisms especially *Salmonella*;

j. Chronic leg ulcers are a common problem and take a long time to heal;

k. Cerebrovascular accident following damage to the cerebral vessels leading to hemiplegia or cranial nerve palsies;

l. Pulmonary hypertension;

m. Splenic sequestration: there is a rapid life threatening reduction in circulating blood volume secondary to red cell pooling in the spleen with a rapidly enlarged spleen;

n. Aseptic necrosis of the femoral head;
o. As with any chronic problem in children it may lead to growth problems and delayed puberty;
p. Acute chest syndrome: fever, increasing dyspnoea, tachycardia, chest pain indicate the possibility. The CXR may show increased bilateral shadowing, with collapse/consolidation. There may be only limited sickling signs — life threatening;
q. Aplastic crisis which is most commonly caused by human parvovirus type B19 (like hereditary spherocytosis) and can last up to 2–3 weeks;
r. Congestive cardiac failure;
s. Blindness caused by retinal infarction and detachment.
   — *Investigations*: See blood film (above) and Hb electrophoresis (above); sickling test identifies patients with about 20% HbS and does not therefore distinguish between carriers and those with the disease.
   — *Treatment*:
   1. Acute treatment of painful crisis involves fluids, analgesics, oxygen and antibiotics.
   2. Blood transfusions (red cells if anaemic or whole blood if sequestration) are limited to selected cases to reduce problems of iron overload and cross-matching problems.
   3. Exchange transfusion is used in two particular cases where there has been an acute chest syndrome or cerebrovascular crisis. Following these crises it is important that these children have regular transfusions to prevent their recurrence. In any life-threatening complication try to reduce the percentage of HBSS to less than about 30%. Problems associated with exchange transfusion are: hyperkalaemia, hypocalcaemia (because of chelation with citrate), hypothermia, circulatory volume imbalance (leading to possible heart failure and arrhthymias) and acidosis (from stored blood). There may be reduced oxygen delivering capacity of the stored blood because of reduced levels of 2,3 DPG (which usually shifts the oxygen dissociation curve to the right).
   4. Chronic treatment involves folate administration, penicillin prophylaxis, Pneumovax vaccine after the age of two.
   5. Parental education: Keep the child well hydrated in the summer, develop the ability to recognise the different types of crises, and so on.
   6. Genetic counselling.
   7. Possible role for bone marrow transplant.

Sudden onset of anaemia in sickle cell disease may be the result of (1) splenic sequestration; (2) hyperhaemolysis secondary to drugs or infection; (3) aplastic crisis.

There are a number of crises in sickle cell disease: (a) haemolytic crisis; (b) splenic sequestration; (c) acute chest syndrome; (d) aplastic crisis; (e) vaso-occlusive crisis (painful).

It is important to know that splenomegaly is often felt in the toddler in sickle cell disease but because of autosplenectomy (arising from repeated infarction episodes) the spleen is not usually felt after the age of about 4–5 years old (but functionally asplenic from the age of about one year). The presence of Howell–Jolly bodies may give a clue to the degree of splenic function (see earlier). **NB**. This auto splenectomy may occur later in the sickle cell variants (such as HbSC and HBS-thalassaemia) so they must be considered in an older child with a palpable spleen.

White cell counts

You may be given questions with differential white cell counts. Don't forget the simple rules:

1. Lymphocytosis is commonly due to viral illnesses such as measles, mumps, rubella, EBV. TB causes lymphocytosis. Acute lymphoblastic leukaemia. Don't forget the association of whooping cough with a lymphocytosis.

2. Monocytosis is found in infections such as tuberculosis and brucellosis as well as in chronic inflammatory states such as juvenile chronic arthritis (JCA).

3. Eosinophilia is found in type 1 hypersensitivity reactions including asthma, eczema and hay fever as well as in parasitic infections such as hookworm; also seen in pulmonary eosinophilia. There is often an increased eosinophil count in premature infants.

4. Basophilia: Chronic myeloid leukaemia (in adults), ulcerative colitis and hypothyroidism.

5. Neutrophilia: (a) infection especially bacterial including septicaemia, abscess formation; (b) trauma — post surgery, burns, fractures; (c) drugs — steroids, adrenaline; (d) haemorrhage; (e) post transfusion; (f) stress: for example, post seizure.

Neutropenia

Increased susceptibility to infection is related to the degree of neutropenia. The clinical consequences of neutropenia are of increased risk of infection from the outside world as well as from sites of the body where there is a high concentration of normal basal bacterial flora which in conditions of neutropenia become invasive and pathogenic. Thus oral infections/ulcers and gingivitis are common, as are pneumonia and perianal infections. Bacterial septicaemia is an additional problem. Treatment depends on severity and involves treating any underlying cause. Barrier nursing in a side room, regular examination of possible sites of infection (for instance mouth, perineum and axilla), four hourly observations and meticulous attention to oral hygiene including antifungals for *Candida* prophylaxis. Treat infections vigorously. Each hospital will have protocols for dealing with a neutropenic fever including antibiotic treatment combinations. Resistant infections might be the result of fungal infections.

Causes of neutropenia (1): *reduced production*

— *Infection*: viral diseases, bacterial diseases such as typhoid, paratyphoid, tuberculosis and in overwhelming bacterial sepsis due to any agent. Remember neonates have a small reserve of neutrophils in the bone marrow and once these have been released neutropenia occurs.

— *Reticular dysgenesis*: AR inheritance. Abnormality in the production of myeloid precursors. Red cell and platelet production is normal (SCID with agranulocytosis).

— *Kostman syndrome* (infantile genetic agranulocytosis): AR inheritance. Abnormality in the maturation of neutrophil precursors. Associated with a monocytosis and eosinophilia. Treatment with granulocyte colony stimulating factor improves survival.

— *Cyclical neutropenia*: Inherited AR, AD or spontaneous. There is a 'cycling' in the neutrophil count that occurs every 14–28 days with an average of 21 days. It affects all cell lines but cycling in production will affect neutrophils (with a half life of approximately six hours) more than red cells (half life 120 days) and platelets (7–10 days). Cycle time is usually constant within an individual. Symptoms tend to improve with age. Diagnose with regular serial full blood counts with differentials.

— *Chronic benign neutropenia of childhood*: moderate reduction in neutrophil count which remains usually unchanged throughout childhood. There is an increased risk of infection in proportion to degree of neutropenia.

— *Diamond–Swachmann syndrome*: inherited as AR condition. (a) Pancreatic insufficiency resulting in malabsorption with subsequent failure to thrive and short stature (second most common cause of pancreatic insufficiency after cystic fibrosis). (b) Deficiency in all myeloid lines especially neutropenia, may also have lower Hb and platelet count. (c) Severe gingivitis which may cause premature loss of teeth and cause infection of adjacent alveolar bone. (d) Hepatomegaly with mild hepatic dysfunction. (e) Renal tubular dysfunction — rare (f) Metaphyseal achondroplasia.

— *Bone marrow infiltration*: leukaemia, solid tumour invasion, glycogen storage diseases, osteopetrosis.

— *Haematinic deficiency* such as vitamin B12 or folate deficiency results in ineffective neutrophil production as well as other cell lines.

— *Drugs*: such as chemotherapy agents but also carbimazole and chlorpromazine.

Causes of neutropenia (2): *increased destruction*

— *Isoimmune neonatal neutropenia* is similar to Rhesus isoimmunisation in theory. Antineutrophil IgG antibodies subsequently cause neutropenia in infants.

— *Drugs*: in addition to affecting bone marrow also immune mediated mechanisms may initiate immune destruction of neutrophils.

— *Autoimmune neutropenia* associated with various conditions such as JCA and SLE or may occur in isolation.

— *Hypersplenism*

Useful investigations in neutropenia are FBC (serial if suspect cyclical neutropenia), blood film, antineutrophil antibodies, bone marrow examination (to look for myeloid precursors and to exclude infiltrative causes).

Qualitative disorders of neutrophil function are discussed in chapter 9.

Thrombocytopenia

A common question relates to the child with thrombocytopenia. You should look up a list of all the possible causes of thrombocytopenia under the headings of (1) reduced production 2) increased destruction. Discussed here are the commoner examination topics.

Idiopathic thrombocytopenic purpura (ITP)

Affects children typically between the ages of 1–5 years old. M:F 1:1. Acute onset of purpura/petechiae, nosebleeds or bruising in an otherwise well child (more rarely haematuria or mucosal bleeding). Evidence of bleeding is only seen in platelet counts less than $20 \times 10^9/l$. Most follow a recent viral illness. Most importantly in the history and examination you should look for the lack of recent weight loss, the absence of lymphadenopathy or hepatosplenomegaly (splenomegaly may indicate leukaemia or lymphoma), and no indicators of other illness. In other words the child with ITP looks clinically well and is in fact well.

You may be given some investigation results as follows: Low platelet count, Hb normal, WCC normal. Antiplatelet antibodies may occasionally be found but are not necessary for the diagnosis. Bleeding time is prolonged.

Bone marrow examination is performed only if there is an atypical presentation, to exclude leukaemia or aplastic anaemia or if it is intended to start steroids which may mask an underlying leukaemia by destroying leukaemic cells, or precipitate a possible tumour lysis syndrome in an inadequately prepared child. Bone marrow will show normal or increased platelet precursors (megakaryocytes) indicating peripheral destruction.

The most severe complication is intracranial haemorrhage which occurs in less than 1%. Chronic ITP — lasting more than six months — occurs in 5–10% of cases. It is commoner in young female adults usually over 10 years of age (beware transplacental transfer of antibodies in a mother with chronic ITP causing neonatal thrombocytopenia). Antiplatelet antibodies are present in about 70% of cases. It has a variable course.

— *Treatment*: Half of all these children will resolve spontaneously by two months of age and 80–90% by six months. In view of this, treatment is controversial and is reserved for platelet counts less than 30 and severe bleeding and consists of (1) IVIG (which blocks Fc receptors in the spleen) improves platelet count within a day for several weeks, although it appears to have no effect on outcome; (2) corticosteroids increase platelet counts and are given for a couple of weeks but yet again there is no effect on overall outcome; (3) splenectomy. Because of the risk of overwhelming infection in this age group, this is reserved only for life-threatening bleeding or failure of response to steroids particularly in the chronic ITP group (20% complete response to steroids, 20% not steroid responsive, 60% partial response). There is a 90% response rate to splenectomy but some (approximately 30%) may subsequently relapse in which case (4) immunosuppressive agents can be used; (5) platelet transfusions may be used in severe bleeding (such as intracranial bleeds) but will be rapidly cleared from the blood by the antibodies.

Causes of neonatal thrombocytopenia

a. *Maternal idiopathic thrombocytopenic purpura.* Look at the mother's platelet count. This is not always reliable and the count may be normal if she has had a splenectomy. Look for antibodies. May last 1–3 months.

b. *Isoimmune neonatal thrombocytopenia.* Theory as for Rhesus haemolytic disease but with anti-PLA1 antibodies passing to the fetus of an anti-PLA1 negative mother. Normal maternal platelet count. Look for antibodies. Can last 1–3 months.

c. *Sepsis* including TORCH syndrome.

d. *Birth asphyxia* caused by depression of bone marrow.

e. *DIC.*

f. *Congenital abnormalities* such as Wiskott–Aldrich syndrome, TAR syndrome.

g. *Haemangioma* causing platelet destruction (Kassalbach–Merritt syndrome — see chapter 12).

h. *Maternal drugs* e.g. some antibiotics.

i. *Tumours* (rarely) caused by leukaemia, neuroblastoma.

Qualitative platelet defects

A number of qualitative platelet defects present in the paediatric patient and their recognition may be tested in an examination question. See Table 8.7.

Other qualitative defects include Wiscott–Aldrich syndrome (small platelets and thrombocytopenia), May–Hegglin anomaly (associated with thrombocytopenia with large platelets and abnormal white cells), Chediak–Higashi syndrome (abnormal platelet function). Uraemia and chronic liver disease may also cause platelet dysfunction.

Table 8.7 A comparison of Glanzmann thrombasthenia and Bernard–Soulier syndrome

	Glanzmann thrombasthenia	Bernard–Soulier syndrome
Inheritance	Autosomal recessive	Autosomal recessive
Appearance and number of platelets	Normal platelet count and morphology	Mild thrombocytopenia and very large platelets
Bleeding time	Increased	Increased
Platelet surface glycoproteins (GP) involved in platelet function	Deficiency in GPIIb and GPIIIa	Deficiency in GPIb and GPV
Platelet aggregation studies	No platelet aggregation with any of the platelet agonists (ADP, collagen and ristocetin).	Platelet aggregation normal with ADP and collagen but abnormal with ristocetin.
Treatment	Treat bleeding episodes with platelet transfusions. Beware isoantibody formation.	Treat bleeding episodes with platelet transfusions. Beware isoantibody formation.

Pattern of anaemia with abdominal pain

The pattern of a child who presents with anaemia and abdominal pain could be caused by the following: sickle cell disease, lead poisoning, glucose-6 phosphate deficiency, bleeding site in GI, vasculitis e.g. Henoch–Schönlein purpura, and chronic disease with GI involvement (such as Crohn disease).

Aplastic anaemia

This will usually present in the form of a pancytopenia. Causes are:

— *Drugs*: Dose-dependent such as chemotherapy agents or idiosyncratic such as chloramphenicol.
— *Chemicals*: Benzene ring solvents. Carbon tetrachloride.
— *Viruses*: Transient in infectious mononucleosis, hepatitis A. Human parvovirus type B19 can produce a transient aplastic anaemia in sickle cell disease and hereditary spherocytosis.
— *Irradiation*
— *Inherited causes*: Fanconi anaemia, Diamond–Swachmann syndrome.
— *Idiopathic*.

Clinically there will be features reflecting a reduction in the red cell, white cell and platelet lines that is, anaemia, increased risk of infection and bleeding. Remember that an important clinical sign to determine is the presence or absence of splenomegaly since this will help differentiate from leukaemia. Investigations are as expected from above: low platelets, low white cell counts and low Hb however with a raised MCV. Reticulocyte count (an indicator of bone marrow function) is low. Bone marrow examination (trephine biopsy or aspiration from two or more sites) will be hypocellular (and in severe cases produce a dry tap).

Treatment is supportive with transfused red cells and platelets, prevention and treatment of infection (see also management of neutropenia above). Androgens, antilymphocyte globulin and high dose steroids are also used. Ideally treatment consists of an HLA matched bone marrow transplant. You should be familiar with the clinical features of graft vs. host disease (a possible grey case scenario) which presents with skin rash, diarrhoea and jaundice as the main features and is treated with cyclosporin. It may also be seen in some conditions where the patient receives non-irradiated blood.

Lymphadenopathy

Whenever you come across lymphadenopathy it is imperative in the clinical examination that you should also look for evidence of sepsis in the region drained by the lymph nodes, hepatosplenomegaly, lymphadenopathy elsewhere and evidence of BCG vaccination (scar on left arm). Other than haematological malignancy and lymphoma you should also think of other causes which include: infectious causes: pyogenic lymphadenitis (e.g. *Staph., Strep.*), tuberculosis, atypical mycobacteria (most often cervical, post auricular or submandibular), typhoid fever, EBV, CMV, toxoplasmosis, cat scratch disease (following a cat scratch typically a papule or pustule develops followed approximately two weeks later by regional lymphadenopathy which is typically unilateral with fever and malaise), sarcoidosis, histoplasmosis, lymphogranuloma inguinale (inguinal lymph nodes) and *Yersinia*.

Other main causes of pancytopenia

1. Hypersplenism. This is an enlarged spleen associated with the reduction of one or more of the blood cellular components resulting in decreases in red cells, white cells and platelets. Causes include: (a) Inflammatory causes such as SLE. (b) Infections for example infectious mononucleosis. (c) Metabolic diseases e.g. Gaucher. (d) Congestive causes that is, any condition causing portal hypertension such as cirrhosis. (e) Lymphoproliferative disorders e.g. leukaemias/lymphomas (see chapter 6).

    In hypersplenism (cf. aplastic anaemia) the reticulocyte count will be normal or increased and the bone marrow if examined would be hypercellular. Splenectomy usually reverses the changes.

2. Infiltration of the bone marrow — leukaemia, neuroblastoma.

3. Pancytopenia may also be seen in haemolytic uraemic syndrome and in disseminated intravascular coagulation.

Acute arthritis and anaemia

Some questions give you a history of a child suffering from acute arthritis and a blood count which shows the child to be anaemic. The causes of this combination include the following:

— Sickle cell disease in an appropriate racial setting.
— Acute leukaemia.
— Neuroblastoma.
— The chronic diseases that have a normocytic normochromic anaemia as part of their presentation such as JCA, SLE, TB arthritis and neoplastic involvement of a joint.

Hyposplenism

The following are associated with hyposplenism: sickle cell disease, ulcerative colitis, Fanconi anaemia, tropical sprue and coeliac disease.

Errors in biochemistry

A common question that is often alluded to in various forms is the errors that one might expect in biochemistry when:

a. Blood is kept for a long period before being sent to the laboratory: raised potassium, phosphate, AST. This is caused by the leaking of these intracellular rich components through the red cell membrane into the extracellular compartment.

b. Blood is haemolysed for example because of a difficult venesecetion: raised potassium, phosphate, AST.

c. There is prolonged venous stasis during venesection: high plasma calcium, increased total and individual protein fractions, increased T4 and increased potassium and phosphate. This is the result of increased hydrostatic pressure causing fluid and electrolytes to leave the vascular compartment, leaving the larger proteins and protein bound ions in the vessel causing their higher concentration in the blood sample.

d. Taking blood from an arm with an infusion running into it: all concentrations will be more dilute and the glucose and sodium and potassium concentrations will approach the concentration of the infused fluid.

Polycythaemia

Some questions will ask you to identify polycythaemia (either in slides, grey cases or data interpretation questions) so you should have a scheme.

Neonatal polycythaemia

Defined as a haematocrit > 65% and can be caused by: IUGR babies, large for dates babies, post-mature babies (last three cases due to intrauterine hypoxia), infants of diabetic mothers, babies with Down syndrome, blood transfusion (twin–twin, delayed clamping of the cord) and congenital adrenal hyperplasia.

There is an exponential increase in blood viscosity above 65% which results in the hyperviscosity syndrome.

— *Skin*: plethoric, cyanosis
— *Neurological*: jittery, intracranial thrombosis, seizures
— *Gut*: NEC
— *Renal*: poor renal perfusion and renal vein thrombosis
— *Metabolic*: hypoglycaemia, hypocalcaemia and hyperbilirubinaemia
— *Haematological*: thrombocytopenia
— *Respiratory*: stiff non-compliant lungs, pulmonary hypertension

Treatment: a PCV of 65–70% and asymptomatic can be treated with increasing fluid intake. Babies with a PCV > 70% or symptomatic with a lower PCV may require a dilutional exchange transfusion.

Polycythaemia in older children

This may have primary and secondary causes. Primary polycythaemia is more common in adults. Secondary causes of polycythaemia are (a) chronic hypoxia e.g cyanotic congenital heart disease, high altitude; (b) ectopic erythropoietin production from tumours such as cerebellar haemangioblastoma, renal hydronephrosis and renal cysts; (c) haemoconcentration (spurious) as a result of dehydration (many causes). Investigations include arterial blood gas PaO_2 estimation and erythropoietin levels as well as any additional tests to exclude a secondary cause. Erythropoietin levels are elevated in secondary and low in primary causes.

Methaemoglobinaemia

A fairly common question relates to the baby or child who has methaemoglobinaemia. Clues to the diagnosis may be given in the history such as the baby who appeared cyanosed but had a completely normal cardiovascular and respiratory examination with a normal CXR and echocardiogram. Arterial blood gas is usually normal. Blood sampling from such a baby reveals blood with a brownish colour; unlike in the normal individual this does not turn red on exposure to air (filter paper test). A persistent brown colour implies a metHb level of more than 10%. Cyanosis develops if the metHb concentration >2 g/dl. Babies may be lethargic, tachycardic and if severe, comatosed.

— *Causes*: It occurs when the iron is in the oxidised ferric (Fe^{3+}) form. This form of haemoglobin cannot bind oxygen and is thus functionally useless. Babies are particularly susceptible to develop methaemoglobinaemia because their antioxidative abilities are not yet fully developed.

— *Congenital*: Caused by (a) an abnormality of the enzymes that keep haemoglobin in the reduced Fe^{2+} state (NADPH methaemoglobin reductase which exists in a heterozygous or homozygous form); or (b) the result of an abnormal haemoglobin molecule that keeps haemoglobin in the ferric form (M haemoglobinopathy — diagnosed on Hb electrophoresis).

— *Acquired*: This occurs when the child is exposed to certain oxidants. Agents include nitrites (sometimes found in high concentration in water from wells), nitrates, aniline dyes, drugs such as sulphonamides, dapsone and primaquine and babies treated with nitric oxide.

— *Treatment*: Removal of possible cause. Oral ascorbic acid. Intravenous methylene blue depending on severity (> 30% metHb = severe. Neonates should not have more than 3–4% metHb).

Carbon monoxide poisoning

An important problem that you should know about. Its sources include motor vehicle exhausts, natural gas combustion devices (especially if there is an enclosed area with poor ventilation), burning charcoal, kerosene or natural gas (for example in heating). Carbon monoxide poisoning is thus commoner in the winter months. Carbon monoxide binds rapidly with haemoglobin with an affinity of about 250 times that of oxygen to produce carboxyhaemoglobin (COHb). This results in blood having a low oxygen content and a shift of the oxygen dissociation curve to the left. Acute symptoms are a result of hypoxia (especially myocardial and neurological) and include headaches, dizziness, nausea (often misdiagnosed as flu). Other people in the environment of the patient may have similar symptoms. In infants vomiting may occur. The classic cherry red skin is very rare, occurring in only about 2% of cases. Cyanosis does not occur and the skin has a pink colour. Syncope and seizures may occur and this is followed by coma and death. Even after recovery from the acute phase sequelae may occur. These include memory disturbance, movement disorders (secondary to basal ganglia involvement) and ataxia. Measure the COHb levels (not a good correlate with the patient's clinical condition or prognosis, which is related to tissue toxicity). In non-smoking individuals a level of COHb more than 5% confirms CO poisoning if the patient has not been given 100% oxygen for more than one hour. Blood gas and oxygen saturation are not useful in determining the patient's level of hypoxia (underestimated). Blood gas is useful to determine the degree of metabolic acidosis which resolves on correcting the hypoxia. Treat with 100% oxygen with a tight fitting mask (reduces half life of carbon monoxide from 5 h to about 1 h). Treat hypotension with fluids and seizures with anticonvulsants. Consider hyperbaric oxygen treatment if severe symptoms or COHb > 40%.

Gum hypertrophy

A possible slide question is a child with gum hypertrophy and you should have a list of possible causes: M4/M5 acute myeloid leukaemia and drugs such as phenytoin and cyclosporin.

Haemorrhagic disease of the newborn

The occurrence of gastrointestinal bleeding in a seemingly well looking newborn baby between the second and sixth days of life should raise the suspicion of haemorrhagic disease of the newborn. It is caused by vitamin K deficiency (see earlier). Babies most at risk are breast-fed babies, asphyxiated babies, premature and small for dates babies and maternal anticonvulsant therapy. Treat acute bleeds with fresh frozen plasma and prevent with oral/i.m. vitamin K. Other causes of haematemesis or PR blood in a well looking baby include swallowed maternal blood at delivery or from cracked nipples during breastfeeding.

Periorbital bruising

A common slide is that of periorbital bruising. You should have a list of differential diagnoses.

1. Bleeding disorder such as haemophilia
2. Leukaemia
3. Neuroblastoma (results in raccoon eyes)
4. Rhabdomyosarcoma
5. Basal skull fracture
6. Non-accidental injury
7. Rarely may be confused with a periorbital cellulitis.

Leukaemia

An important topic, as it is the cause of about 30% of all childhood cancers. It is caused by the proliferation of a single bone marrow stem cell that has undergone malignant transformation.

Symptoms and signs arise as a result of bone marrow infiltration with leukaemic cells resulting in the effects of pancytopenia, infiltration of other tissues of the body and an increase in the basal metabolism sustaining a large tumour mass.

Acute lymphoblastic leukaemia (ALL) is the commonest leukaemia of childhood peaking at 3–4 years of age. Acute myeloid leukaemia (AML) is the commonest acute leukaemia in adulthood but both can occur at any age. Chronic leukaemias are very rare in children (85% ALL, 14% AML, 1% CML).

In acute leukaemia there is an increased amount of blast cells in the peripheral blood whereas in chronic leukaemia there is an increased amount of normal-looking leucocytes.

Presentation

For the sake of the exam be familiar with the modes of presentation: a short history of being unwell with symptoms related to anaemia (pallor, tiredness), thrombocytopenia (bleeding) and leucopenia (increased infections). Bone pain (common in children with leukaemia because of blast accumulation in marrow), recent weight loss, lymphadenopathy and hepatosplenomegaly (more common in ALL than AML), anorexia, headache, dizziness and blurred vision; nausea and vomiting are accompaniments to CNS involvement (which is commoner in ALL than AML, occurring in up to 75% of patients). Cellular hyperviscosity syndrome can occur with blast counts > $100 \times 10^9/l$ and can cause headache, confusion and focal neurological signs. This complication may be partly protected by the pancytopenia but may be precipitated following a transfusion.

Investigations

White cell count can be normal, increased or decreased with a normochromic, normocytic anaemia with the presence of large numbers of lymphoblasts (in

ALL) or myeloblasts (in AML). Platelet count is low. In AML one may see Auer rods in the leukaemic cells which are cytoplasmic inclusion bodies (pathognemonic of AML). The bone marrow is hypercellular packed with blast cells and it is essential to sample the CSF looking for blast cells indicative of CNS involvement.

Prognostic factors in acute leukaemia

Prognosis worse if: (a) male (b) WCC > 30 at presentation; (c) age less than one year or older than 10 years at presentation; (d) morphology: L2, L3 worse prognosis than L1; (d) abnormal chromosomes present with translocations; (e) cytogenetics — haploidy a worse prognosis than polyploidy; (f) B cell worse prognosis than T cell; (g) CNS involvement at presentation; (h) bulky disease with hepatosplenomegaly and lymphadenopathy; (I) failure to induce a remission within 14 days; (J) black children generally have a worse prognosis.

Classification of ALL

The classification of ALL can be remembered as **MICE**.

Morphology: Refers to the morphology of the lymphoblasts and called L1, 2, 3 (85% of ALL are L1).

Immunological markers: Describes from which type of progenitor cell the malignancy derived: B cell, T cell (older boys), non-B, non-T ALL, null type. Eighty per cent are from the common non-B, non-T cell type.

Cytogenetics: This describes the number of chromosomes in the leukaemic cells which is usually above the normal 46 component. The greater the number the better the prognosis.

Enzyme studies: Terminal transferase present in 95% of ALL.

There is a morphological classification for AML (M1-M7) that you should know exists.

Treatment for ALL

This is only a broad outline since protocols are continually evolving and changing.

Supportive measures include correction of anaemia and thrombocytopenia with transfusions and treatment of dehydration as well as the prevention and treatment of infections (cotrimoxazole for PCP prophylaxis).

— *Induction of remission*: Chemotherapy for weeks 1–4. A combination of four drugs is used such as prednisolone, doxorubicin, asparaginase and vincristine. The combination will vary according to the prognostic types of the leukaemia. The aim is to eliminate blast cells from the bone marrow. A 95% remission rate with return of normal blood counts with normal haemopoiesis and elimination of the leukaemic clone.

— *Intensification/consolidation*: In order to remove any remaining malignant blast cells further combinations are given often using some of the same drugs used in induction.

— *Maintenance*: This involves weekly methotrexate and daily 6-mercaptopurine (both orally as an outpatient), in addition to monthly pulses of vincristine. This treatment is given for about two years.

— *CNS prophylaxis:* Cranial irradiation and intrathecal methotrexate usually post remission. Regular assessment for relapse is essential. This includes looking for bone marrow relapse (poor prognosis consider BMT), CNS relapse and in boys testicular relapse.

Complications of treatment

1. Chemotherapy-induced bone marrow suppression pancytopenia with risks of infection and bleeding.

2. Tumour lysis syndrome. It is commonest in those with the highest white cell counts and bulky tumours. It occurs following the rapid destruction of the leukaemic cells. This destruction is accompanied by release into the circulation of large amounts of potassium, uric acid and phosphate. In a data question look out for the biochemical features of: hyperkalaemia, hyperphosphataemia, hyperuricaemia and hypocalcaemia occurring usually within 24 h of starting chemotherapy. There is a potential for renal obstruction secondary to uric acid and calcium phosphate precipitation in the kidneys (more likely in acid conditions). Prevent with hyperhydration and alkalinisation (sodium bicarbonate) of the patient before commencing chemotherapy and administration of allopurinol until the WCC has stabilised (various regimens exist, the aims of which are to reach an ideal urinary specific gravity, urinary volume and urinary pH). Closely monitor U&Es, calcium, phosphate, urine output, pH and specific gravity regularly during treatment.

3. Second malignancy.

4. Cranial irradiation can damage the pituitary gland and hypothalamus resulting in growth failure and other consequences of pituitary dysfunction. Spinal irradiation may cause stunting of spinal growth.

Immunology 9

Immunology is an important topic since several questions ask you to recognise particular immunodeficiency diseases and patterns, and discuss their investigation and management. This chapter attempts to cover the main immunodeficiencies emphasising in particular the theory and points that are commonly referred to in the examination.

BASIC IMMUNOLOGY

Definitions

— *Immunogenicity:* The capacity to drive an immune response.

— *Antigenicity:* This is the property of being recognised by an antibody.

— *Epitope (determinant):* This is the smallest/minimal part of a molecule with which an antibody or cell can interact.

— *Hapten:* This is too small to be immunogenic but has the potential to be epitopic if it is coupled to a carrier molecule.

— *Specificity:* This describes the ability to detect very small differences between foreign bodies.

— *Memory:* This describes the immunological phenomenon that develops from previous exposure to foreign material. This response is made use of in vaccinations.

— *Primary response:* This occurs on first exposure to an antigen. Characteristically there is a delayed response which is of short duration and weak potency. It consists of an IgM response.

— *Secondary response:* This occurs on subsequent exposure to the antigen. It is of rapid onset, greater potency and longer duration as compared to the primary response. It consists of an IgG antibody response.

— *Self-tolerance:* This is the ability of the body to recognise self as self and not mount an immunological response against itself.

TYPES OF IMMUNODEFICIENCY

There are three main types of immunity, namely humoral (B cells and antibody production with GMADE antibody subtypes); cell-mediated (T lymphocytes); and non-specific immunity (for example, phagocytes and complement system).

Immunodeficiency is subdivided into primary (the rarer inherited causes) and secondary causes. The secondary causes include malnutrition, stress (for example post surgery), burns, post irradiation, autoimmune disease, malignancy, infection associated (HIV, rubella, TB), drug associated (corticosteroids and cytotoxic drugs among others) and syndromes such as Down syndrome.

When should immunodeficiency fall into your differential diagnosis? It should be suspected in a child who develops recurrent infections (more than the expected average), which may be accompanied by failure to thrive. In addition if the child develops recurrent infections that become chronic, or if atypical organisms are grown from infected sites, or if opportunistic infections caused by usually non-pathogenic organisms occur, then one should suspect a possible immunodeficiency. Suspicion should also be high if there is a positive family history. Other clues may be present in the question, for example the presence of bulbar telangiectasia in ataxia telangiectasia.

Abnormalities of antibody-mediated immunity

IgG is the only antibody type that crosses the placenta to the fetus from the mother. Thus it is IgG that confers immunity on the fetus during the first few months of life. The full complement of IgG is reached by three years of age. The transplacental transfer of antibody occurs after about 30 weeks' gestation only, and therefore a baby born prematurely before this time will not of course receive this conferred immunity. Since there is no IgM transfer across the placenta any IgM antibody found in the cord blood or neonatal blood sample at birth can be assumed to be caused by an intrauterine infection (that is, produced by the baby in response to the infection). The full complement of IgM is reached by one year of age.

Antenatally acquired IgG in the baby decreases to very low levels by about four months of age. Infant IgG and IgM increase only slowly from birth. Thus there is a period between approximately 4–6 months when the baby has low antibody levels (awaiting infant immunoglobulin production) and is relatively immunodeficient. This time period is referred to as transient hypogammaglobulinaemia of infancy.

IgA is the major antibody of bodily secretions found in saliva, tears, nasal secretions, breast milk and sweat. The full complement of IgA is reached by 14 years of age. IgD is present in minute concentrations in blood and other bodily fluids. IgE binds to Fc receptors on the surface of mast cells and basophils. When the IgE molecules are complexed with a specific antigen there is a triggering of the release of inflammatory mediators (degranulation) and this is the basis of the type I hypersensitivity reaction.

There will be clues in the history that should point you in the direction of a humoral immunodeficiency. The disorders of antibody-mediated immunity usually present themselves after 4–6 months, since before this time the child is protected by maternal transplacental transfer (as discussed above). As a general rule antibody deficiencies predispose the child to infections caused by extracellular encapsulated organisms such as *Haemophilus influenzae*, *Streptococcus pneumoniae* and *Staphylococcus aureus*. Infections of the paranasal sinuses, lungs and otitis media therefore account for about 70% of the infections. Gastrointestinal infections (commonly *Giardia lamblia* but also *Salmonella*) account for about 20% and meningitis, septic arthritis, skin sepsis (such as impetigo and cellulitis) cause the remainder. Failure to thrive and death during childhood is not common compared to T cell disorders.

The commonest primary humoral immunodeficiencies (excluding transient hypogammaglobulinaemia of infancy) include: Bruton disease, common variable immunodeficiency and selective IgA immunodeficiency (see Table 9.1).

Disorders of cell-mediated immunity

Strictly speaking severe disorders affecting T cell function also have an affect on humoral immunity since antibody production is partially T cell dependent. Abnormalities in T cell function typically cause an increased susceptibility to viral, fungal, protozoal and TB infections. Symptoms are generally more severe than with humoral defects. Failure to thrive is commoner than with humoral disorders, and these disorders may often be fatal in childhood.

Severe combined immunodeficiency (SCID)

There are a number of questions that relate to SCID so it is important that you recognise the usual clinical pattern.

There is a failure of differentiation of stem cells into T and B cells. Inherited as (a) X-linked (50%); and (b) autosomal recessive (50% — Swiss-type). Fifty per cent of the AR inherited SCID type have an adenosine deaminase deficiency.

Table 9.1 Comparison of the main humoral immunodeficiencies

	Infantile sex-linked hypogammaglobulin-aemia (Bruton disease)	Common variable immunodeficiency (CVI)	Selective IgA immuno-deficiency
Pathophysiology	X-linked inherited condition with males affected only. Abnormality in B lymphocyte differ-entiation leading to absent B cells and normal T cells. Absent plasma cells in bone marrow, lymph nodes and gut. Very low levels of serum Ig.	Abnormality in ability of B cells to produce antibodies. Normal circulating levels of B and T cells. Reduced antibody levels especially IgG and A with normal IgM. In addition T cell function is abnormal.	Most common primary immunode-ficiency (1:700). Circulating B cells are normal. Normal T cell function. Normal concentrations of other circulat-ing classes of antibodies. IgA levels usually less than 5 mg/dl.

Table 9.1 Continued

	Infantile sex-linked hypogammaglobulin-aemia (Bruton disease)	Common variable immunodeficiency (CVI)	Selective IgA immuno-deficiency
Clinical features	Onset after few months. Recurrent infections especially of the lungs and paranasal sinuses (sinopulmonary). Most common pathogens are *Staph. aureus*, *Strep. pneumoniae*, *Haemophilus influenzae*. There is relatively little lymphoid tissue in comparison to the frequency of infections.	Clinical features appear in later childhood even up to the second decade. Chronic and recurrent sinopulmonary pulmonary infections occur. In addition chronic diarrhoea is common, often secondary to *Giardia lambia* (malabsorption and villous atrophy possible). Lymphadenopathy and splenomegaly occurs (cf. Bruton disease). Increased autoimmune disorders (haemolytic anaemia, ITP and pernicious anaemia) and risk of malignancies (non-Hodgkin's lymphoma, gastric carcinoma).	Asymptomatic or mild symptoms generally. Some patients have an increased incidence of sinopulmonary infections, gastrointestinal infections (such as with *Giardia*), allergies and autoimmune diseases (rheumatoid arthritis, SLE and pernicious anaemia).
Treatment	Early diagnosis to prevent chronic lung disease. IVIG (intravenous immunoglobulin). Aggressive antibiotic treatment of infections.	Early diagnosis and aggressive treatment of infections as for Bruton disease.	Symptoms are usually so mild as not to require treatment. Children should not be given IgA in any form since sensitisation can occur and may lead to anaphylaxis. This includes ordering IgA deficient blood for transfusions.

It presents usually in the first few months of life (usually < three months), and there is a failure to thrive. Respiratory infections are common and an opportunistic infection such as with *Pneumocystis carinii* or CMV is typical. Gastrointestinal infections are common with chronic diarrhoea, chronic GI candidiasis, *Giardia* and *Cryptosporidium* infections. Chronic skin infections are also typical with cutaneous candidiasis, *Herpes* and *Varicella* infections. These children have no lymphoid tissue and an absent thymus (compared with Bruton disease where there is little lymphoid tissue but the thymus is present). Thus there is no hepatosplenomegaly or lymphadenopathy in response to infection compared with common variable immunodeficiency.

Most infants have lymphopenia (a possible clue in the question). In addition there will be reduced T cell populations and reduced CD4 helper cells compared to normal as well as reduced numbers of B cells. Abnormal T cell function tests and reduced G, A and M antibodies will also be found.

Treatment consists ideally of a bone marrow transplant which provides the only possibility of cure. Aggressive treatment of infections. Prophylaxis with amphotericin (against *Candida*) and cotrimoxazole (against *Pneumocystis*). Intravenous immunoglobulin is given intermittently. The child should not receive any live vaccinations. All blood products given must be CMV negative and irradiated. The latter is done to prevent graft vs. host disease — GVHD — caused by the introduction of functional lymphoid cells into a child who is immunodeficient. Features of GVHD are hepatosplenomegaly, lymphadenopathy, skin rash and diarrhoea.

Wiscott–Aldrich syndrome

This is inherited in an X-linked fashion and there is a combined B and T cell defect. This syndrome consists of immunodeficiency, chronic eczema and thrombocytopenia (with very small platelets that are rapidly destroyed by the spleen) as its main features. IgA and E are raised and IgM is low. There is a poor antibody production response to polysaccharide antigen and thus the children are prone to infection with encapsulated organisms such as *Haemophilus* and *Streptococcus pneumoniae* usually in the form of sinopulmonary disease. The co-existing T cell abnormality gives rise to an increased incidence of infections with viruses such as herpes, CMV and *Pneumocystis carinii*. There is also an increased risk of lymphoma and autoimmune diseases.

Treatment involves aggressive treatment of infections. Intravenous immunoglobulin is sometimes used. Splenectomy can increase platelet counts but a matched bone marrow transplant will reverse most of the abnormalities. A possible slide question is of a child who is described as having recurrent infections who has widespread eczema and possibly petechiae (from thrombocytopenia).

Ataxia telangiectasia

This is inherited in an autosomal recessive fashion: it is a combined B and T cell defect. The syndrome consists of cerebellar ataxia starting in the first five years, oculocutaneous telangiectasia starting usually after three years of age, recurrent sinopulmonary infection often leading to bronchiectasis, mental retardation with growth failure in later childhood and immunodeficiency that affects cell-mediated and humoral immunity. There is an increased susceptibility to malignancy especially to lymphoma, leukaemia and medulloblastoma. Patients display radiation sensitivity of their DNA with increased chromosomal breakage (which can be observed in cultured leucocytes and fibroblasts). Bloom and Fanconi syndromes are other syndromes that demonstrate chromosomal fragility. Typically one finds low levels of IgA and E with the presence of low molecular weight IgM and very low levels of IgG2. Alpha-fetoprotein is raised as is CEA. In some cases where IgG2 is low IVIG may be used with some success. Aggressive treatment of the lung infections will slow the pulmonary deterioration.

DiGeorge syndrome

There are a number of abnormalities that result from abnormal development of the third and fourth pharyngeal pouches during intrauterine life. There is a spectrum of severity of disease. There is thymic hypoplasia (T cells are reduced to less than 30% of the total circulating lymphocytes — normally 40–80%) leading to increased susceptibility of infections. Hypocalcaemia results from absent parathyroid glands and usually presents in the first few days or weeks classically as hypocalcaemic tetany. Typical DiGeorge facies include hypertelorism, low-set malformed ears, antimongoloid slant to the eyes, micrognathia, carp-shaped mouth and cleft palate. Cardiac abnormalities occur commonly and these are usually truncus arteriosus and interrupted aortic arch. B cell and antibody function is intact. Treatment may consist of a fetal thymus graft. Blood products should be irradiated. A possible slide question may consist of a child with typical DiGeorge facies and a mid-sternotomy scar from a cardiac correction. Another slide may be of a CXR film of a neonate who has no thymic shadow and has a concurrent infection. Here the possibilities include SCID and DiGeorge syndrome.

Chronic mucocutaneous candidiasis

This is a T cell abnormality with a resulting cell-mediated immunity defect to *Candida*. This results in chronic *Candida* infection of the skin, mucous membranes and nails. Some have a family history. In about half of all cases there is an associated immunological disorder such as IDDM, Addison disease, pernicious anaemia and hypoparathyroidism so that their corresponding features may be superimposed. Humoral immunity is in tact. Treatment consists of topical and systemic antifungal agents in addition to management of any associated endocrine disorder.

Job syndrome (hyperimmune IgE syndrome)

Inherited in an autosomal dominant fashion, there is a combined B and T cell defect. Serum IgE levels are very high and in addition there is a raised eosinophil count. Characteristic features consist of coarse facial features, recurrent skin sepsis with abscess formation (*Staphylococcal*), chronic dermatitis and sinopulmonary disease (lung abscesses may occur).

Phagocytic disorders

These disorders present in the first few months of life. Neutrophil disorders are divided into either qualitative or quantitative abnormalities. (Quantitative neutrophil defects are described in chapter 8.)

Leucocyte adhesion deficiency (lazy leucocyte syndrome)

Inherited as autosomal recessive disorder. It is thought to be caused by abnormalities in the intercellular adhesion molecules (ICAM) that neutrophils use in order to move and adhere to surfaces. It may present with delayed separation of the umbilical cord at birth (as a manifestation of global impaired wound healing), repeated soft tissue infections with absent pus (caused by failure of neutrophils to accumulate in sites of infection) and gingivitis. Granulocytosis (neutrophilia) is a constant finding (granulocytes produced but not reaching their destination) and in some cases the granulocytosis may be so high in a bacterial infection that it may resemble a leukaemoid reaction on blood count. Treatment is with antibiotic prophylaxis and bone marrow transplant.

Chediak–Higashi syndrome

Inherited in an autosomal recessive fashion, there is an abnormality in neutrophil chemotaxis and degranulation thus predisposing to recurrent infections. The complete syndrome consists of partial oculocutaneous albinism, characteristic giant cytoplasmic inclusion bodies in the neutrophils and a mild bleeding disorder caused by defective platelet aggregation. There may be a progression to an accelerated phase in the second decade of life with organomegaly and bone marrow infiltration and this is often fatal.

Chronic granulomatous disease (CGD)

This condition is rare with a 75% X-linked inheritance and 25% autosomal recessive inheritance. There appears to be an abnormality in the NADPH oxidase subunits in the neutrophil membrane. This results in a failure of the neutrophils to produce superoxide radicals as part of their killing mechanism (the radicals include hydrogen peroxide, hydroxyl free radical and superoxide).

Children present in the first year of life with particular types of infections. These are caused by organisms described as catalase positive. Hydrogen peroxide is produced by many organisms. In catalase positive organisms the catalase destroys the hydrogen peroxide (produced by the organism) leaving no excess hydrogen peroxide which can be used by the phagocyte (which is defective) and thus cannot kill the organism. This is in contrast to catalase negative organisms where excess hydrogen peroxide (not catabolised by catalase) can be incorporated into the metabolic pathway of the defective neutrophil in order to compensate for its lack of endogenous production so that in effect the organism helps in its own suicide.

Catalase positive organisms include *Staph. aureus*, *Salmonella*, *E. coli*, *Serratia marcessans* and fungi such as *Candida* and *Aspergillus* (the latter is the most serious lung disease in CGD). Be familiar with the spectrum of infection. The most common presentation is with severe infections of the skin and lymph nodes (often cervical) with abscess formation which is often recurrent and becomes chronic and suppurative with time. Lung involvement consists of pneumonia with lung abscess formation and empyema. There is osteomyelitis especially of small bones, hepatic and perianal abscesses. Chronic diarrhoea, hepatosplenomegaly and failure to thrive are common. In addition obstruction is a particular problem especially affecting the gastric antrum, ureters and sinuses as a result of granuloma formation.

Investigations

a. Nitroblue tetrazolium test (NBT). In this test colourless/yellow NBT is reduced to a deep blue colour when exposed to normal neutrophils which are able to produce a respiratory burst during phagocytosis. Thus in CGD the NBT remains colourless/yellow. Carriers may have intermediate transitions

b. Absent chemiluminesence.

c. ESR is often raised and there are usually raised levels of Igs G,A and M.

Treatment includes treating the infection adequately with antibiotics and surgery. Prophylactic cotrimoxazole is given. Gamma interferon may reduce the frequency of infections. White cell count transfusions are given for life threatening infections. Consider bone marrow transplant.

Glucose 6-phospate dehydrogenase deficiency
Rarely G6PD deficiency may also affect neutrophil metabolism and function (as well as erythrocyte function). See chapter 8.

Myeloperoxidase deficiency
Autosomal recessive inheritance. There is a deficiency of myeloperoxidase in phagocytes. Symptoms are generally mild requiring no treatment.

Disorders of complement pathway

The clinical effect depends on which component is missing. You should have a rough picture of what you remember of the classic and alternative pathways of the complement pathway. In summary, deficiencies in complement components C1–C4 result in increased susceptibility to infection by encapsulated bacteria (*Haemophilus influenzae, Streptococcus pneumoniae* and so on). There is also an increased incidence of connective tissue disorders such as SLE (secondary to immune complexes). Deficiencies in the C5–C9 components result in an increased susceptibility to *Neisserial* sepsis such as meningococcal and gonococcal infections.

Treatment involves prophylaxis (antibiotics and vaccination) and aggressive treatment of infection.

Hereditary angio-oedema:
This is included here as a defect in complement (no immunological features).

Inherited in an autosomal dominant fashion. It is caused by a deficiency of C1 esterase inhibitor (C1INH). This usually inhibits the activation of the C1 complement component. There are two types: (1) 85%: reduced levels of C1INH. (2) 15%: normal levels but defective function. It is rare before puberty but increases in incidence afterwards.

Clinically it presents as recurrent episodes of angio-oedema principally affecting the face, extremities, airway (hoarseness, stridor) and intestine (abdominal pain, D and V, acute abdomen). The angioedema is typically painless, non-pruritic, non-pitting and non-erythematous compared with urticaria. There may be a serpiginous border and therefore may mimic erythema marginatum. Precipitating factors are common and include a sudden change in temperature, menstruation, stress and infection.

— *Investigations:* If asked for an investigation say that you would like to measure C1INH levels. There are reduced C1INH and C4 levels during an attack and between attacks. C2 is reduced during an attack but is normal between attacks. Remember C1INH levels may be normal if there is a functional problem (in 15%) so also perform a functional assay if in doubt.

— *Treatment* consists of the basic principles of resuscitation in an acute attack especially if airway is involved. An androgen such as danazol is given to increase the synthesis of C1INH. Antifibrinolytic agents also can be used (for example E-aminocaproic acid).

INVESTIGATION OF IMMUNOLOGICAL DISORDERS

You may be asked in some questions to list some investigations that you may want to carry out in order to make your diagnosis.

1. Full blood count including white cell differential. Cultures if infection is suspected (many immunodeficiencies have typical infections), ESR and CRP.

2. Split T cell subtypes. (CD3/CD4/CD8).

3. Complement. CH50 is a non-sensitive screening test for the classic complement pathway. Include C3 and C4 in a complement component screen. A reduction in any of these will lead you to perform assays on individual complement components.

4. B cell function can be assessed by measuring immunoglobulin levels IgG, M, A, D and E. B cell function can also be assessed by measuring antibody production responses to antigens such as measuring antibody levels against DTP. In addition isohemagglutinin levels such as anti-A, anti-B may be measured.

5. T cell function can be assessed using delayed type hypersensitivity skin tests against for example mumps antigen, *Candida* antigen and *Tetanus* toxoid. A positive skin test makes a T cell abnormality very unlikely. T cell proliferation studies may also be performed: here T cells are cultured with mitogens such as phytohaemagglutinin and the proliferative response assessed (the latter is significantly reduced in T cell abnormalities).

6. Tests of phagocyte function. Nitroblue tetrazolium test (NBT) — see earlier description.

7. CXR is helpful in the newborn period if one suspects a T cell abnormality since it may be associated with an absent thymus shadow (e.g. DiGeorge syndrome, SCID). A CXR may also indicate pulmonary infection, a common accompaniment of immunodeficiency states.

PAEDIATRIC AIDS

AIDS in the paediatric population is usually acquired by vertical transmission (80–90%). The remainder are accounted for by blood transfusion, blood products such as for leukaemia, sexual activities/abuse and i.v. drug abuse). Blood products are now properly screened but children may still be at risk if they received products before about 1996. It seems that the vertical risk of transmission is greater if the mother has a low CD4 cell count, if the baby is below 34 weeks' gestation, if the baby is second born (rather than first born) and if the baby is born by a vaginal delivery. The vertical transmission rate is estimated to be about 14%. Breastfeeding increases the risk of vertical transmission by a further 14%. Thus babies tend to be delivered by caesarian section and parents are advised against breastfeeding. The latter is not the case in Third World countries where the risk of death from malnutrition is greater than that from AIDS.

Clinical features of AIDS

It appears that the pattern of illness falls into two separate categories. Babies who acquired the HIV prenatally appear to have a short incubation period with symptoms developing at about 4–6 months of life. Those who acquired HIV peri- or postnatally tend to have a longer incubation period with symptoms starting at about 2–3 years. These children account for about 80% of cases and they tend to have a better prognosis.

Infants may come to the attention of paediatricians because of non-specific features such as failure to thrive, pyrexia of unknown origin, generalised lymphadenopathy and/or hepatosplenomegaly (the latter two more common than with adult HIV infection). Other non-specific features include parotid gland enlargement, chronic dermatitis, chronic *Candida* nappy rash as well as persistent oral candidiasis; recurrent otitis media is also common.

They may present with infection secondary to immunodeficiency. B cell dyfunction may present with features discussed earlier such as *Streptococcal, Haemophilus* and *Staph. aureus* infections and recurrent severe pyogenic infection is common. These may be severe and recurrent and difficult to treat. Opportunistic infections include *Pneumocystis carinii* pneumonia (diagnosed by broncheolar lavage and specific Ag staining), *Mycobacterium avium-intracellulare, Candida* (gastrointestinal candidiasis), *Cryptosporidium* (chronic diarrhoea), *Cryptococcus neoformans* (meningitis) and *Herpes simplex* and *Varicella zoster* infections of the skin. *Pneumocystis carinii* occurs at a relatively early stage in the illness compared to adults with AIDS. In those infants who have a short incubation period this can even be their presenting illness, which in some cases can be fatal.

Lymphocytic interstitial pneumonitis (LIP) describes a type of chronic lung disease which is caused by infiltration of the lungs with lymphocytes and plasma cells. There are few symptoms early in the disease. It affects about half of the children affected with HIV infection. The CXR shows bilateral reticulonodular shadowing. Later in the disease the children may develop gradually increasing dyspnoea, cough, wheeze, hypoxaemia, mediastinal lymphadenopathy and clubbing sometimes complicated later with an opportunistic infection. Those children with initial LIP presentation have a longer survival compared to those with an initial opportunistic infection presentation.

HIV infection affects the central nervous system causing an encephalopathy (more commonly than adults) and can cause failure of brain growth with resulting microcephaly, developmental delay and an array of other neurological disturbances with a very variable expression such as spasticity and ataxia. CT shows characteristic enhancement of the frontal lobes and basal ganglia with possible calcification, cerebral atrophy, ventricular enlargement and white matter attenuation. CNS tumours are uncommon in paediatric AIDS (cf. adults) and supra added infections such as *Cryptococcus* may occur. The course of HIV encephalopathy is very variable.

Tumours such as the common skin tumour Kaposi sarcoma are rare in children with AIDS.

There are many immunological changes noted in AIDS children and these include T cell abnormalities (decreased CD4 cell count, decreased IL-2 production and IFN-G production and decreased proliferative responses to antigens) and B lymphocyte abnormalities (polyclonal B cell activation resulting in hypergammaglobulinaemia, production of auto antibodies and immune complexes with for example a positive Coombs' test and positive ANA). The increased production of auto antibodies is responsible for the increased incidence of autoimmune diseases seen in AIDS.

Investigation of AIDS

— *Anti-HIV IgG* (by ELISA and confirmed by Western blot techniques). The problem of identifying these antibodies in the infant is that it is possible that the baby may have acquired them from the mother through the placenta. These antibodies can last for 18 months. Thus detection of the antibody in the infant only after this age makes the diagnosis positive. The presence of anti-HIV IgA antibodies (which cannot cross the placenta) are also a method of making a positive diagnosis.

— *Polymerase chain reaction* is a method of HIV DNA amplification and is a method used to detect HIV virus in the blood.

— *P24 antigen* detection can be used.

— *Viral culture* of white cells remains the gold standard for detection of the virus.

Management of AIDS

This involves many aspects. See Table 9.2.

Table 9.2 Summary of management principles in paediatric AIDS

Infections	Early diagnosis and aggressive treatment of infections.
Immunisations	Should receive almost all vaccinations. Not live polio but killed (including co-habitants). No BCG. Should receive Pneumovax, influenza vaccination, Hep. B vaccination. Passive Ig if exposed to measles or chicken pox.
Antibiotic prophylaxis	Cotrimoxazole is given to HIV infected children when CD4 cell counts drop below certain levels as a protection against PCP.
AZT (zidovudine)	Reverse transcriptase inhibitor. Standard therapy in children, though not started in children who are asymptomatic. Beware bone marrow suppression and hepatotoxicity side effects. DDI (dideoxyinosine) and DDC (dideoxycytosine) are used in children unresponsive to AZT. Use of AZT during pregnancy decreases the risk of HIV transmission to baby significantly. Continue postnatally in baby for six weeks.
Regular follow up	To check for growth and development, worsening symptoms and side effects of treatment.
Psychosocial support	This involves caring and educating the family as well as the child, some of whose members may themselves be HIV positive. Assessment of coping strategies. Ultimately terminal care.

Metabolic diseases 10

In this chapter we will cover the commoner metabolic disorders that are frequently asked about in the examination as well as some of the rarer ones that are also exam favourites.

Although direct questioning about inborn errors of metabolism is relatively rare some knowledge about the commoner disorders is expected, and have come up in the grey cases and data interpretation questions in the past. In addition, the presentation and management of such disorders could well be asked about in the clinical examination. You should have a reference to simplified metabolic pathways as you read through the inborn errors of metabolism.

HYPONATRAEMIA

Causes

1. Saline depletion hyponatraemia
Obviously simultaneous salt and water loss will not affect plasma sodium concentration. However when volume depletion is sufficient to cause ADH release then water retention will lead to hyponatraemia (overriding osmotic control). In renal causes of salt loss the ADH response is often inadequate and an increase in volume is achieved by thirst and drinking.

— *Causes:* Vomiting, diarrhoea, intestinal fistula, sweating, excess diuretics, adrenal insufficiency and renal disease. Clinical signs will be those of volume depletion and treatment will involve fluid replacement.

2. Dilutional hyponatraemia
There is in essence an excess of water. This may be due to excess ADH production or a result of the renal inability to dilute urine.

— *Causes:* Excessive fluid intake (rare), renal failure, cardiac failure, cirrhosis, nephrotic syndrome, iatrogenic hypotonic intravenous infusion, syndrome of inappropriate ADH production (SIADH). SIADH is caused by lung disease, for example pneumonia, ventilation, CNS disease such as trauma, meningoencephalitis, tumour; pain for example post-operative; drugs such as chlorpropamide, carba mazepine, morphine, rifampicin, vincristine. Ectopic production is rare.

The general treatment of dilutional hyponatraemia involves fluid restriction but if fluid overloaded i.v. mannitol can induce a diuresis and eliminate water. For a detailed description of SIADH see chapter 7.

3. Increased number of osmoles in the plasma

For example, glucose. This increases the extracellular fluid (ECF) osmolality causing water to pass into the ECF from the ICF decreasing the ECF sodium concentration. In addition to this, the increase of ADH caused by the osmolar load causes water retention with a corresponding fall in aldosterone production and a natriuresis.

4. Pseudohyponatraemia

This is where there is hyperproteinaemia or hyperlipidaemia that decreases the fractional water content of plasma.

The plasma osmolality will thus be increased in cause (3), will be normal in cause (4) and reduced in (1) and (2). In (1) there will be signs of ECF volume depletion, in SIADH there will be a normal ECF volume and in the other dilutional causes there will be an increase in ECF volume (raised JVP, oedema, ascites and pulmonary oedema).

NB Osmolarity is calculated and osmolality is measured. Osmolarity (mOsmol/kg) = 2 × (Na + K) + urea + glucose. If the measured osmolality is significantly greater than the osmolarity (for example by 10 mOsm or so), referred to as an osmolar gap, then one should suspect that there are osmotically active components other than those mentioned in the above equation.

Sodium deficit in an individual with hyponatraemic dehydration (not in dilutional hyponatraemia) may be calculated by the following equation:

— Sodium deficit = 0.6 × body weight (kg) × (normal plasma sodium i.e 135 — patient's plasma sodium).

— The mmol required to raise the plasma sodium by X mmol/l (acutely) = 0.6 × body weight × rise wanted in mmol/l. Beware of acidosis during rapid correction.

HYPERNATRAEMIA

Causes

— Isolated water depletion: diabetes insipidius
— Iatrogenic: via hypernatraemic i.v. infusions and drugs
— Conn syndrome (with low potassium)
— Combined water and sodium loss with water loss predominating.

It is important to remember that signs of volume depletion will not be as obvious as they are in hyponatraemic dehydration since there is a shift of fluid from the ICF to the ECF and thus weight loss is the most reliable indicator. The skin may have a 'doughy' texture.

HYPOKALAEMIA

Clinically presents as weakness, paralytic ileus, urinary retention (both secondary to effects on smooth muscle), polyuria and metabolic alkalosis. See chapter 2 for ECG changes.

Causes of hypokalaemia

— Reduced intake

— Increased losses

   Renal: diuretics, osmotic diuresis (for example glycosuria), hyperaldosteronism, renal tubular acidosis.
   Gastrointestinal: vomiting, diarrhoea, laxative abuse, villous adenoma (which produce a lot of mucus).

— Movement of potassium into the cell: insulin administration (or following a glucose infusion), metabolic alkalosis, catecholamines, drugs such as salbutamol infusion.

Urinary potassium excretion is useful to know since a urinary potassium excretion of more than 20 mmol/l potassium implies renal loss, and a urinary excretion less than this less implies extrarenal losses. Treat the underlying cause and give potassium supplements.

HYPERKALAEMIA

Clinically presents as weakness and cardiac arrhythmias (see chapter 2 for ECG changes).

Causes of hyperkalaemia

— Reduced renal excretion: renal failure, hypoaldosteronism (Addison disease), potassium sparing diuretics (e.g. spironolactone) and hypovolaemia.

— Movement out of cells: Hypoinsulinism, acidosis, rapid cell lysis for example tumour lysis syndrome, trauma and burns.

— Increased intake in particular if there is abnormal renal function.

— Pseudohyperkalaemia: Leaving cuff on arm for too long before venepuncture. Haemolysis if there is a difficult venepuncture or if the needle is too small. Stored blood.

Treatment consists of treating the underlying cause and stabilising the heart with calcium gluconate, using bicarbonate or insulin/glucose infusions, salbutamol nebulisers/infusions, exchange resins, diuretics and dialysis.

METABOLIC DISORDERS

The presentation of lethargy, poor peripheral perfusion and a metabolic acidosis in a neonate should immediately lead you to think of the three most likely causes which are: sepsis, congenital heart disease and a metabolic disorder. Remember that the presence of a metabolic acidosis together with hypoglycaemia should strongly suggest to you a metabolic disorder. Sepsis commonly produces a metabolic acidosis but is usually accompanied by hyperglycaemia.

In any metabolic disorder you should look for clues in the history such as previous neonatal deaths, family history and precipitating factors. Precipitating factors include birth (the placenta acting as a dialyser in utero is no longer present), changing feeds, giving fruit juice for first time and weaning. Has there been another triggering agent such as infection, trauma or surgery that has precipitated a decompensation now?

A useful initial metabolic screen would involve performing a blood gas, sending urine and blood for organic and amino acids, blood lactate, pyruvate and an ammonia level.

The commonest causes of acute encephalopahy in the neonate

Acute encephalopathy in the neonatal period (see Table 10.1) usually presents as lethargy, hypotonia, poor feeding, vomiting, apnoea, seizures, poor peripheral perfusion, metabolic acidosis, hypoglycaemia and possibly coma.

Treatment of any of these conditions in Table 10.1 involves general measures acutely such as careful fluid and electrolyte balance, treating hypovolaemic shock and hypotension and preventing a catabolic state and treating hypoglycaemia with a dextrose infusion (including stopping feeds). Care must be taken to prevent the neonate from becoming acidotic with bicarbonate infusions and possibly dialysis in an attempt to remove the excess accumulated molecules.

Table 10.1 Commoner neonatal causes of acute encephalopathy

Inborn error of metabolism: example	Metabolic defect	Presentation	Investigation	Treatment
Amino acidopathy: Maple syrup urine disease (MSUD)	Deficiency of alpha ketoacid dehydrogenase resulting in increased branched chain amino acids (leucine, isoleucine and valine).	AR inheritance. Acute encephalopathy within the first month. Maple syrup odour urine.	Hypoglycaemia, metabolic acidosis. Urine and blood amino acid screen (raised leucine, isoleucine and valine).	Reduce branched chain acid intake to minimum required for growth. Reduce catabolism to minimal (dextrose infusions, treating infections effectively), peritoneal dialysis.

250

Table 10.1 Continued

Inborn error of metabolism: example	Metabolic defect	Presentation	Investigation	Treatment
Organic acidaemia: Propionic acidaemia, methyl malonic acidaemia.	Propionyl CoA carboxylase and L-methyl malonyl CoA mutase are involved in branched chain amino acid degradation. Increased organic acids result in inhibition of urea cycle with subsequently increased ammonia levels.	AR inheritance. Acute encephalopathy.	Metabolic acidosis, hypoglycaemia, hyperammonaemia, white cell count and platelets often low. Increased blood lactate. Urine organic acid screen.	As above. Biotin (a cofactor) can be given in methylmalonic acidaemia.
Fatty acid oxidation defects: Medium chain acyl CoA dehydrogenase deficiency (MCAD), carnitine deficiency (fatty acids are beta-oxidised in mitochondria for energy production).	There is defect in the conversion of fatty acids to ketone bodies. This may involve long, medium and long chain acyl CoA dehydrogenase or mitochondrial carnitine transfer. Ketones are necessary for gluconeogenesis and thus hypoglycaemia occurs and hyperammonaemia results from secondary inhibition of the urea cycle.	Fasting results in depletion in hepatic glycogen, and the brain and muscle thus relies on ketone bodies (produced from fatty acid oxidation). Thus acute hypoketotic hypoglycaemic encephalopathy when fasting. Hepatomegaly, skeletal and cardiac myopathy. MCAD associated with SIDS (cot death).	Fasting non-ketotic hypoglycaemia, reduced carnitine levels, free fatty acid levels, urinary organic acid screen.	Prevent prolonged starvation. Carnitine administration increases the elimination of toxic organic acid intermediates by the kidney.

Specific interventions for each disorder may also be required and are discussed in Table 10.1. However, usually only general measures are employed initially until confirmatory investigations have returned. Long term management such as diet and regular review should be carried out by experts in the field of metabolic disorders.

Table 10.1 Continued

Inborn error of metabolism: example	Metabolic defect	Presentation	Investigation	Treatment
Urea cycle defects: Ornithine transcarbamylase (OTC) deficiency.	There is a defect in the conversion of ammonia (a neurotoxic byproduct of amino acid metabolism) to urea resulting in raised ammonia levels. Some excess ammonia is converted to orotic acid. Other causes of hyperammonaemia include: aminoacidopathies, organic acidopathies, fatty acid oxidation defects, transient hyperammonaemia of newborn (THAN) seen in premature babies with respiratory problems often from birth.	OTC deficiency (sex-linked, others AR). Males often die early and females are generally well but will suffer symptoms during catabolic states e.g. infection. Generally acute encephalopathy after the first day, hyperventilation leading to a respiratory alkalosis secondary to excess NH_3. Association with pulmonary haemorrhage.	Blood ammonia, urinary orotic acid excretion increased, blood amino acids and urinary organic acids and amino acids. Specific liver enzyme assay.	Acutely hyperammonaemia is an emergency. Prevent catabolism with i.v. dextrose infusions. Gut bacteria elimination (to reduce production of ammonia by urease). Administration of urea cycle intermediates. Dialysis (haemo/peritoneal). Long term reduce protein-intake, keep catabolic states to a minimum, sodium benzoate and phenylacetate help in the elimination of ammonia.

MARFAN SYNDROME AND HOMOCYSTINURIA

This is an exam favourite and you should be aware of the clinical similarities and differences (Table 10.2).

Homocystine is an important intermediate in the conversion of methionine to cystine. CBS deficiency results in increased homocystine in the blood.

Table 10.1 Continued

Inborn error of metabolism: example	Metabolic defect	Presentation	Investigation	Treatment
Lactic acidosis: Glucose-6 phosphatase deficiency (von Gierkes disease) also called type 1 glycogen storage disease (GSDI).	Cannot produce glucose from gluconeogenesis or glycogenolysis. Inability to produce glucose results in accumulation of pyruvate and thus lactate. Other causes of lactic acidosis include: defects in the citric acid cycle or pyruvate metabolism and defects in mitochondrial electron transport.	Fasting hypoglycaemia leading to encephalopathy, hepatosplenomegaly, later developing central obesity, failure to thrive and round doll facies. Many go on to develop benign hepatic adenomas. (GSD III resembles GSD I but is less severe — caused by deficiency of amylo 1,6 glucosidase).	Increased lactate, increased triglyceride and cholesterol levels, ketoacidosis, hyperuricaemia, specific liver enzyme assay. Administration of glucagon results in increased lactate and not glucose. Also oral glucose test reduces lactate levels to normal.	Administration of glucose initially. Correct the acidosis and prevent hypoglycaemia with frequent feeding such as 1–2 hourly feeds and overnight NG feeds. In addition augment feeding with starchy foods that release glucose slowly and help maintain steady blood glucose concentrations.
Non-ketotic hyperglycinaemia	Problem in breakdown of glycine in the brain resulting in very high levels of cerebral glycine.	AR. Severe hypotonia in neonates, myoclonic seizures, apnoea and hiccoughs.	Glycine levels are high in the blood and urine but extremely high in the CSF.	No treatment exists.
Pyridoxine deficiency	Mechanism unknown	Presents as fits in first few days of life. Suspect if no obvious cause or if inadequate control of fits with anticonvulsants.	Pyridoxine levels	Administer i.v. pyridoxine.

METABOLIC DISEASES THAT AFFECT RENAL FUNCTION

Chapter 4 discussed renal tubular disorders and mentioned some of their causes: some of these include metabolic diseases. The most common renal tubular defect caused by metabolic disorders is the Fanconi syndrome which is seen in cystinosis, galactosaemia, hereditary fructose intolerance, tyrosinaemia, Wilson disease and Lowe syndrome. Other common consequences of metabolic disorders on renal function include renal stone production such as seen in cystinuria.

Table 10.2 Comparison between homocystinuria and Marfan syndrome

	Homocystinuria	Marfan syndrome
Aetiology	Cystatathionine B-synthase (CBS) deficiency*	Defect in protein linking collagen fibres together
Inheritance	AR	AD (15% spontaneous mutation rate)
Height	Tall	Tall
Mental retardation	Present in most	Normal intelligence
Musculoskeletal	Arachnodactyly, pectus excavatum, high arched palate, kyphoscoliosis	Arachnodactyly, pectus excavatum, high arched palate, kyphoscoliosis, increased risk of pneumothorax, increased incidence of hernias
Cardiovascular system	Aortic and mitral regurgitation, coronary artery thrombosis	Dilated aortic root with possibility of aortic dissection. Aortic and mitral valve regurgitation
Ophthalmology	Myopia, lens dislocation (down and outwards) – ectopia lentis, retinal detachment	Myopia, lens dislocation (up and inwards) – ectopia lentis, retinal detachment
Vascular thrombosis	Increased risk of thrombosis (responsible for increased risk of stroke, MI and mental retardation)	No increased risk of vascular thrombosis
Bone density	Osteoporosis	Normal
Joints	Joint stiffness	Joint laxity
Investigation	Homocystine in urine. Cyanide nitroprusside test (goes purple) positive	No homocystine in urine
Treatment	Oral pyridoxine (vitamin B6) and folate to increase the co-factor for CBS. Betaine reduces levels of homocystine by stimulating resynthesis of methionine from homocysteine. Low methionine diet. Early recognition and treatment of complications	Early recognition and treatment of complications

*Methionine → Homocysteine → Cystine + serine
　　　　　　　　　　　　　CBS

Cystinosis

This is a lysosomal storage disease caused by a defect in the transport of cystine across the lysosome resulting in its accumulation in the reticuloendothelial system and in other organs around the body. Its clinical features are dominated by Fanconi syndrome with a hyperchloraemic hypokalaemic metabolic acidosis (type 2 RTA) with failure to thrive, polyuria, polydipsia and hypophosphataemic rickets (see chapter 4). Eventually renal failure ensues by the end of the first decade (a milder adolescent form exists with renal involvement occurring later). Eye involvement is a result of cystine crystal deposits in the cornea causing photophobia, and in the retina causing the so called 'salt and pepper' retinopathy. Deposition in the thyroid gland causes hypothyroidism. Children with cystinosis are often described as 'miserable children' (especially in grey case or data interpretation questions) probably as a result of CNS involvement.

Diagnosis is made by (a) slit-lamp examination of the cornea to identify crystals; (b) reticuloendothelial (bone marrow, lymph node) or rectal biopsies; (c) white cell cystine levels. Treatment consists of use of cysteamine which combines with intralysosomal cystine to produce a disulphide combination which can be eliminated by an alternative pathway. Using this method early in the disease, children have an improved height profile and less renal damage. It can also be applied to the eyes in the form of drops to rid the cornea of the cystine crystals.

Lowe syndrome (oculocerebral renal syndrome)

This is inherited in an X-linked fashion and affects the kidney (Fanconi syndrome), eyes (cataract and glaucoma), CNS (microcephaly, hypotonia and mental retardation).

Proteinuria with an absent red reflex

— *Causes:* Galactosaemia, Wilson disease, Lowe syndrome, nephrotics treated with long term steroids.

LYSOSOMAL STORAGE DISEASES

These are common slides and clinical cases. The most common types are the mucopolysaccharidoses (MPS).

The mucopolysaccharidoses

There are a number of different types of MPSs but essentially they are characterised by defects in the enzymatic breakdown of glycosaminoglycans that subsequently accumulate in various tissues of the body.

Somatic features
Coarse facial features (large skull, large tongue, thick lips, small irregular teeth, broad nasal bridge), short stature, hepatosplenomegaly, dysostosis multiplex (comprising dolicocephaly, oar-like ribs, kyphoscoliosis, thick and coarsely trabeculated bones, anterior beaked vertebrae, bullet-like small bones of hands and feet and reduced joint mobility), cardiomyopathy, hypertrichosis, umbilical and inguinal hernia and deafness.

Neurological features
These are usually developmental delay and mental retardation.
  The MPSs vary in their predominance of somatic or neurological features.

a. Hurler (AR) and Hunter (X-linked) — Both somatic and CNS features present. Hurler have cloudy corneas and Hunter have clear corneas.

b. Sanfillipo — Mainly CNS features with severe mental retardation and behavioural abnormalities and only mild somatic involvement. It is the commonest MPS.

c. Morquios, Maroteaux–Lamy and Scheie present with mainly somatic features and a normal CNS.

Morquios is associated with pectus carinatum that can cause breathing problems.

— *Investigations:* There is increased accumulation and subsequent excretion in the urine of the glycosaminoglycans heparan sulphate and dermatan sulphate (except in Morquios where keratan sulphate is excreted). In addition white cell and fibroblast culture together with lysosomal enzyme assay will provide accurate diagnosis. Alder–Reilly bodies are seen in white cells. Management involves treating the individual complications and bone marrow transplant has some success in some of the mucopolysaccharidoses.

Other lysosomal storage diseases

Tay–Sachs
A gangliosidase commoner in Ashkenazi Jews. Caused by a deficiency of hexosaminidase A and thus the accumulation of gangliosides which produces progressive neurological deterioration from infancy and is eventually fatal. It produces paralysis, hyperaccusis, blindness, dementia and the cherry red spot in the retina caused by the accumulation of gangliosides in the retinal cells (that are as a result pale) surrounding a normal fovea (the so-called cherry red spot). Cherry red spots are also seen in Niemann–Pick and Farber disease — a common slide question.

Gaucher disease
The commonest storage disease is caused by a glucocerebrosidase deficiency. An infantile form (neuronopathic form — rare) may present with nuchal rigidity, opisthotonus and strabismus and is fatal. The adult and juvenile forms (non-neuronopathic) are of variable severity and result from accumulation of glucocerebrosidases in various tissues causing hepatosplenomegaly, bone involvement with pain, pancytopenia, thinning of the cortex and flaring of the ends of the long bones. Diagnosis is on bone marrow examination showing the classic Gaucher cells (wrinkled tissue) and on white cell or fibroblast culture with enzyme assay. Treatment involves splenectomy for possible hypersplenism or discomfort, and BMT.

Niemann–Pick disease

Caused by the accumulation of sphingomyelin and commoner in Jews. Hepatosplenomegaly, skin pigmentation and mental retardation are common. Investigation shows typical foam cells in the bone marrow and a culture of white cells or fibroblasts and enzyme assay will make the diagnosis. Treatment is as for Gaucher.

OTHER DISORDERS ASSOCIATED WITH CNS INVOLVEMENT

Phenylketonuria (PKU)

This is caused by increased blood phenylalanine levels as a result of a deficiency of phenylalanine hydroxylase in the liver (or more rarely a defect in tetrahydrobiopterin — a phenylalanine hydroxylase co-factor — causing a more severe disease). This prevents the conversion of phenylalanine to tyrosine. Babies are normal postnatally, but phenylalanine is toxic to the brain and if not detected and treated early results in mental retardation, microcephaly, cerebral palsy, eczema and a 'mousy' smell of the urine. Phenotypically they often have fair/blond hair and blue eyes.

All babies are screened for PKU with the Guthrie test (a bacterial inhibition test) taken from the baby's heel usually between the fifth and 14th days (after feeding is well under way). The diagnosis is confirmed by measuring serum phenylalanine levels in the infant. Remember also to measure tyrosine since transient tyrosinaemia in the newborn can result in raised levels of phenylalanine.

Treatment involves a diet low in phenylalanine at least until puberty (controversial). Some dietary phenylalanine is needed for normal growth since it is an essential amino acid. Phenylketonuric females wishing to have children should be on a low PA diet from before conception to prevent the offspring from developing mental retardation.

Lesch–Nyhan syndrome

Inherited in an X-linked recessive fashion. There is a deficiency of hypoxanthine guanine phosphoribosyl transferase (HPRT) resulting in excess uric acid production. Consequences of this are male babies normal at birth who later go on to exhibit developmental delay in the first few months, followed by hypotonia and choreoathetoid movements, spasticity and dysarthria: the characteristic self-mutilatory behaviour then develops (up to this point children have often been diagnosed as having cerebral palsy). Self-mutilatory behaviour consists of finger or lip biting (a common exam slide), or head banging. Uric acid nephrolithiasis and gout may later develop.

Investigations include finding a raised serum uric acid level. The diagnosis is confirmed by finding increased urinary uric acid/creatinine ratio levels and performing an enzyme assay from cultured white cells or fibroblasts. Treatment is with allopurinol.

NB Other diseases associated with self-mutilatory behaviour include: lead poisoning, Riley–Day syndrome and leprosy.

Menkes kinky hair disease

Inherited in an X-linked fashion. There is a defect in the utilisation of ingested copper. It results in abnormal coarse facies with fragile hair, which show increased spiral twisting (pili torti). Mental retardation and developmental delay are also common. There may also be lax ligaments, osteoporosis, hernia, arterial dilatation and dissection and a predisposition to hypothermia. Investigations demonstrate a low plasma copper and caeruloplasmin level and treatment involves giving early parenteral copper which does not always improve the prognosis.

METABOLIC DISEASES CAUSING HEPATITIS

These infants often present with jaundice (conjugated and unconjugated), hepatomegaly, hypoglycaemia and the Fanconi syndrome. You should be familiar with them as a cause of prolonged jaundice in the neonatal period.

It is useful to know the monosaccharide components of the dissacharides.

Lactose (main milk carbohydrate) = glucose + galactose, maltose = glucose + glucose and sucrose = glucose and fructose.

Galactosaemia

This is caused by a deficiency of galactose-1-phosphate uridyl transferase (GALPUT) — galactose cannot therefore be converted into glucose. Babies may present with lethargy, poor feeding, vomiting, diarrhoea, hepatomegaly and a mixed jaundice as well as abnormal liver enzymes with later cirrhosis. In addition there is hypoglycaemia and Fanconi syndrome. Lamellar cataracts may develop. *E. coli* sepsis is found in 25–50% of cases. Later mental retardation develops. To confirm the diagnosis (a) reducing substances in the urine which if positive (that is, clinitest +ve and clinistix –ve) you should go on to perform (b) red cell GALPUT levels to confirm the diagnosis. Treat by eliminating all milk products from the feeds and change to a lactose and galactose free diet throughout childhood (which reduces the complications). **NB** The combination of hepatomegaly with jaundice and cataracts can be seen also in congenital rubella.

Fructose intolerance

Deficiency in fructose-1-phosphate aldolase deficiency. Symptoms develop soon after ingestion of fructose or sucrose, for example fruit juices or sugar. Vomiting and diarrhoea followed by hepatomegaly, jaundice and hypoglycaemia. Fanconi syndrome may occur. Hypophosphataemia occurs early. Diagnose by liver biopsy and enzyme assay (the loading test is dangerous).

Tyrosinaemia type 1

Caused by famaryl acetoacetate hydrolase (FAH) deficiency. It causes liver disease and Fanconi syndrome and presents early (often fatal) or late (less severe). Investigation involves finding raised AFP and raised succinylacetone in the urine. Treatment is with a low tyrosine and phenylalanine diet.

Acid lipase deficiency

Presents in the neonatal period with hepatomegaly, progressive liver disease and neurological deterioration. Adrenal calcification is often present on a plain AXR. No treatment is available.

Glycogen storage disease type 4

The result of a brancher enzyme deficiency causes liver disease progressing to cirrhosis at a few months of life and death usually by 2–3 years of age. Liver transplant in selected cases.

Alpha-1 antitrypsin deficiency causes liver disease in early infancy and Wilson disease causes liver disease in later childhood. Both are discussed in chapter 6.

Causes of a positive Clinitest are

— *Presence of reducing sugars:* glucose, lactose, galactose, fructose, pentose (not sucrose).
— *Drugs:* salicylates, phenothiazines, cephalosporins.
— *Vitamin C* (high dose), homogentisic acid (in alkaptonuria).

Clinistix is specific for glucose.

METABOLIC DISEASES THAT AFFECT MUSCLE

Glycogen is a storage carbohydrate in the body mainly formed in the liver and muscles. When muscles are exercised, initially glucose (from glycogen) is used to fuel the work. If the exercise is maintained however, then fatty acids become the main fuel for the muscles (during anaerobic exercise). If there is a failure of these fuel supplies to meet these requirements then skeletal muscle is affected with resulting muscle weakness and wasting, muscle cramps and rhabdomyolysis (with increased CPK) and myoglobinuria which has the potential to cause renal failure.

Glycogen storage disease type V (McCardle disease)

There is a defect in the phosphorylase enzyme, thus preventing the breakdown of glycogen to glucose and therefore failing to supply muscle with fuel during the initial period of work. It presents in late childhood. The muscle symptoms (described above) are developed at the beginning of exercise, however the symptoms gradually subside as exercising continues. Investigations include lack of increase in lactate concentration during exercise (often performed with the forearm exercise test using an inflated blood pressure cuff to stop blood supply) as a result of diminished glycolysis. Alternatively a muscle biopsy is performed. Treatment involves avoidance of exercise and prevention of myoglobinuria-induced renal failure with hydration and keeping the urine alkaline. They tend to have normal life expectancy.

Carnitine palmitoyl transferase deficiency

Here the problem is in supply of fatty acids to the muscle so that symptoms occur after sustained exercise and not early on during exercise. Investigations are as with McCardle disease but here there is a normal rise in lactate after exercise.

Glycogen storage disease type II

This is caused by alpha glucosidase. It affects skeletal muscle causing extreme hypotonia with thickened muscles in infancy (including hypoglossia). It also affects the heart causing severe cardiomegaly. CXR shows obvious cardiomegaly and the ECG shows characteristically very large QRS complexes in all the leads with a short PR interval. Death is likely within the first year although there are milder variants that occur later in childhood.

Fatty acid oxidation defects

There are a number of defects in fatty acid metabolism, for example carnitine palmitoyl transferase I and II deficiency (distinct from those described earlier in acute encephalopathy) and ketone body formation that can cause fasting hypoglycaemia, muscle weakness and cardiomyopathy.

Glycolytic disorders and mitochondrial electron transport chain defects

These disorders can also produce muscle weakness. Mitochondrial disease presents with a multisystem disease that affects the main energy-requiring organs and tissues. Thus these patients tend to present with short stature (impaired growth), hypotonia, weakness, encephalopathy, developmental delay, myoclonic epilepsy, ataxia, dysphagia, deafness, blindness and opthalmoplegia. Cardiovascular involvement includes cardiomyopathy and arrhythmias and renal involvement may cause the Fanconi syndrome. There is an interesting inheritance pattern.

a. Mitochondrial proteins derived from the nuclear genome. Thus inheritance is AR or X-linked recessive.

b. Mitochondrial proteins derived from the mitochondrial chromosome (mainly the respiratory chain). Because inheritance of the mitochondria is through the mother, mutations in the mitochondrial chromosome have a maternal pattern of inheritance with males and females both equally likely to develop the condition.

Examples of type (a) include Leigh syndrome. *Examples of type (b)* include MERRF which stands for mitochondrial myopathy, encephalopathy (and) ragged red fibres. MELAS stands for mitochondrial myopathy, encephalopathy, lactic acidosis and stroke-like episodes. Others include LHON (Leber hereditary optic neueropathy).

Mitochondrial disease can be identified by finding raised lactate levels in the blood and CSF. Muscle biopsy usually provides the diagnosis.

PEROXISOMAL DEFECTS

This includes a group of fatal diseases that are caused by defects in peroxisomal metabolism. They have various clinical features in common. These include various degrees of: abnormal facies, progressive CNS deterioration with mental retardation, hypotonia, deafness, retinopathy, neonatal seizures, hepatomegaly, cirrhosis and calcific stippling of epiphyses. They are all inherited in an AR fashion except X-linked adrenoleukodystrophy.

The classic example is of Zellweger syndrome where there are no peroxisomes present (see chapter 14). Death usually occurs within six months. Other examples include diseases where peroxisomes are present but certain peroxisomal enzymes are deficient, such as X-linked adrenoleukodystrophy which presents with features of white matter degeneration and adrenal insufficiency, the child dying at around 10 years of age. Another example is rhizomelic chondroplasia punctata.

Diagnosis is made by liver biopsy with electron microscopy looking at the presence and morphology of peroxisomes, as well as fibroblast culture and enzyme assay.

RICKETS

Rickets is a qualitative defect of bone caused by deficient bone mineralisation of osteoid (the bony matrix). It is equivalent to osteomalacia in adults. It results from deficiencies of calcium or phosphate. Clinical presentation: craniotabes (soft skull like a ping-pong ball), caput quadratum (square head), frontal bossing, rachitic rosary (caused by swelling at the costochondral junctions), Harrison sulci, epiphyseal cartilage swelling at the wrists and ankles (and other joints), delayed closure of the anterior fontanelle, bowing of the legs or knock knees, muscle weakness, delayed teeth eruption, kyphoscoliosis and increased tendency to fracture.

X-ray appearances of a joint in a child with rickets shows widening of the joint space and cupping, irregularity and a ragged flaring metaphyseal surface ('cupping, splaying and fraying'). A summarised description of vitamin D metabolism can be seen in Fig. 10.1.

Causes of rickets

Abnormalities in vitamin D utilisation (PTH increased)

1. Reduced intake of vitamin D either through the diet or through reduced exposure to sunlight. This may occur in babies who are breast-fed alone especially if there is a poor maternal diet. It is also seen more commonly in dark-skinned people.

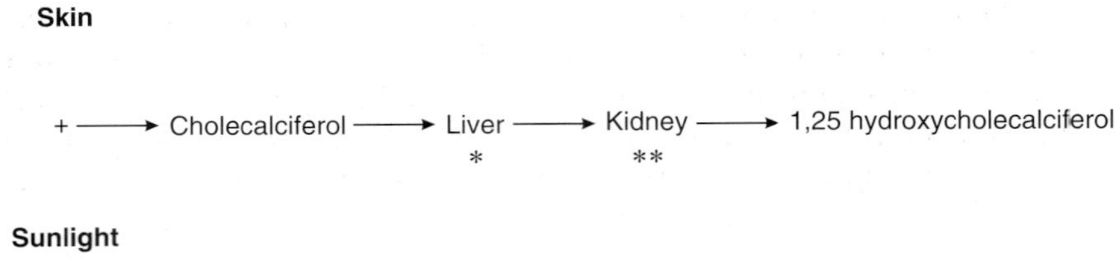

Skin

+ ⟶ Cholecalciferol ⟶ Liver ⟶ Kidney ⟶ 1,25 hydroxycholecalciferol
                                    *   **

Sunlight

* 25 Alpha hydroxylase enzyme

** 1 Alpha hydroxylase enzyme

Fig. 10.1 Vitamin D metabolism.

2. Malabsorption of vitamin D. Remember that vitamin D is a fat soluble vitamin so that any cause of fat malabsorption will cause vitamin D malabsorption such as obstructive jaundice or proximal bowel pathology (such as coeliac disease).

3. Liver disease as a result of obstruction to bile and thus fat malabsorption, but also due to the defective 25 hydroxylation of cholecalciferol. Treat with 25 hydroxycholecalciferol.

4. Renal disease resulting in defective 1 alpha hydroxylation of 25 hydroxycholecalciferol (renal rickets). Treat with 1 alpha hydroxycholecalciferol (alphacalcidol) or 1,25 hydroxycholecalciferol.

5. Vitamin D dependent rickets type 1 is caused by renal deficiency of the 1 alpha hydroxylase enzyme (presenting at around four months of age and treated with very high levels of vitamin D or 1 alpha cholecalciferol). Type 2 is due to an abnormality in the vitamin D receptor (commoner in Arab populations and associated with alopecia). Type 2 does not respond well to treatment.

Abnormalities in phosphate metabolism
These result in reduced available phosphate. PTH normal. Low phosphate.

1. X-linked (dominant) hypophosphataemic rickets (a common data interpretation question). Males are much more commonly affected than females and essentially there is severe phosphate wasting from the renal tubules resulting in extremely short stature and rickets. There will be normal vitamin D levels, ALP in some will be mildly to moderately elevated and there will be a very low phosphate.

2. Fanconi syndrome (see chapter 4).

3. Post renal transplant. This occurs because before the transplant the chronic hypocalcaemia resulted in a secondary hyperparathyroidism. Because of the non-functioning kidneys the tubules did not respond to the PTH. With new functional transplanted kidneys, however, the tubules are responsive to the raised PTH and result in excessive renal loss of phosphate.

4. Neonatal rickets in premature babies (osteopenia of prematurity). Results from inadequate phosphate intake sufficient for growing bones (and increased renal phosphate loss). Babies should be given phosphate and if unresponsive, vitamin D and calcium should be added. An X-ray of the wrist shows generalised opsteopenia and wrist changes as described above (if severe, fractures may be seen). The ALP will be elevated.

In addition to the above causes, dietary deficiencies of calcium or phosphate may very rarely be responsible for rickets.

Rarely in a child treated with anticonvulsants there may be induction in the hepatic enzymes responsible for vitamin D metabolism resulting in rapid elimination of vitamin D from the body.

In questions you must look for a cause such as diet or evidence of chronic renal failure.

Investigations

Apart from the radiological features discussed above, the biochemistry of rickets shows a low calcium, low phosphate and raised alkaline phosphatase levels. PTH levels may be high or low depending on the cause (see above). Performing vitamin D derivative levels will aid the diagnosis of the aetiology of the rickets. In nutritional rickets 25 hydroxycholecalciferol is low. In vitamin D dependent rickets type 1 1,25 hydroxycholecalciferol is low and 25 hydroxycholecalciferol is normal. In type 2 dependent rickets 1,25 and 25 hydroxycholecalciferol levels are in the normal range (or 1,25 hydroxycholecalciferol levels are high). 1,25 and 25 hydroxycholecalciferol levels are normal in x-linked hypophosphataemic rickets. Remember that in vitamin D deficient rickets calcium levels may be normal as a result of a secondary hyperparathroidism (however phosphate levels may consequently be low). Renal function, liver function, urinary phosphate and calcium levels may also be useful. A venous gas should be performed to exclude RTA. Antigliadin antibodies may be performed to exclude coeliac disease.

THE PORPHYRIAS

This is a rarely asked question but will be a common differential diagnosis in many clinical scenarios and may come up in a grey case. They are a group of disorders that are caused by mutations in the production of enzymes necessary for haemoglobin synthesis and the clinical features are the result of an accumulation of precursors (see Table 10.3). You will not of course be expected to memorise individual enzyme defects but you should be familiar with the patterns of illness that they may cause.

If asked in a question for investigations required, you will probably get away with simply sending urine, faeces and blood to the laboratory for porphyrin measurement: however you may not get away with this in a data question. The commonest porphyria tested for in the exam is AIP. During an attack there is an increase in urinary delta aminolaevulinic acid and porphobilinogen. The same may be seen in variegate porphyria together with an increase in faecal porphyrins. **NB** Note that lead poisoning which can also present with abdominal pain and neurological symptoms has increased

Table 10.3 Comparison of the porphyrias in the paediatric population

Type of porphyria	Clinical features
Congenital erythropoietic porphyria	Rarer. AR. Onset usually within the first year. *Cutaneous features:* Bullae, urticaria, purpura on sun-exposed regions leading to scarring, hypertrichosis and pigmentation. *Haemolytic anaemia:* sometimes associated with splenomegaly. *Other:* Dark urine. Red staining of teeth (erythrodontia). No acute episodes.
Erythropoietic porphyria	Commoner. AD. Onset before puberty. *Cutaneous features:* as above. *Liver disease:* gallstones, jaundice, hepatitis, liver failure.
Acute intermittent porphyria (AIP) — Swedish type	Commoner. AD. Attacks start after puberty. F > M. Precipitated by drugs (barbiturates, sulphonamides, phenytoin, oral contraceptive pill etc.), infections, dieting, female sex hormones. *Abdominal symptoms:* pain, vomiting, constipation. *Neurological:* seizures, change in personality, peripheral neuropathy, paralysis. *Autonomic neuropathy:* abdominal pain, labile blood pressure, tachycardia. *Other:* Hyponatraemia (SIADH caused by hypothalamic involvement), urine goes deep red on standing.
Variegate porphyria (South African type)	Rarer. AD. Onset after puberty. Very similar to acute intermittent porphyria except that cutaneous features are common. *Cutaneous features:* photosensitive lesions as above.
Hereditary coproporphyria	Rare. AD. *Neurological features:* as above. *Cutaneous features:* as above.

Porphyria cutanea tarda (the remaining porphyria) is an adult disease.

urinary delta aminolaevulinic acid, increased urinary coproporphyrin and a normal porphobilinogen. Know the other differential diagnoses of abdominal pain with neurological features (see chapter 6).

ACID-BASE QUESTIONS

These are usually in the form of interpretation of blood gases (see chapter 3). Use is however sometimes made of anion gap in the interpretation of a metabolic acidosis. If you are given pH, sodium, potassium, bicarbonate and chloride ion concentrations, then determine the anion gap. Anion gap = $[Na + K] - [HCO_3 + Cl]$ usually between 10–14 mmol/l.

Metabolic acidosis with a raised anion gap

— Lactic acidosis (type A secondary to poor tissue perfusion and type B a result of inborn errors of metabolism). Blood lactate > 5 mmol/l
— Ingestion of acid, ethanol, methanol
— Drug ingestion for example salicylate

— Renal failure
— Metabolic disorder such as organic acidaemia.

Metabolic acidosis with a normal anion gap

This implies a raised chloride ion concentration.

— Renal tubular acidosis
— Addison disease
— Drugs such as acetazolamide (a carbonic anhydrase inhibitor)
— Ingestion of chloride-containing acid: for example, HCl
— Uraemia (unusual)
— Severe diarrhoea
— Post ureteric diversion into large bowel.

Metabolic alkalosis

— Vomiting
— Cushing disease, Conn syndrome
— Diuretics
— Hypokalaemia.

HYPERLIPIDAEMIA

The clinical presentation of hyperlipidaemia is uncommon in the paediatric population. In the examination you are likely to encounter only two of the long list of causes. These are:

Familial hypercholesterolaemia

Inheritance AD. Carrier frequency of 1:500 in the population. There is a defect in the hepatic LDL receptor that takes up LDL from the peripheral circulation resulting in reduced clearance and increased production of LDL (since lost negative feedback control). Heterozygotes present with tendon xanthomas between the ages of 10–20 years usually on the extensor surfaces of tendons, particularly the Achilles tendon. Serum cholesterol is typically between 8–12 mmol/l. There may be a history of premature death (before the age of 50) from atherosclerosis in the family history. After the age of 20 patients develop arcus senilis, xanthelasma (around the upper and lower eye lids) with clinical signs of coronary artery disease in the 40–50 year age group. Homozygotes are affected to a greater extent with evidence of coronary artery disease in the teenage years. Serum cholesterol is usually above 18 mmol/l. Treat with a low fat diet and lipid lowering agents such as cholestyramine (a resin).

Familial chylomicronaemia

Inheritance AR presenting in childhood. It is caused by a deficiency in the lipoprotein lipase enzyme (or apoprotein C-II which activates lipoprotein lipase) present in adipose tissue and muscle. Chylomicrons cannot therefore be converted to chylomicron remnants which can not then be taken up by the liver. This results in elevated triglyceride levels (in the range of 20–80 mmol/l) and elevated cholesterol levels (in the range of 8–12 mmol/l). Clinical features consist of acute abdominal pain secondary to recurrent pancreatitis, eruptive xanthomatas, hepatosplenomegaly and lipaemia retinalis (not atherosclerosis). The serum appears milky. Treatment consists of a low fat diet and fish oils containing Omega-3 fatty acids.

Secondary causes

In addition to the primary hyperlipidaemias you should also know the secondary causes of hyperlipidaemia which include:

— *Raised cholesterol:* hypothyroidism, IDDM, cholestasis.

— *Raised triglycerides:* obesity, renal failure, alcohol excess (adults).

— *Raised cholesterol and triglycerides:* nephrotic syndrome, glycogen storage disease type 1, diet, drugs: oral contraceptive pill, beta-blockers and thiazide diuretics.

DRUG POISONING

This topic is extremely important in the exam since it should be included in many differential diagnoses of many common presenting clinical scenarios. Accidental poisoning is common in paediatric clinical practice and is most common in children aged between 1–3 years of age. Boys are commoner culprits than girls. Many non-pharmaceutical products are ingested by children and these in addition have their own associated morbidities and mortalities, however here we will concentrate on drugs since the questions also concentrate on this area.

It is beyond the scope of this book to describe the modes of treatment of individual poisonings but what is intended is that you will have an understanding of how different poisonings may present in children and thus recognise these features in a question on the topic. In clinical practice it is not uncommon for children to present with poisoning without a history of ingestion so you must always think of it as a possible cause.

Presenting features fall into the following categories: (1) coma; (2) metabolic acidosis: look for an increased anion gap for example with ethanol overdose; (3) cardiac arrhythmia; (4) GI symptoms — anorexia, nausea, vomiting, abdominal pain, diarrhoea; (5) seizures. The presence of any of these in a clinical case scenario should lead you to think of drug ingestion as a differential diagnosis.

If you suspect drug intoxication in a grey case then your investigation of choice is a blood and urine toxicological screen. See Table 10.4.

There are often clues given in clinical cases as to the likelihood of drug ingestion. The family may be known to social services, since lack of parental supervision is associated with accidental drug ingestion. Don't forget the possibility of Münchausen by proxy as a cause of drug intoxication in some children. A history of parental psychiatric illness or marital disharmony may also

Table 10.4 Comparison of the presenting features and investigations in the commoner drug ingestions

Agent ingested	Clinical features	Investigations
Iron ingestion	Symptoms start between 30 min to 6 h after ingestion. In general < 40 mg/kg Fe ingestion is safe. *Stage 1*: GI irritation: vomiting, abdominal pain diarrhoea (may be bloody), metabolic acidosis, shock. *Stage 2*: Silent phase: starts 10–15 h after ingestion and lasts about 24 h. *Stage 3*: Shock, encephalopathy, hepatic impairment. *Stage 4*: This may occur 2–6 weeks following ingestion: GI strictures (especially pyloric and small intestine) leading to GI obstruction, CNS damage and hepatic failure.	Remember iron tablets are radio-opaque and an AXR may help diagnosis in uncertain cases. FBC, G&S/crossmatch (depending on severity), U&E, glucose (may produce hyperglycaemia). Serum iron levels 2–4 h post ingestion.
Paracetamol	Paracetamol is converted to N-acetylbenzoquinoneimine (NABQUI) which is very toxic and rapidly conjugated with reduced glutathione. In excess, reduced glutathione is depleted and the unconjugated NABQUI binds covalently to hepatocytes causing necrosis. Symptoms are minimal immediately post ingestion except for some possible nausea. This period is followed about 36 h later by hepatic necrosis and liver failure if severe. Renal failure secondary to ATN may also occur.	Blood taken for paracetamol levels at least 4 h after ingestion. Also LFTs and PT time. Look up normogram for levels at 4 h or more if presentation is late. This will give indication for need for treatment. If poisoning is severe measure LFTs including prothrombin time for the first few days to pick up liver damage.
Salicylates e.g aspirin	Anxiety, sweating, fever, tachycardia, hyperventilation (secondary to metabolic acidosis caused by the salicylate itself) leading to a respiratory alkalosis (and later acidosis), ketosis, tinnitus, nausea and vomiting, abdominal pain, hyperglycaemia, vertigo, confusion and eventually coma.	Take blood salicylate levels at 4–6 h. Salicylates induce gastric stasis and may still be recoverable up to 12 h after ingestion. Again consult normogram. Treat if > 3.5 mmol/l. Forced alkaline diuresis

Table 10.4 Continued

Agent ingested	Clinical features	Investigations
Tricyclic antidepressants	*Anticholinergic effects*: dilated pupils, decreased bowel sounds, dry mouth, warm dry flushed skin, tachycardia and other arrhythmias, hyperthermia, urinary retention, ataxia and seizures. *Myocardial membrane effects*: AV block, widened QRS complexes, atrial/ventricular arrhythmias, hypo/hypertension. *Alpha blockade*: postural hypotension. *NA uptake inhibition*: agitation, drowsiness, coma.	ECG monitor. Toxicology screen to confirm.
Phenothiazines	Miosis. Alpha blockade: see above. Myocardial membrane defects: see above. Tremor, convulsions. *Extra pyramidal effects*: oculogyric crisis, opisthotonus, back arching, trismus, tongue protrusion.	Cardiac monitor. Toxicology screen to confirm.
Lead poisoning	See chapters 5 and 6.	
Alcohol	Drowsiness dysarthric, ataxic, hypoglycaemia — common in children following excess alcohol ingestion (secondary to inhibited gluconeogenesis).	Blood alcohol level. Blood glucose level.
Antihistamines	Anticholinergic features: see above.	
Benzodiazepines	Hypothermia, hypotension, bradycardia, hyporeflexia, respiratory depression, coma.	Antidote = flumazenil
Opiates	Small pupils, drowsiness, cardiorespiratory depression, coma.	Antidote = naloxone

be mentioned in the question. Other clues include that one or other of the parents is being treated pharmacologically for a particular medical condition. Thus the child has a ready access to the medication.

Glue sniffing/solvent abuse is seen mainly in boys in the 10–16 year age group. It can be recognised by the following features: typical erythematous facial rash, dizziness, dysarthria, visual hallucinations, cerebellar syndrome (caused by cerebellar degeneration), peripheral neuropathy, renal tubular acidosis and haematuria and proteinuria, aplastic anaemia, rhabdomyolysis (with myoglobinuria and thus possible acute renal failure), myalgia and optic atrophy. CT may show ventricular enlargement. Cardiac arrhythmias may be caused by propellent components of the solvent (freons). The main aromatic hydrocarbon solvent in glue is benzene.

Rheumatology

In this chapter we will discuss the collagen vascular diseases that commonly come up in the examination as well as the diseases that primarily affect the musculoskeletal system.

THE CAUSES OF ARTHRITIS

Monoarthritis and polyarthritis

— *Trauma:* Commonest cause. Accidental or non-accidental.

— *Sepsis:* Septic arthritis (most often in the lower limbs). Organisms are most commonly *Staph. aureus, Streptococcus, Salmonella* (in sickle cell disease), tuberculosis, viral causes for example mumps, and in neonates Group B *Streptococcus* and Gram-negative bacilli. There may be an adjacent osteomyelitis which may be secondary to the arthritis or may be the primary cause. Lyme disease infection is caused by *Borrelia burgdorferi* from bites from infected Ixodes ticks which may cause arthritis usually affecting large joints. Gonococcal arthritis is a pauciarticular erosive arthritis associated with sexual activity, often with a pustular skin rash on the palms and soles.

— *Reactive arthritis*: There is a sterile arthritis that occurs following viral illnesses such as mumps, infectious mononucleosis, mycoplasma or following viral gastroenteritis. Most commonly it causes a polyarthritis. Reiter syndrome: conjunctivitis, urethritis and arthritis (usually knees and ankles).

— *Henoch–Schönlein purpura* (HSP): Associated with purpuric rash on legs and buttocks. Arthritis may precede onset of rash and occurs in about two-thirds of all cases of HSP, most commonly affecting the lower limb (see chapter 4).

— *Juvenile chronic arthritis*: see later.

— *Other collagen vascular diseases*: SLE (usually a migratory symmetrical polyarthritis most commonly affecting small joints and very destructive);

rheumatic fever (migratory arthritis mainly affecting large joints following a Group A beta haemolytic *Streptococcal* infection – Jones major criteria, look for other criteria).

— *Sickle cell disease*: Arthritis may be caused by a sickle crisis or as mentioned before a *Salmonella* septic arthritis.

— *Bleeding disorders*: such as haemophilia following an intra-articular bleed.

— *Psoriatic arthropathy*: occurs in about 10% of psoriasis cases. In the majority of cases there is a large joint monoarthritis and less commonly a symmetrical small joint arthritis. It may occur in the absence of active skin disease.

— *Inflammatory bowel disease*: This most commonly causes a symmetrical arthropathy affecting the large joints. May precede the bowel symptoms. Sacroileitis is more common in UC.

— *Malignancy*: Osteosarcoma most commonly affects the region around the knee joint and can present as a swollen knee.

Investigations

— FBC looking for evidence of a raised WCC. Include a differential count looking for a lymphocytosis or neutrophilia. Remember that a raised platelet count is a common accompaniment to inflammatory conditions during the active phase.

— Erythrocyte sedimentation rate (ESR): this will indicate active inflammatory disease. Also CRP.

— Blood culture: looking for evidence of a bacteraemia in a possible septic arthritis.

— Viral serology: acute and convalescent titres.

— Throat swab (especially for suspected *Streptococcal* disease) and ASOT.

— Immunology: C3, C4, CH50.

— Joint aspiration and fluid sent for MC&S.

— X-ray of joint looking for damage to the bone. Widening of the joint space may indicate effusion/blood.

— Ultrasound will help confirm the presence of fluid in the joint (and can sometimes differentiate pus from clear fluid) and joint aspiration can be performed via ultrasound guidance.

JUVENILE CHRONIC ARTHRITIS (JCA)

Many questions will be based on the topic of juvenile chronic arthritis. It is a much loved topic of examiners owing to the variety of presentations and somewhat tricky diagnostic evaluation. Patients are usually fairly well and may have excellent clinical signs and thus make a very likely short or long case. It is a diagnosis of exclusion and arthritis has to be present for at least six weeks. Other causes of arthritis must have been excluded by history, examination and investigations. The disease progression over the first six months from presentation will determine into which of the three diagnostic categories the child can be placed. See Table 11.1.

— *Systemic onset JCA*: Systemic symptoms are common.
— *Pauciarticular JCA*: This type affects four or less joints.
— *Polyarticular JCA*: Five or more joints are involved.

It is important to know the differential diagnosis of systemic onset JCA since these conditions must be considered and eliminated in every case: acute leukaemia, neuroblastoma, infections (e.g infectious mononucleosis,

Table 11.1 Comparison of the three main types of JCA

	Systemic onset JCA	Pauciarticular JCA	Polyarticular JCA
Proportion of all JCA	10%	60%	30%
Age at onset	Throughout all childhood but commonest under 5 years	Type 1: 1–5 years Type 2: Over 8 years	Type 1: (90%) Rh. Factor –ve. Mean: 6 years Type 2: (10%) Rh. Factor +ve. Mean: teenagers
Male/female ratio	M = F	Type 1: F > M Type 2: M > F	Type 1: F > M Type 2: F > M
Joint involvement	Not a prominent initial feature but later produces a chronic polyarthritis.	Type 1: Lower limb joint, non-erosive arthritis esp. knee and ankle. Asymmetrical. Type 2: Lower limb joints, including the hips, sacroileitis. Asymmetrical.	Type 1: Any joint involvement especially small joints of hands and feet. Type 2: More aggressive destructive arthritis with similar distribution to type 1. Worse prognosis.
Extra-articular features	Classically relapsing and remitting. Intermittent daily high fevers, blotchy pink non-itchy erythematous rash often accompanying the fever, lymphadenopathy, hepatosplenomegaly, serositis (pericarditis, pleuritis, peritonitis). Growth retardation is common.	Type 1: One-third of patients have chronic iridocyclitis (esp. if ANA positive). Type 2: Malaise, fatigue, constitutional upset, enthesopathy*, episodes of acute uveitis occur.	Both types may have extra-articular features such as fever and malaise but less severe than systemic onset JCA. Growth retardation is common in the more severe disease.

Table 11.1 Continued

	Systemic onset JCA	Pauciarticular JCA	Polyarticular JCA
Investigations	Normochromic normocytic anaemia. Increased platelet count. Increased WCC (usually neutrophilia). Increased ESR. Rheumatoid factor and ANA negative. Complement levels may be increased.	Type 1: Normal. 80% of those with uveitis are ANA +ve. Rh. factor –ve. Type 2: Normal except raised acute phase reactants and ESR in constitutional upset. Rh. factor –ve	Type 1: Rh. factor –ve. ANA +ve in 25%. Type 2: Rh. factor +ve, ANA +ve in 50%.
Prognosis	Chronic erosive arthritis in 25%. Most have self-limiting disease.	Type 1 arthritis often resolves spontaneously. Uveitis must be managed early before ocular damage occurs. Type 2 especially HLA-B27 haplotype may go on to develop a seronegative arthropathy such as ankylosing spondylitis.	Type 1 generally good prognosis with most outgrowing disease. Type 2 poorer prognosis with more severe disability and more likely to continue into adulthood.

*Enthesopathy refers to inflammation at the point of insertion of tendons or ligaments into bone resulting in pain (there may be some calcification later). It is a common feature of adult seronegative arthritides. Examples include Achilles tendinitis and plantar fasciitis.

Streptococcal infection — rheumatic fever) as well as of course other causes of an arthritis mentioned in the list at the beginning of the chapter.

The overall prognosis for JCA is that between 60–70% of children will outgrow their disease but the individual prognosis will depend on which diagnosis the child has. The course during childhood is typically that of relapses and remissions.

Treatment

Treatment involves a multidisciplinary approach.

1. Initially NSAIDs — a response may take some time.

2. Second-line drugs/disease modifying drugs include sulphasalazine, hydroxychloroquine, gold and D-penicillinamine. Monitor for toxicity.

3. Steroids. These are useful for controlling systemic symptoms especially in systemic onset JCA. Severe inflammatory arthritis may be helped with intra-articular steroids (such as triamcinolone following joint aspiration).

Steroids do not appear to halt the progression of arthritis. Sudden relapses and flare-ups (including systemic symptoms) may be aborted with courses of i.v. prednisolone pulses. Uveitis is usually treated with topical steroid eye drops (and rarely systemic steroids) and mydriatics.

4. If the above has failed to control symptoms then methotrexate can improve symptoms and inflammation of the joints but has little effect on the systemic symptoms. Cyclosporin has also been used.
5. Physiotherapy. Patients should have a full physiotherapy assessment and detailed programme of daily exercises in order to maintain maximal function, increase muscle bulk and strength and reduce the development of flexion contractures. Hydrotherapy is very helpful.
6. Splints: often both day and night time splints are specially made.
7. Occupational therapy: help for activities of daily living in more restricted patients including a home assessment.
8. Surgery may become necessary in the form of soft-tissue releases and joint replacement.
9. In pauciarticular arthritis regular opthalmological assessment with slit-lamp every six months in ANA +ve children and yearly in ANA –ve children to diagnose uveitis so that treatment can be offered early to prevent permanent damage.

DISTINGUISHING BETWEEN MECHANICAL AND INFLAMMATORY PAIN IN ARTHRITIS

It is important to know the features in a history that help you to distinguish between an arthritis that is caused by mechanical factors or by inflammation (such as JCA).

— *Pain and stiffness*: In inflammatory conditions children often describe pain and stiffness being worse in the morning. It takes a few hours for the stiffness to wear off (often described as having glue in their joints). Patients find it difficult to get out of bed in the mornings. In mechanical pain the pain is usually worst at the end of the day.

— *Exercise and rest*: In inflammatory diseases the pain is improved by exercise and made worse after a period of inactivity. In mechanical arthritis the pain is worse after exercise.

ORTHOPAEDICS AND RHEUMATOLOGY IN RADIOLOGY

The range of X-rays that can be used as slides or question prompts in the clinical examination is huge. Here we will try and cover the most likely possibilities.

It is important to know something about the development of the skeletal system so that you can interpret X-rays correctly. You should know the normal anatomy of a bone with the diaphysis, metaphysis and epiphysis.

Between the metaphysis and the epiphysis is an avascular strip of cartilage called the epiphyseal growth plate (physis) which is responsible for longitudinal bone growth. By the time of birth most epiphyses have not started to ossify and therefore cannot be seen on an X-ray and fractures at these sites at this age are diagnosed largely from clinical observation. As the child ages these epiphyses ossify in a predictable fashion so that X-rays of the epiphyses of a child help us to determine the maturity of the epiphyseal centres and thus estimate the age of the child using bone age (in particular the number, size shape and density of the epiphyseal centres). Usually the left hand and wrist are used for standardisation. Comparing bone age with chronological age can help in investigating various metabolic, endocrine and other disorders.

As the child ages the epiphyses continue to ossify but it is only at puberty that the epiphyseal growth plates also begin to ossify. Epiphyseal closure occurs later when final adult height is reached. Of course damage to bones in the vicinity of the epiphyseal growth plate may affect further growth.

— You may be shown *a supracondylar fracture of the humerus* which occurs when a child falls back on an outstreched arm whilst it is extended. Complications include Volkmann's ischemic contracture arising from damage to the brachial artery as well as damage to the median and ulnar nerves.

— A *Greenstick fracture* describes the common type of fracture in children when the fracture line does not cross both sides of the bone margin because of the thick and elastic periosteum.

— *Perthes disease* is an avascular necrosis of the femoral head where bone resorption is followed by revascularisation. There is an initial increase in bone density of the femoral head and this is followed by fragmentation and mushrooming of the femoral head. There is often interspersed sclerosis and radiolucent areas. It is almost always unilateral and if bilateral an epiphyseal dysplasia should be suspected. Other causes of such fragmentation of the femoral head include: sickle cell disease, post traumatic, septic arthritis and TB of the hip.

— *Slipped upper femoral epiphyses* (SUFE). Here there is a separation of the epiphyses from the femoral neck through the growth plate resulting in medial displacement of the femoral head in relation to the femoral neck (actually posteriorly and inferiorly). In 25% of cases the condition is bilateral. Under normal circumstances one can follow a smooth curve following the medial side of the femur under the femoral head on to the pelvic bone. This is characteristically lost in SUFE. A frog-legged lateral X-ray is the best X-ray for diagnosis.

— *Osgood–Schlatter disease*. There may be soft tissue swelling in the region of the tibial tubercle. Alternatively there may be distortion and fragmentation of the tubercle.

— *Congenital dislocation of the hip*. Often the acetabulum is shallow and dysplastic and the femoral head is hypoplastic and located laterally and superiorly to its expected position. The angle of the acetabulum is greater than normal. Remember that you will not be able to see the femoral head until about 3–6 months of age by which time ossification begins in the femoral head.

— *Dysplastic femoral epiphyses* may be seen occasionally in hypothyroidism.

— *Radial aplasia*. Once seen never forgotten. Its appearance is characteristic with absence of the radius and radial angulation of the hand and wrist. Know a list of associations: TAR syndrome, Fanconi anaemia, VATER syndrome and the Holt–Oram syndrome.

— Know the characteristic features of *osteoarthritis* which consist of loss of joint space (loss of joint cartilage), subchondral cysts, osteophytes and subchondral sclerosis. It may be seen in any cause of arthritis such as repeated haemarthrosis.

— *Osteosarcoma*. It is found most commonly around the knee joint (metaphysis cf. Ewing sarcoma where it is more common in diaphysis). There is cortical bone destruction. Soft tissue swelling occurs secondary to invasion by tumour and sometimes one can see elevation of the periosteum with accompanying subperiosteal new bone formation (Codman triangle). On occassions one can see radiating bone spicules in the mass (sun-ray appearance).

— *Osteopetrosis* manifests itself on X-ray as generalised increased bone density and loss of the normal trabecular pattern of bone. As the condition progresses the ends of long bones may develop flask-shaped deformities. AR/AD. Features consist of (a) pancytopenia as a result of bone marrow involvement (may give a dry bone marrow tap); (b) extramedullary haemopoiesis leading to hepatosplenomegaly; (c) nerve compression leading to blindness, deafness and other cranial nerve palsies. Treatment is supportive but improvement can be expected with steroids and bone marrow transplant.

— Chronic disease may manifest itself on X-ray as linear horizontal growth arrest lines and metaphyseal lucencies. This is seen especially in ALL.

— *Multiple skull lesions* are seen in histiocytosis X, leukaemia and neuroblastoma.

— *Wormian bones* are seen in Down syndrome, cleidocranial dysostosis and hypothyroidism.

CLINICAL SCENARIOS

The child with a limp

This is important clinically and many questions will expect you to recognise the typical features for grey cases. Limps can be subdivided according to whether they are painful and painless.

— *Painful limp* (most common in childhood): the child usually has a reduced stance phase (foot down on ground) called an antalgic gait so that the affected limb is used as little as possible. A reduced swing phase may be seen in an arthritis where the joint is stiff or painful.

— *Painless limps* produce a typical waddling gait (Trendelenburg gait). It may be seen in congenital dislocation of the hip, proximal muscle weakness and with weak hip abductors. Steppage gait is caused by inadequate foot dorsiflexion (for example lateral popliteal nerve damage) and leads to excessive knee flexion so that the toes clear the ground during the swing phase.

An examination should consist of a rheumatological and neurological examination.

Pain at any age

In children it is vital to examine all the joints of the lower limb even if the child complains of pain in only one joint. This is because referred pain is very common. In children hip pain is commonly referred to the knee, thigh and groin. The following list includes acute and chronic conditions.

— Common miscellaneous disorders: ingrowing toenail, uncomfortable shoes (e.g. pebble).
— Trauma.
— Septic arthritis/osteomyelitis.
— Reactive arthritis.
— Joint involvement in: haemophilia, Henoch–Schönlein purpura.
— Juvenile chronic arthritis and other rheumatic conditions.
— Osteochondritis: Osgood–Schlatter disease, chondromalacia patellae and Perthe disease (see later).
— Tendon or ligament damage including enthesitis.
— Sickle crisis.
— Tumours (primary and secondary).
— Neurological problems (cerebral tumour, hemiplegia, myopathy, spinal disorder and drug intoxication).

Particular causes of limp that affect special age groups

Perthe disease

There is segmental avascular necrosis of the femoral head. Look in the history for the signs of a typical case. The child is more commonly male (M:F 5:1), between the ages of four and ten, and shorter than expected for his age. There is generalised retarded bone age, presenting with a limp that may or not be painful (classic painless limp). There may be referred knee and groin pain. On examination there is reduced abduction and internal rotation. Extensive involvement of the epiphyses may result in a permanent femoral head deformity. X-ray appearances as described above. MRI may be useful in early diagnosis. A bone scan will show reduced uptake in the femoral epiphysis. Treatment consists of the principle of containment (aiming to keep the healing femoral head in the acetabulum during femoral head remodelling). This can be accomplished by abduction bracing and possibly osteotomy. Healing can take up to two years. Complications include femoral head deformity and arthritis of the hip (especially in older children).

Slipped upper femoral epiphyses (SUFE)
This involves a posterior separation of the femoral epiphysis from the metaphysis through the growth plate. It tends to occur in two distinct types of children usually between the ages of 10–15. Obese hypogonadal children (with low circulating sex hormones) and tall thin children often boys (often post growth spurt, thus younger in girls). This implies a possible endocrine basis for the condition (there is an association with hypothyroidism). It is bilateral in 25% of cases. It presents with a painful limp. Acutely all hip movement is painful. If there has been a gradual slippage there will be limited medial rotation and the hip will be externally rotated. Radiological features are discussed earlier. The condition should be considered an emergency and requires epiphysiodesis (with a screw) for mild slips and possible open reduction and fixation or osteotomy for bigger slips.

Transient synovitis (irritable hip)
This is the commonest cause of a limp in children. It is commoner in boys and occurs between the ages of 2 and 12 years. If often occurs following an upper respiratory tract infection. There is a history of a sudden onset of a limp and there may be pain in the hip (which may be referred to the knee) and the child may refuse to weightbear. There are no signs of inflammation (such as localised swelling, heat or erythema) and hip movement is painful. Septic arthritis produces a more acutely painful immobile joint cf. transient synovitis. In transient synovitis there may be pain and restriction to abduction, internal rotation and extension. There may be some tenderness to palpation over the anterior aspect of the hip joint. To help differentiate it from septic arthritis the ESR and white cell count (including differential) are usually normal or mildly elevated. X-rays and ultrasound may show fluid in the joint space but less than one would expect in septic arthritis. Ultrasound may sometimes differentiate clear fluid and pus. If one cannot exclude a septic arthritis then the joint fluid is aspirated. It may be cloudy, but in septic arthritis it is purulent. The condition usually improves within a couple of weeks with bed rest, analgesics and possibly some skin traction. A later diagnosis of Perthe disease is made in about 6% of cases of initially diagnosed transient synovitis.

Investigations in a child with a limp will be guided by history and examination but initially will consist of: FBC, ESR, blood culture (if febrile or other evidence of septic arthritis or osteomyelitis), X-ray and ultrasound. Then joint aspiration (+/− ultrasound guidance), isotope bone scan and tuberculin test.

Possible slide questions
— You may be shown a slide of an X-ray of *congenital dislocation of the hip (CDH)*. It is associated with a positive family history, commoner in girls, breech presentation, oligohydramnios and first baby. Be familiar with the

clinical correlates of a positive Ortolani and Barlow test. The consequences of a missed CDH are: asymmetrical thigh skin folds, shortened leg length, tendency to falling, limping and a limited abduction of the hip.

— A common slide in the examination is that of swollen hands with swollen fingers in a black child. The diagnosis is usually *sickle dactylitis* but the differential diagnoses include juvenile chronic arthritis and other connective tissue disorders.

— You may be shown a slide of a child or X-ray of *scoliosis*. Scoliosis means a lateral curve of the spine. Eighty per cent are found in girls. Postural scoliosis corrects with an adjustment of posture (as opposed to structural scoliosis). It may be noticed by finding one shoulder higher than the other or a prominent scapula. The scoliosis in the thoracic region is usually convex to the right (higher right shoulder) and to the left in the lumbar region. It is checked by asking the child to bend forwards since this makes the scoliosis more pronounced as a result of vertebral rotation. About 80–85% are idiopathic, the remainder are caused by congenital spinal disorders such as hemivertebrae, neuromuscular disorders such as muscular dystrophies, and syndromes such as Marfan and mucopolysaccharidoses. Severe scoliosis should be referred for assessment for possible surgical correction.

Bone tumours

Some questions will expect you to pick up on typical clinical features.

Osteosarcoma

Its peak incidence is during the growth spurt of puberty. It arises in the metaphysis of long bones mainly, with half of these around the knee joint. It can present with pain, limp, deformity and pathological fracture. X-ray appearance is described above but CT scan will also be useful. Biopsy provides the diagnosis. Treatment consists of preoperative chemotherapy (usually), then surgery followed by repeat chemotherapy. Regular surveillance is required to diagnose possible pulmonary metastases early so that these can be treated with pulmonary resection and further chemotherapy. The prognosis is better the further the tumour is from the trunk.

Ewing sarcoma

This is the second most common malignant bone tumour of childhood and tends to occur at a slightly younger age than osteosarcoma. Presentation is similar to osteosarcoma (except that systemic symptoms are commoner) and X-ray findings show more periosteal bone formation compared with osteosarcoma. Treatment consists of combined chemotherapy and radiotherapy.

Osteoid osteoma

This is a benign tumour that occurs in childhood. It is commoner in boys and may affect any bone (but is commonest in the femur and tibia). Characteristic features include extreme sensitivity over the site of the tumour and nocturnal pain. The X-ray is classic with a small osteolytic lesion of about 1 cm surrounded by an area of osteosclerosis. Bone scan is useful in localisation. The pain is said to be very sensitive to aspirin. Treatment is surgical removal. Bone cysts may come up as a slide and are usually located in the metaphysis of long bones and may cause bone pain and pathological fracture.

Osteochondroma

Commonest between 10–20 years of age and appears as a bony outgrowth which may be single or multiple.

Neuroblastomas

These commonly metastasise to bone.

Craniosynostosis

This is a common slide question. There is premature fusion of the sutures (sagittal, coronal and/or lambdoid sutures) that can be idiopathic or associated with various syndromes, secondary to hypothyroidism (commonest cause), over treatment with thyroxine therapy, hypophosphataemia, uncontrolled rickets and hypercalcaemia. A skull X-ray may show loss of suture lines as a result of their premature fusion.

Complications include: raised intracranial pressure, cranial nerve palsies especially deafness and strabismus, exophthalmos and cosmetic deformity. When craniosynostosis occurs there is reduced growth of the skull perpendicular to the line of fusion of the sutures which results in the structural abnormalities.

Crouzon syndrome

AD. There is premature fusion of all three sutures. This results in a deformed skull with reduced anteroposterior diameter, prominent forehead, hypertelorism, proptosis, beaking of the nose, low-set ears, prominent ridges at the sites of suture fusion and usually normal intelligence.

Apert syndrome

AD inheritance and a high mutation rate. There is premature fusion of the coronal suture which results in a reduced AP diameter, prominent forehead, flattened occiput and high vertex (called tower head, acrocephaly or turricocephaly). It is associated with syndactyly.

Carpenter syndrome

A similar AR condition to Apert syndrome with polydactyly as a feature.

Scaphocephaly (dolicocephaly)

There is premature fusion of the sagittal suture resulting in increased AP diameter of the skull.

Brachycephaly

This results from premature fusion of the lambdoid sutures and produces a flat occiput. Management involves referral to a specialised team consisting of plastic surgeons, orthopaedic and neurosurgeons who attempt to reconstruct the skull to reduce complications and improve cosmetic appearance.

Sprengel deformity

A possible slide question is of a child with Sprengel deformity. With the child's back towards you one scapula can be seen to be small, hypoplastic and higher than the other one. There is reduced scapular movement. It arises from the failure of the scapula to descend to its correct final position during fetal life. Associated with Klippel–Feil syndrome. In severe forms a bone (omovertebral bone) may bridge the gap between the scapula and the cervical vertebra.

Torticollis

Torticollis is a common presentation in children. It may be congenital or acquired. Congenital causes may be as a result of intrauterine positioning. A sternomastoid haematoma (sternomastoid tumour) may be seen after a traumatic delivery and may fibrose later on, causing contracture of the ipsilateral sternocleidomastoid muscle. Acquired causes include: neurological causes such as basal ganglia disorders and tumours. Musculoskeletal causes include cervical spine bony abnormalities, tumours or infection. Post traumatic causes. Retropharyngeal abscess. Ocular causes such as ocular imbalance and strabismus. Rarely associated with severe gastro-oesophageal reflux (Sandifer syndrome) sometimes with back scratching.

Arthritis and anaemia

Know the clinical pattern of arthritis and anaemia. The differential diagnosis includes: sickle cell anaemia, acute leukaemia, neuroblastoma (secondary to bone marrow invasion), juvenile chronic arthritis, TB arthritis, connective tissue disease such as SLE, any chronic arthropathy treated with NSAIDs which can cause GI bleeding. Methotrexate can also cause bone marrow suppression and is sometimes used in treating JCA.

Pes cavus

Know the causes of pes cavus which you might be presented with in a slide question or a short case. Causes include: Friedreich ataxia, Duchenne muscular dystrophy, spina bifida, tethered cord syndrome, Charcot–Marie–Tooth disease, idiopathic and familial.

Caffey disease

Caffey disease or infantile cortical hyperostosis is usually seen in the first year of life and produces a tender swelling of flat bones (such as the mandible) and tubular bones (such as ulna and radius). X-ray shows an intense periosteal reaction thought to be caused by inflammation. Treatment may be required in the form of steroids. It may sometimes be mistaken for healing fractures as a result of physical abuse or osteomyelitis.

Lyme disease

Be aware of the child who presents initially with an erythematous annular lesion in association with neurological, cardiac and/or joint symptoms. Think of Lyme disease which is caused by the spirochaete *Borrelia burgdorferi* released by bites from Ixodes ticks. It is found in the USA, Australia and in various parts of Europe, so look for travel abroad in the history. Lyme disease presents with a gradually enlarging erythematous annular lesion usually on the trunk, thigh or buttocks called erythema chronicum migrans which can occur up to three weeks following the initial bite (present in about 80% of cases and at this stage may be confused with erythema marginatum, erythema multiforme or a cellulitis). Accompanying the skin lesion or immediately following it headache, malaise and fever are common.

After a few weeks to months neurological signs may develop and cause a meningoencephalitis, cranial nerve palsies, peripheral neuropathy and a Guillain–Barré-like syndrome. Cardiac problems include a pancarditis and various conduction defects. Arthritis develops in about 50% of patients with inflammation involving the knees in particular but other joints may be involved. Soft tissue swelling can be considerable. Arthritis is often recurrent.

Investigations include serology for *B. burgdorferi*. Treatment involves penicillin and NSAIDs for symptoms. Differential diagnosis includes JCA, rheumatic fever and Reiter syndrome (combination of urethritis, arthritis and conjunctivitis often following enteric infections such as *Shigella*, *Campylobacter* and *Salmonella*).

Dermatomyositis

A common exam question both in the grey cases and slides. It presents at all ages of childhood and is commoner in girls. In children the condition demonstrates marked vasculitis of skin, muscles and internal organs. There may be a gradually worsening or acute onset of a symmetrical proximal myopathy which may be mild or be severe enough to make the child bed-bound, develop the Gower manoeuvre, affect the muscles of swallowing and speech and possibly result in respiratory depression.

Skin features (often seen in slides) consist of non-pitting oedema, periorbital oedema, violacious/purple heliotrope around the eyes and cheeks which may extend down to the upper trunk (shawl distribution). Pink scaly-like lesions are found on extensor surfaces such as knuckles, elbows, knees and ankles (Gottron patches). Look for the characteristic telangiectasia in the nailbed. You should know that it is common to get calcinosis in the skin, joints and subcutaneous tissues (possible X-ray slide).

The vasculitis affects in particular the gastrointestinal tract and may present as abdominal pain (possible acute abdomen), bleeding or perforation.

Diagnosis is made by finding a raised ESR, raised CPK, characteristic EMG (polyphasic short motor potentials with spontaneous fibrillations), muscle biopsy (inflammatory changes). An MRI is sometimes performed at a particular site to define the degree of inflammation and to follow its course accurately with treatment. Treatment involves physiotherapy and oral or i.v. steroids depending on the severity. Resistant cases may require methotrexate, gammaglobulin and possibly immunosuppressives.

Systemic lupus erythematosus (SLE)

Seen in children of all ages and is commoner in girls (especially after menarche) and in the Afro-Caribbean population. It may present with generalised symptoms such as malaise, fever, weight loss, lymphadenopathy or splenomegaly. Arthritis typically causes a symmetrical small joint polyarthritis. Skin features are varied and may include the typical malar butterfly rash (differential diagnoses include dermatomyositis, malar flush of mitral stenosis, eczema or contact dermatitis), photosensitivity, nail-fold infarcts, splinter haemorrhages and possibly Raynaud phenomenon. Renal involvement is common (commonest presentation of lupus in children) and frequently presents as a nephrotic syndrome but nephritis may also occur (or there may be a slow progression to chronic renal failure). CNS involvement may cause peripheral neuropathies, nerve palsies, fits or changes in behaviour and even psychosis. Cardiac involvement can produce a pericarditis, cardiac failure and non-bacterial vegetations on the mitral and aortic valves (Libman–Sacks endocarditis). Haematological abnormalities result from autoimmune phenomena and include leucopenia, thrombocytopenia and a Coombs' positive haemolytic anaemia. Lung involvement includes a bilateral lower lobe alveolitis and pleuritis +/- effusion.

Drug-induced lupus syndrome is seen with hydralazine, isoniazid, propylthiouracil and produces a lupus-like syndrome without the typical malar rash, renal and CNS involvement and complement levels are normal. Antihistone antibodies are often seen.

Investigations include: raised ESR, antinuclear antibodies are positive in 95% of cases. Seventy-five per cent of cases will have antidouble-stranded DNA antibodies. Rheumatoid factor is positive in 30%. Low levels of CH50, C3 and C4 (especially if renal involvement). Renal biopsy in suspected renal involvement.

Treatment consists of supportive measures such as transfusion, analgesics, antibiotics, steroids and possibly immunosuppressive agents (if steroid resistant or for steroid sparing properties). Plasmapharesis may be used in some patients.

Neonatal lupus

Maternal SLE results in the transplacental transfer of IgG antibodies which cause the following: skin rash (transient) with pink macules or papules — half the babies will have complete heart block (permanent and noted in the postnatal examination as a bradycardia). Thrombocytopenia and anaemia (both transient). The neonate (and mother if asymptomatic) should be investigated for antinuclear antibodies, antiRo antibodies (associated with complete heart block) and anti-La antibodies (associated with the rash). Maternal SLE is also associated with recurrent miscarriage and stillbirth.

Kawasaki disease

Know about the criteria for diagnosing Kawasaki disease. Five out of the following must be present:

a. Fever for more than five days.
b. Polymorphous rash (various types from maculopapular to urticarial can occur).
c. Cervical lymphadenopathy (often unilateral).
d. Mucosal involvement: dry red chapped lips, strawberry tongue, oropharyngeal erythema.
e. Involvement of extremities: indurated, erythematous and oedematous hands and feet (palms and soles). Fingertip and toe desquamation (usually after about ten days).
f. Conjunctivitis: bilateral non-suppurative inflammation.

Other systems to be affected include:

— CVS: Coronary artery aneurysms and thrombosis (with consequent myocardial ischaemia) usually develop between 2–4 weeks from onset. In addition there may be a myocarditis and pericarditis. Vasculitis may be severe.

— CNS: aseptic meningitis, nerve palsies.

— GUS: Sterile pyuria, urethritis.

— Musculoskeletal: arthritis.

— GI: Diarrhoea, vomiting and hepatitis (usually mild) and gallbladder hydrops.

Investigations show: raised white cell count, thrombocytosis (with risk of coronary artery thrombosis) usually increases in second to third week, increased ESR, increased CRP, increased ANCA (indicative of the vasculitis), sterile pyuria and increased liver enzymes. ECG: For arrhythmias and myocarditis. Echocardiogram should be performed to look for aneurysms at diagnosis and repeated at regular intervals since aneurysms can occur many weeks following the illness.

Treatment involves:

a. Intravenous gammaglobulin as a high dose single infusion (or lower dose over 4–5 days) which helps to reduce the incidence of coronary artery aneurysms if given in the first ten days.
b. Aspirin should be given for the first two weeks at high dose and then at a reduced dose for six months (in an attempt to reduce the likelihood of platelet aggregation and thrombosis occurring).
c. If coronary artery aneurysm with thrombosis occurs treatment with streptokinase and prostacyclin.

Prognosis: Less than 50% of children (untreated) will develop coronary aneurysms but over half of these will resolve spontaneously within a couple of years.

The prognosis is better in children who are female, aged more than one year, who have fusiform aneurysm compared to saccular aneurysms with a diameter of less than 4 mm and a low platelet count.

Non-accidental injury (NAI)

You should be familiar with the characteristics of fractures in children that lead one to suspect non-accidental injury. These are bucket handle metaphyseal fractures (of long bones), spiral fractures (caused by twisting of long bones), mid-shaft fractures (caused by direct impact), fractures on X-ray that appear to be of differing ages and fractures particularly of the ribs, skull and pelvis. Other features that should lead you to the diagnosis are many significant bruises in an infant below the age of one year (after which time a certain amount of bruising is expected from attempts at walking and so on). If there are many bruises at several different stages of resolution (unreliable) or if bruises have characteristic patterns such as fingertip bruising, hand-slap marks, bite marks or bruises in unexpected places such as the perineum or ears then you should suspect non-accidental injury. In addition look for cigarette burns, scalds, retinal haemorrhages, subdural effusions, torn frenulum and the characteristic 'frozen watchfulness' of the child (which describes the alert but somewhat anxious appearance). There may be failure to thrive, under-achievement at school and developmental delay.

Other features in the history that may lead you to suspect NAI are any delay in seeking medical attention, inconsistencies in the history, inappropriate parental concern (either too much or too little), abnormal affect of the parents and anger at the thought of admission of the child. Parents may accuse or protect each other's stories; the child may try to cover up for what his parents might have done. Sexual abuse may come to light by the child confiding in someone, by the presentation of vaginal bleeding or discharge, recurrent abdominal pain or the development of sexually transmitted diseases such as warts or through pregnancy in an adolescent girl. Reflex anal dilatation occurs in sexual abuse but also in children with chronic constipation. The commonest presentations of Münchausen by proxy is with recurrent apnoeas, failure to thrive, haematuria, recurrent fever or with multiple unlinked presentations.

In the case of bruising and fractures, bleeding and clotting problems should be excluded as well as underlying conditions such as osteogenesis imperfecta. A skeletal survey (and possibly a bone scan) and clotting studies should then be performed.

In all these cases described above the paediatrician's main concern is the wellbeing and safety of the child. A detailed history and examination should be performed and clearly documented and injuries should be treated appropriately. If suspicion is high then the child must be admitted. The 'at risk' register should be looked up and social services should be contacted. A case conference should be organised as soon as possible.

Dermatology 12

There are many paediatric dermatological conditions: there are however particular ones that make regular appearances in the examination and you should be familiar with them. A large number of questions relating to dermatology turn up in the slides section of the written part of the examination; be aware that although this is a test of recognition, the slides are usually accompanied by questions testing basic knowledge about the condition. Dermatology problems may of course turn up in the clinical examination as well as elsewhere. This chapter covers the commoner dermatological conditions and tries to pinpoint possible areas of questioning.

NAPPY RASH

You should be familiar with these rashes and able to distinguish between them.

Napkin dermatitis

This is sometimes called ammoniacal dermatitis and is commonly caused by inadequate frequency of nappy changing. This causes bacterial conversion of urine to ammonia which is an alkaline irritant leading to erythema and ulceration. There is characteristic sparing of the flexures. Treat with frequent changing, exposure, zinc and castor oil cream and careful washing with each change.

Candidiasis

This can occur on its own or following napkin dermatitis. It appears as bright red areas which involve the flexures. It often spreads from the anus. Characteristic satellite lesions may be seen in the area. May follow a course of antibiotics. Inspection of the mouth for oral candidiasis is essential. Treat with topical nystatin.

Infantile seborrhoeic dermatitis

This is a common self-limiting rash in the first 2–3 months of life appearing as erythematous and scaly lesions. It especially affects the skin folds of the groin, neck and scalp (the latter causing yellow crusting and greasy scales — cradle cap). Treatment involves a mild steroid and antiseptic cream. It may be mistaken occasionally for atopic eczema. Cradle cap is treated with an antiseborrhoeic shampoo and removal of the scales with a mineral oil.

ECZEMA

The following are characteristic features of eczematous lesions:

— Inflamed skin which is hot and erythematous.
— Spongiosis (separation of keratinocytes secondary to oedema causing intradermal vesicles to appear).
— Weeping of fluid on to the surface with crusting and excoriation which chronically leads to a thickening and lichenification of the skin.
— Secondary infection can occur in the broken skin.

Atopic eczema has a genetic component (if both parents were affected there is a 60% risk that the child will be also), a dietary component (some children find that certain foods cause exacerbation, for example milk and eggs) and additional exacerbating factors such as contact with woollen clothing, humidity and excessive drying of the skin. Half of all patients with eczema will commence symptoms in the first year of life and 90% by five years. It is usually self-remitting with 50%, and 90% of patients symptom-free at 13 and 18 years respectively. Peak onset is at 2–6 months of age.

— *Infantile eczema*: There is usually crusting, scaling and weeping starting on the face. The nappy area is not usually affected. Extensors are then affected and later there is a gradual spread of lesions on to the flexures.

— *Childhood eczema*: The exudative weeping lesions diminish and give rise to the lichenification especially on the flexures. Sago grain vesicles may be seen in the palms and soles of the feet.

— *Adult phase*: Seen in teenagers and is similar to the childhood phase with more lichenification seen. You should be familiar with the complications. Skin infections are common and may be bacterial (commonly *Staph. aureus*) or viral (esp. *Herpes simplex* causing eczema herpeticum). Severe atopic eczema patients may develop growth retardation (approximately 10%): whether this is a result of the disease itself, steroid treatment or a combination of these factors is not certain.

— *Treatment*: Involves education of the parents and the child. Avoid exacerbating factors. Use emollients to prevent dry skin (used as soaps, bath oils and applied to the affected skin after baths). Topical corticosteroids are applied twice daily to affected areas (not more than 1% hydrocortisone applied to children's faces of less than one year old). Stronger ones (such as betnovate and dermovate) can be used on the hands and feet. Antibiotics are sometimes used since some flare-ups are associated with *Staph. aureus* overgrowth. Sedative antihistamines can reduce nocturnal itching and help with sleep. Bandaging can be used in the form of zinc oxide impregnated cotton bandages. Weeping lesions can best be treated by soaking the affected lesions in 1/8000 potassium permanganate solution. For more severe, extensive and topical treatment-resistant disease, systemic steroids can be used. Chinese herbal teas also have reported success.

— *Differential diagnosis*: Includes seborrhoeic dermatitis (less than 3–6 months old), scabies (look for burrows especially in the finger webs), napkin dermatitis and tinea corporis (which looks like large scaly rings). Intertrigo occurs at flexural creases and appears as a moist erythematous rash often in tubby infants.

PSORIASIS

The commonest chronic form of psoriasis — psoriasis vulgaris — with which we are familiar in adults is very uncommon below the age of 15 years. The commonest form of psoriasis in paediatric populations is guttate (drop-like) psoriasis occurring over the trunk and limbs 10–14 days following a group B *Streptococcal* infection and lasting 2–3 months. The lesions are small (< 1 cm) and ovoid in shape, pink in colour with silvery scales.

Other forms include psoriasis vulgaris which is commoner in older teenagers. It is a chronic form of psoriasis with a predeliction for the scalp, extensor surfaces of the knees, elbows and lumbosacral areas. Classic lesions consist of well circumscribed raised erythematous, salmon-pink plaques with silvery scales.

Pustular psoriasis is localised to the palms and soles and consists of itchy sterile vesicles. Napkin psoriasis affects the perineum. Nail psoriasis (seen in 5% of those with skin disease) consists of onycholysis, nail pitting and oil droplet formation. Psoriatic arthropathy (seen in 7% of patients with skin disease) often with distal interphalangeal joint involvement or as a monoarthritis which may precede the skin changes. Psoriasis demonstrates the Koebner phenomenon where lesions occur on sites of previous trauma (also seen with warts, lichen planus and vitiligo).

Treatment

This includes topical dithranol in Lassar's paste (zinc oxide and salicylic acid), coal tar preparations in the form of creams and shampoos, topical corticosteroids, calcipotriol (a vitamin D derivative), UVB, PUVA (combination of a photosensitiser called psoralens and UVA) and systemic treatments such as methotrexate, etretinate and cyclosporin.

CLINICAL SCENARIOS

Adenoma sebaceum

A possible question relates the child who is referred to the dermatologist because of acne that is not responding to treatment. You are told that the child is on anticonvulsants and is behind at school. These should be sufficient clues to lead you to think of the possibility of a misdiagnosis of adenoma sebaceum for acne, and the diagnosis of tuberous sclerosis. Adenoma sebaceum is common in tuberous sclerosis and usually starts between the ages of two and five.

They are angiofibromas which are red or brown papules, often in a butterfly distribution around the nose (often resembling acne). Remember the other dermatological manifestations of tuberose sclerosis: ash-leaf spots which are hypopigmented macules (seen with Wood's) that may be present from birth; shagreen patches which are leathery in nature often in the lumbosacral area and buttocks, beginning at 2–5 years; and finally subungual fibromas that usually appear from puberty. Café au lait macules are seen rarely.

Port wine stains

Port wine stains (nevus flammeus) are flat (not palpable) pink/red macular vascular lesions caused by dilated capillaries under the skin and occur alone or in association with certain syndromes. Growth occurs in proportion to the child. Port wine stain questions usually appear in two guises. Firstly the child who has Sturge–Weber syndrome with a port wine stain in the ophthalmic division of the trigeminal nerve together with a vascular abnormality in the ipsilateral cerebral cortex and meninges (see chapter 5). The second possibility is where a port wine stain overlies hypertrophy of the underlying soft tissue and bone, especially limbs (usually affecting extremities). This association is referred to as the Klippel–Trenaunay syndrome. Port wine stains can be treated with laser therapy.

Langerhans cell histiocytosis

A possible question may describe a child with a nappy rash that is not responding to treatment. A slide may show you a nappy area which resembles seborrhoeic dermatitis. Think of Langerhans cell histiocytosis (previously called histiocytosis X). There are several forms.

— *Eosinophilic granuloma* (the most benign form) usually presents between the ages of 20–40 with well defined lesions in the skull, vertebrae and ribs. It presents with localised swelling and bone pain.

— *Hand–Schuller–Christian* disease presents in early childhood as a more widespread disease. As a result of infiltration, one may encounter proptosis, diabetes insipidus (caused by infiltration of the pituitary gland with possible growth failure), lytic bone lesions, hepatosplenomegaly, chronic draining otitis media and honeycomb lung. Other causes of a chronic discharge from the ear include chronic otitis externa, cholesteatoma and chronic discharging otitis media.

— *Letterer–Siwe disease* is the most severe form and presents in the first couple of years with fever, anaemia, generalised lymphadenopathy and a seborrhoeic dermatitis-like rash. A skin biopsy, lymph-node biopsy, bone curettage for biopsy with histological analysis (Birbeck granules seen on electron microscopy) and possible skeletal survey may be needed. There is a high spontaneous remission rate. Prognosis depends on age — children under two at presentation have a worse prognosis — and degree of organ involvement. Treatment involves chemotherapy.

Haemangiomas

Haemangiomas are divided up into two types (a) strawberry naevi which are superficial (also called capillary haemangioma); and (b) cavernous haemangiomas which are deeper in the skin. Strawberry naevi are bright red, raised, lobulated lesions with distinct borders. They are common (occurring in 10% of infants) and usually start growing in the first few weeks of life and rapidly thereafter until about six months to a year of age. Thereafter involution takes place so that most lesions have completely disappeared after the age of six or seven. Cavernous haemangiomas, since they are deeper in the skin, may be skin coloured or bluish/purple in colour and have irregular borders.

Complications include bleeding, infection, functional impairment (if around the orbit), Kassabach–Merritt syndrome (platelet sequestration which may result in thrombocytopenia) and high output cardiac failure secondary to AV shunting (the latter two only in extensive lesions). Treatment is conservative except where lesions compromise function such as periocular lesions (which may lead to amblyopia), near the airway or the Kassabach–Merritt syndrome. Treatment here involves a short course of systemic steroids to help involution or laser/surgery. Remember that the presence of a haemangioma should prompt the search for additional haemangiomas on the skin and possible further investigation for internal or visceral haemangiomas. The baby with stridor and cutaneous haemangiomas should undergo laryngoscopy for detection of laryngeal haemangiomas.

Mongolian blue spot

Never mistake the appearance of a Mongolian blue spot which is a grey/blue macular discoloration usually seen on the lumbosacral region, but also seen on the limbs and buttocks. It is especially common in babies of Asian or black descent (seen in approximately 80% compared with 10% of white children). They usually fade spontaneously but this may take many years. Differential diagnosis in a slide would include non-accidental injury.

Pigmented naevi

A common slide is that of pigmented naevi. Congenital melanocytic naevi are present at birth. Size is very variable and they are referred to as giant naevi if they are more than about 20 cm. They are often associated with hair appearing on their surface. They grow in proportion to the child's growth. The main concern is the development of melanoma in the larger lesions (approximately 7% lifetime risk). Management involves regular examination and follow up (including comparison photos), possible full thickness excision and grafting and dermabrasion (cosmetic only).

Erythema multiforme (EM)

This often comes up in the slide section: there are major and minor types. The minor types are usually symmetrical target-shaped lesions (pale centre and red surrounding) most commonly on the hands, feet and extensor surfaces of the limbs. There is another vesicular/bullous type in which the bullae are central or around the periphery of the lesion. They are non-pruritic (unlike urticaria). Lesions usually evolve over a couple of weeks and settle spontaneously over 4–6 weeks (unlike urticaria which is in the differential diagnosis).

Causes: 50% idiopathic. Infections: *Herpes simplex* (think of herpes if attacks are recurrent), *Mycoplasma*, EBV, *Histioplasmosis*. Drugs: penicillins, sulphonamides. Systemic diseases: collagen vascular disease. Stevens–Johnson syndrome is the extreme from of erythema multiforme (EM major) and is a severe bullous condition, which involves at least two out of three of the following mucosal surfaces: oral, eye (conjunctivitis, corneal ulceration and uveitis) and genital ulceration. There is a severe systemic upset and associated polyarthritis, pneumonia and severe fluid and electrolyte imbalance can occur (mortality 5–20%). Treatment of EM is removal of the causative agent if possible. Steroids are controversial. Stevens–Johnson syndrome is managed with mouthwashes, antibiotics to prevent secondary infection and careful fluid and electrolyte balance. In addition an ophthalmological opinion should be obtained.

Erythema nodosum

Another exam favourite. It presents as painful erythematous nodules up to 4–5 cm in diameter on the shins that develop over a few days and fade to leave possible pigmentation of the skin. It usually presents mainly over the age of five. Causes include infections: *Streptococcal*, TB, cat-scratch disease, leptospirosis; drugs: penicillin, tetracyclines, sulphonamides, oral contraceptives; systemic disease: inflammatory bowel disease (10% of IBD), sarcoidosis, connective tissue disease. Recurrent erythema nodosum is associated with IgG2 deficiency. Treatment is conservative with pain relief. In children the nodules often go unnoticed and are commonly mistaken for other conditions such as: insect bites, bruises, thrombocytopenic purpura and NAI.

Scalded skin syndrome (Ritter syndrome)

Caused by *Staph. aureus* phage group 2 which produces toxic epidermal necrolysis via an exfoliative toxin. Large blisters develop which burst leaving a red raw underlying skin. Skin displays the Nikolsky sign where gentle pressure applied to a bulla results in its extension. There is also usually a fever and general malaise. Treatment is with antibiotics.

Impetigo

Can be caused by *Staph.* or *Strep.* infections. The natural history is from papules to thin-walled pustules or bullae which rupture leaving a shallow erythematous base. It is almost always associated with the characteristic orange/honey-coloured crusting which you should look for in a slide to make the diagnosis. It is most often found on the face in children. If bullae predominate call it bullous impetigo. Remember that impetigo can give rise to serious complications including osteomyelitis and pneumonia. The source of recurrent impetigo may be from the nose of a child who may be a carrier of the offending organism. In this case topical antibiotic applications to the nostrils may help.

Toxic shock syndrome

This is caused by toxic shock syndrome toxin (TSST-1). It occurs most commonly in older children (15–20 years) with high fever, myalgia, malaise, headache, abdominal pain, vomiting and diarrhoea and hypotension. Renal failure, thrombocytopenia and hepatitis are possible sequelae. Skin manifestations include a diffuse macular erythema which often desquamates usually from the palms and soles of the feet after about ten days (in a similar way to Kawasaki disease and scarlet fever). It has been associated with the use of hyperabsorbent tampons which have been in situ for excessive periods (in vaginas colonised with the toxin producing *Staph.*). Treatment is with resuscitation, antibiotics and removal of precipitating factors.

Peutz–Jehgers syndrome

A common slide is of a child with perioral pigmentation with accompanying symptoms that may include abdominal pain and gastrointestinal bleeding. This may be caused by hamartomatous polyps usually in the small bowel (but may also be present in the large bowel) (AD inheritance).

Dermatophyte infections

Common in paediatrics. They invade keratinised tissue of the skin, hair and nails. The species include *Microsporum*, *Epidermophyton* and *Trichophyton*. The condition is described according to the site affected — thus tinea corporis affects the body. Lesions are usually annular and scaly with raised borders that expand peripherally, with small vesicles on the advancing border and central clearing (and hence called ringworm). Tinea capitis involves the scalp resulting in scaling, hair loss, a kerion — a boggy inflammatory mass caused by an intense immunological reaction to the fungus with overlying hair loss. The cause is *Microsporum canis* which fluoresces green in Wood's light. Tinea pedis affects the feet causing athlete's foot especially on the soles of the feet and in the toe webs. Tinea unguim affects the nails. Tinea cruris affects the groin area (often seen in males with chronic dermatophyte foot infection). Diagnosis of dermatophyte infections are made by taking scrapings from skin, hair or nails and dissolving them in potassium hydroxide (keratolytic) and then microscopically trying to identify hyphae. Culture is also available. Treatment consists of topical antifungals (imidazoles, nystatin) for localised infection and oral agents (griseofulvin, itraconazole) for widespread infection, nail and scalp involvement.

Tinea versicolor

A common fungal infection in children is tinea versicolor caused by *Pityrosporum orbiculare (Malassezia furfur)*. It affects mainly the upper trunk and arms and sometimes the face. A slide will be recognised by multiple macules, often slightly scaly, that appear either hypopigmented (often in tanned skin) or hyperpigmented (often in fair skin). Diagnosis is made by skin scrapings and culture or by fluorescence with Wood's light where it appears orange. Treat with topical antifungal creams. Do not confuse with the hypopigmented, often symmetrical, annular areas of vitiligo. It presents a convex edge to the normal skin. It is associated with autoimmune disease and therefore consider a thyroid autoantibody screen and blood glucose (for diabetes). Other causes of depigmentation in paediatrics includes tuberous sclerosis (ash-leaf macules), following burns, scars, following infections and bullous skin disorders (post inflammatory inflammation is also known as pityriasis alba).

Erythema marginatum

This may come up as a slide as it has a characteristic appearance. It occurs in about one-fifth of all cases of rheumatic fever. It is found transiently mainly on the trunk and limbs. The rash is flat, non-painful and consists of normal pale areas of skin surrounded by red rings with serpiginous borders. It occurs during acute rheumatic fever (major criteria). Subcutaneous nodules, also seen in rheumatic fever, are small, painless, pea-sized nodules found under the skin mainly over the tendons and joints.

Urticaria

Know what this looks like. It is simply the result of dermal oedema resulting from vasodilatation and increased capillary permeability (because of mast cell release of histamine and other vasoactive substances). Urticaria describes local wheals (with pale centres) and erythema, while angio-oedema involves deeper loose subcutaneous structures (such as feet, hands, lips and upper airway) as well as the dermis. The lesions are pruritic and fade spontaneously over minutes to hours (differentiating them from erythema multiforme). Urticaria may be idiopathic, IgE mediated such as in atopy, allergic (including drugs and food), secondary to infections and stings, complement mediated such as hereditary angio-oedema (see chapter 9), physically mediated such as with UV light, cold, dermographism and cholinergic types of urticaria. Urticaria may be seen in some systemic diseases such as JCA, Behçet disease and SLE. Urticaria is a common rash seen in the prodromal phase of hepatitis B infection. Urticaria lasting more than six weeks is referred to as chronic urticaria and the cause is only found in the minority of cases.

Hand, foot and mouth disease

If you are shown a slide of pustules or vesicles on the hand with a history of similar lesions on the feet, or vesicles or ulceration in the mouth then think of hand, foot and mouth disease. The pustules are usually surrounded by mild erythema. The child may be slightly unwell and there may be a history of contacts with similar lesions. It is caused by Cocksackie virus and resolves spontaneously. I have seen some confusion in slides with herpetic whitlow pustules which may look similar. If faced with a slide of a hand with a pustule in the site of expected paronychia I would go for herpetic whitlow. This is found in children who suck their thumbs and bite their nails a lot (remember also nosocomial infection — common in nurses and thus may spread in a ward.)

Scabies

This is caused by a mite (*Sarcoptes scabei*) that can be spread by close direct contact. The mite burrows in the skin depositing the eggs (which hatch larvae in a few days) in the stratum corneum of the skin and it is the parasites themselves that cause an inflammatory reaction. The burrows can be seen as fine, wavy dark lines up to 1 cm in length with a small papule at one end (not always easy to see because of secondary excoriation). Papules alone are more common in infants compared to linear burrows (which are commoner in older children and adults). Scabies occurs more commonly in immunocompromised children and children with Down syndrome. An erythematous papular rash tends to occur especially in the finger webs and the flexor surface of the wrists and elbows. Although in adults the face tends not to be affected it can be in children. Treatment involves a single application of 1% lindane lotion below the face, to be left on for 12 hours. Alternatively, benzyl benzoate 25% emulsion can be applied and left on for 24 h. Remember that these products are very irritant.

Acrodermatitis enteropathica

A child who develops an acute mucocutaneous perioral or perianal rash (usually eczematous with pustules or bullae) soon after weaning from breast milk (or earlier in bottle-fed babies) must be investigated for the possibility of acrodermatitis enteropathica. It is an AR inherited disease and is caused by defective intestinal zinc absorption. It is also associated with diarrhoea, failure to thrive and hair loss. Low levels of serum zinc and ALP are found. Treatment is with oral zinc supplements which rapidly reverse the symptoms.

Molluscum contagiosum

You may be shown a slide. Lesions are classically single or multiple, dome shaped, flesh coloured, up to 3 mm in diameter and have a characteristic central umbilication. It is caused by the *Pox* virus. Lesions resolve spontaneously but treatment is often given to prevent spread. Treatment includes pricking the centre of the lesion with a sharp-ended instrument dipped in liquid phenol. Alternatively curettage or cryotherapy may be used.

Diabetic skin lesions

Diabetes is associated with the following skin lesions: necrobiosis lipoidica diabeticorum, candida infection, granuloma annulare, lipoatrophy/hypertrophy, stiff joints, waxy skin, eruptive xanthomata and recurrent skin abscesses.

Blistering lesions

Seen in infections (for example, *herpes simplex* infection, *varicella zoster* infections, impetigo), dermatitis herpetiformis, erythema multiforme, epidermolysis bullosa and porphyria (porphyria cutanea tarda, variegate porphyria and congenital erythropoietic porphyria).

NAI

Some slides will show lesions on the skin that do not look as if they were caused by natural phenomena. Sometimes one can make out buckle, whiplash, cigarette butt marks, bite marks, immersion burns or fingertip bruising around the face (caused by squeezing the face). The answer to these slides should mention the possibility of non-accidental injury (NAI). On the subject of unnatural well dermarcated looking lesions, bracelets, necklaces or watchstraps can cause contact dermatitis if they contain chemicals to which the person is sensitised (a common example is nickel allergy). Itching and vesicle formation are common; they improve when contact with the skin is terminated.

Pityriasis rosea

Thought to be caused by a virus since it often occurs in clusters. It is most common in the spring and autumn and is preceded by a herald patch, which is a single circular or oval scaly lesion usually seen on the trunk, abdomen or scapular area. A couple of weeks later there is an eruption of smaller oval scaly macules on the trunk and sometimes upper limbs often following a Christmas tree distribution (following the lines of the ribs). It usually clears after about a month.

Cutis marmorata

A possible slide is bluish mottling/marbling of the skin which can occur normally in neonates as a result of cooling of the skin, or in babies who are peripherally shutdown. Cutis marmorata is also recognised in a number of conditions. These include Down syndrome, Edward syndrome, congenital hypothyroidism and Cornelia de Lange syndrome.

Hirsutism and hypertrichosis

You must know the distinction between these two. Hirsutism refers to the growth of androgen dependent hair whereas hypertrichosis refers to the growth and thickening of hair (which can be anywhere on the body).

Skin and gut lesions

The association of skin and gut lesions occurs in a number of conditions including Peutz–Jegher syndrome, inflammatory bowel disease, hereditary haemorrhagic telangiectasis and Gardener syndrome (colonic premalignant polyps, osteomas of the skull and jaw and dermoid/epidermal tumours).

Scarlet fever

Caused by a group A *Streptococcal* infection that produces an erythrotoxin. There is usually an associated pharyngitis. The rash is a diffuse blanchable punctate erythema commonly seen on the trunk, abdomen and in skin folds. The texture of the rash is often likened to sandpaper. Pastia's lines are dark red lines seen in the skin creases. There is a flushed facial appearance with typical circumoral pallor, and a typical 'strawberry tongue'. After the rash fades there may be a period of skin peeling from the hands and feet. Confirmatory evidence from a throat culture or ASOT titre may be helpful. Do not forget the complications of rheumatic fever and post-*Streptococcal* glomerulonephritis following *Streptococcal* infections.

Granuloma annulare

A relatively common benign self-limiting condition that is found mainly over the extensor tendons on the hands, fingers, feet and legs. It consists of flesh-coloured papules or nodules that spread peripherally forming a ring. The centre is usually slightly depressed and may have a yellowish discoloration. Unlike in adults there is no association with systemic diseases (DM association in adults).

Warts

Warts are caused by the human papilloma virus and are usually flesh coloured, well circumscribed papules and are described according to their site. Verrucas involve the hands and feet. Verrucae plantaris involve the soles of the feet. Condylomata accuminata are genital warts and appear as soft, fleshy polyps or pedunculated lesions: their presence should alert the paediatrician to the possibility of sexual abuse, but they may be transmitted at birth through contact with an infected birth canal.

Incontinentia pigmentii

A very rare X-linked dominant condition that occasionally turns up in the exam. It affects females only (since lethal to males in utero). There are three phases:

1. *Bullous phase*: In first weeks of life bullae/vesicles develop on the trunk and extremities (they contain intradermal eosinophils). Differential diagnosis includes *H. simplex*, bullous impetigo, epidermolysis bullosa.

2. *Papular phase*: Linear streaks of irregular red papules (self-remitting in months). Differential diagnosis includes warts and other papular conditions.

3. *Hyperpigmented stage*: This is the most characteristic phase (thus a possible slide question).
   Whorling/streaky pattern of pigmentation (blue-grey) seen on the trunk and extremities lasting several years and resolving to leave hypopigmented areas.

— *Complications*: One-third have CNS involvement (seizures, UMN signs), two-thirds have delayed dentition/pegged teeth, cardiac and skeletal abnormalities and ophthalmic complications include cataracts and blindness.

Albinism

Inherited in an AR fashion, and characterised by white skin, white hair and blue/pink eyes (nystagmus, photophobia and refractive errors are also common). It is caused by a defect in tyrosine metabolism. In PKU there is failure to convert phenylalanine to tyrosine and hypopigmentation of the skin, hair and eyes results. Mental retardation in a child with blond hair and blue eyes could be a result of Angelman syndrome (see chapter 14).

Icthyosis

Consists of four separate disorders. They all tend to produce fish-like scaling.

— *Icthyosis vulgaris* (AD): Onset in childhood. Produces fine white scales on the skin especially back and extensor surfaces.

— *X-linked icthyosis*: (X-linked recessive). Collodian membrane surrounding baby, later generalised dark scales over the body except palms and soles, possible corneal opacities and a placental enzyme defect that can cause poor uterine contraction in the mother.

— *Lamellar icthyosis*: (AR) Collodion membrane at birth (most common icthyosis with collodion membrane presentation at birth). Later thick dark plate-like coarse brown scales. Nails are often absent.

— *Epidermolytic hyperkeratosis*: (AD). Presents at birth with generalised erythroderma and later develops thick warty scales and recurrent bulla formation.

Treatment involves the advice of a dermatologist. In any icthyosis emollients are very important.

Epidermolysis bullosa

A very rare skin disease that you should know about for the examination. There are different forms that occur depending on which layer the bullae develop in the skin.

— *Epidermolysis bullosa simplex*: (AD) Mild and severe forms exist. Scarring does not occur. Blisters develop within the first year especially over contact areas of skin such as the knees and palms when crawling commences. Localised or generalised blistering occurs in the basal cell layer of the epidermis.

— *Junctional epidermolysis bullosa*: (AR) Presents at birth with bullae or blisters in a generalised distribution. Ranges from mild to severe (potentially fatal with infection and fluid loss). Blistering occurs at the junction of the dermis and epidermis.

— *Dystrophic epidermolysis bullosa*: Two forms exist. Both produce scarring. AD form produces less scarring, is milder and tends to develop with the onset of crawling (knees especially). AR form (EB letalis) can be very severe with mucous membrane involvement, intraoral blistering is common, nail loss and dystrophy, syndactyly, oesophageal strictures, and generally the prognosis is guarded. Blistering occurs in the upper part of the dermis.

Congenital teeth

Sometimes seen in slide questions. They may be secondary to a syndrome such as Ellis van Creveld syndrome or occur on their own. Consultation with a dentist is required, and removal may be necessary if there is a risk of them falling out (with subsequent aspiration) or if they are interfering with breastfeeding.

Discoloured teeth

You may be given a slide of discoloured teeth. Fluorosis may cause a brownish discoloration caused by excessive exposure to fluoride. Tetracyclines may accumulate in bones and teeth producing a brown-yellow discoloration of the teeth: these drugs should not be used before eight years of age (by which time the permanent dentition is fully enamelled).

Dermatitis herpetiformis

An extremely pruritic chronic blistering condition occurring usually after 15 years of age (itching may precede the onset of the rash). It is symmetrical and small vesicles and papules appear on extensor surfaces. Excoriation may mask the lesions. It is associated with gluten-sensitive enteropathy. Treat with dapsone and a gluten-free diet.

Viral exanthemems

Viral exanthemems — being so common — may come up in the examination. See Table 12.1.
Mumps included for completeness.

Table 12.1 Comparison of some exanthemems in children

Disease	Incubation, prodrome and rash	Complications
Measles	Incubation of 8–12 days, followed by cough, coryza and conjunctivitis and Koplik's spots on the inside of the cheeks (short lived). Fever and lymphadenopathy then develop. Then a maculopapular rash develops (initially blotchy and later confluent) which spreads down from around the ears and reaches the legs by day 3 when the face begins to clear. Infectious from onset of prodrome until a week after onset of rash.	Bronchopneumonia and otitis media are common. Abdominal pain (possibly because of mesenteric adenitis) may occur. Lymphopenia may occur. SSPE 5–10 years following measles presents with neurological deterioration (behavioural and intellectual) and myoclonic seizures (disease is fatal). Encephalitis (1/1000) presents with headache, lethargy, vomiting and focal neurological signs (mortality 15%). Prophylaxis with immunisation. Measles has a much worse prognosis in the Third World with a more severe course.
Mumps	Incubation 2–3 weeks, followed by fever and swelling of one or both parotid glands (sometimes tender to palpation). Earache, pain on eating sour juices e.g. lemon; Stensen's duct may be inflamed. Submandibular glands may be involved. Sternal oedema may be seen. Infectious from three days before until nine days after onset of parotid swelling.	Meningo-encephalitis, orchitis (mostly after puberty), oophoritis and acute pancreatitis.
Rubella	Incubation 2–3 weeks. Prodrome of mild coryza or malaise. Generalised lymphadenopathy with suboccipital lymphadenopathy (often painful lymphadenopathy). Fine pink lacy maculopapular rash starting on the face and spreading to the rest of the body. Rash usually lasts three days total. Infectious until seven days after onset of rash.	Encephalitis, thrombocytopenia, small joint arthritis most commonly in older girls. Infection during the first trimester may cause IUGR, microcephaly, CVS defects (most commonly PDA), sensorineural deafness, congenital cataracts, meningoencephalitis, 'salt and pepper retinitis'.

If a non-immune pregnant woman comes into contact with *Varicella* she should be given *Varicella* immunoglobulin (ZIG). If a pregnant woman develops chickenpox a week before or after delivery then the baby should be given ZIG. Acyclovir should be given as soon as the baby develops

Table 12.1 *Continued*

Disease	Incubation, prodrome and rash	Complications
Chicken pox (Varicella)	Incubation period of 10 days–2 weeks. Followed by fever and malaise. The rash develops first usually on the trunk and then spreads elsewhere. Macule to papule to vesicle ('teardrop' on erythematous base) to pustule. Crusting then occurs. There will always be skin lesions at various stages of healing. Mucous membranes may be involved. Infectious from three days before the onset of rash until all the vesicles have crusted (isolation for six days after the vesicles first appeared).	Pneumonia (may result in calcification). Encephalitis (1/1000 often with cerebellar involvement) presenting usually within a couple of weeks from the onset of the rash. Transverse myelitis and nerve palsies may occur. Reye syndrome may develop 3–8 days after onset of rash. Secondary bacterial infection (commonly *Staph.*) A severe haemorrhagic rash may be seen in immunodeficiency states. *Varicella zoster* or shingles occurs after reactivation of the virus that remains dormant in the dorsal root ganglion after primary *Varicella* infection. Blistering lesions on an erythematous base with a dermatomal distribution, which dry and crust usually towards the end of the week. Most common in thoracic region. Pain may be severe. Ophthalmic zoster may occur. Ramsey–Hunt syndrome is caused by involvement of the geniculate ganglion. There may be pain in the ear followed by facial paralysis. Look for vesicles in the external auditory meatus.*
Roseola Infantum (Exanthem subitum) Human herpes virus type 6	Most commonly affects children under two years. The child usually has a high fever for 3–4 days with no obvious source. The fever then subsides giving rise to a diffuse truncal (which later spreads elsewhere) macular rash which usually disappears after a day. Initial neutrophilia may later gives rise to neutropenia.	Febrile convulsions may occur during the febrile period.

the rash (chickenpox in neonates can be very severe). A newborn baby who comes into contact with chickenpox is protected if the mother has previously had the disease. If unsure then you need to check mother's and baby's immune status.

Table 12.1 *Continued*

Disease	Incubation, prodrome and rash	Complications
Erythema infectiosum (Human parvovirus type B19)	Incubation period of one week. Then a 'slapped cheek' rash appears on the face. There may be a fine, diffuse maculopapular rash on the trunk and limbs. It fades with central clearing giving a characteristic lacy pattern.	Intrauterine infection may give rise to fetal hydrops. May give rise to aplastic crisis especially in children with haemoglobinopathies (especially sickle cell disease) or red cell membrane defects (especially hereditary spherocytosis).

*First trimester *Varicella* infection may result in the baby having microcephaly, IUGR, cerebellar hypoplasia, cutaneous scars, often in a dermatomal distribution, limb hypoplasia, muscle hypoplasia, cataracts and choroidoretinitis.

Miscellaneous clinical scenarios

— *Salmon patches* (nevus simplex) — also called stork marks — appear as faint pink macular stains over the eyelids, glabella, forehead, nape of the neck and occiput in many neonates. They are caused by dilated capillaries and resolve spontaneously over months to years although the ones over the back of the head and neck may persist.

— You should be able to recognise what a *cephalhaematoma*, *subaponeurotic haemorrhage* and *chignon* look like on a slide and how you would manage these conditions.

— A *pseudomonas-infected skin lesion* consists of a necrotic centre with an erythematous leading edge. A typical site for such a lesion is following a penetrating foot injury through a shoe.

— Beware of *dermatitis artefacta* — it does not fit into a classic dermatological pattern and is actually caused by the child herself — usually by intense scratching. They tend to be seen as part of attention seeking behaviour in adolescent females with an underlying personality disorder.

— The association of *mouth and genital lesions* is seen in Behçet's disease, lichen planus, Stevens–Johnson syndrome and Sjogren syndrome.

— *Dermatomyositis* has a number of classic skin changes which may be shown to you in slides, clinical cases or alluded to in grey cases (see chapter 11).

— *Depigmentation* is associated with vitiligo, pityriasis versicolor, leprosy, albinism, post-burns phenylketonuria, Chediak–Higashi syndrome and hypopituitarism (the last four cases produce a more generalised picture).

— *Nail pitting.* Seen in psoriasis, lichen planus and alopecia areata.

— The differential diagnoses of *purpura* include thrombocytopenic purpura (decreased production or increased loss) or non-thrombocytopenic purpura such as HSP and *Meningococcal* septicaemia.

— *Café au lait macules* are seen in a number of conditions including neurofibromatosis, Russell–Silver syndrome, Turner syndrome, tuberous sclerosis and the McCune–Albright syndrome.

— Pigmentation of the skin creases, pigmentation in previous scars and pigmentation of buccal mucosa are typical of *Addison disease*. Generalised pigmentation may also be seen.

— *Cushing disease* is associated with acne, purpura, thinning of the skin, purple striae, buffalo hump and a protuberant abdomen (see chapter 7).

CLINICAL DERMATOLOGY

It is quite possible for a child with a chronic skin condition to be invited to appear in the short cases (or long cases). It is equally possible for a child to be brought down from the ward with an acute skin sign providing they are reasonably well. In either case you should have a simple system for dealing with a dermatology case.

— Firstly make yourself familiar with the dermatological definitions so that you can use them confidently.
— Remember that your main tools in dermatological cases are your observational skills.
— Make sure you can see all the skin: that is, undress the child (maintaining dignity).
— Then describe the lesion as follows:

1. Site. Is the lesion localised to one part of the body or is it generalised? Note symmetry.

2. Shape. Are they all of a similar shape? Round, oval, varying shapes etc.

3. Border. Well defined, irregular, serpiginous (erythema marginatum)?

3. Colour. Describe the colour. Is the colour uniform, variegate? Is there hyperpigmentation or hypopigmentation?

4. Size. Are the lesions of a similar size or varying?

5. Are the lesions at different stages of their natural history such as chickenpox (vesicles, pustules and crusting)?

6. Many paediatric skin conditions are itchy, so make a point of looking for marks of excoriation.

7. Feel the lesion. You must first ask the child or parent if the lesion is painful before attempting to touch the lesion. This is unlikely to give you additional information in the majority of conditions since a lesion can be seen to be raised or flat usually without palpation and sometimes the texture of the lesion can also be deduced visually.

8. Finally, no dermatological examination is complete without examining the hair, nails and mucous membranes.

9. Now formulate your differential diagnosis.

Vision and hearing

VISION

Questions relating to vision are rare in the written parts of the examination but relatively common in the slides. It is important that you are able to recognise slides and to list a few a causes in each case. I have listed the commoner ones.

Ptosis

This implies a drooping of the upper eyelid caused by a weakness of the eyelid elevator muscles or their innervation. Here is a list of causes:

— *Horner syndrome:* Ptosis, miosis, enophthalmos and ipsilateral anhydrosis of face. May accompany birth trauma. Caused by disruption of sympathetic fibres anywhere from the hypothalamus.

— *Third nerve palsy:* There may be a complete ptosis. The affected eye looks downwards and outwards (unable to elevate and adduct the eye). The pupil is dilated.

— *Myopathies:* These usually produce a bilateral ptosis: myaesthenia gravis, dermatomyositis and myotonic dystrophy.

— *Familial ptosis:* AD. Smith–Lemli–Opitz syndrome.

— *Pseudoptosis:* Upper eyelid drooping caused by surrounding pathology e.g. tumour pressing the eyelid down.

Proptosis

This is a common slide question and you should have a list of possible differential diagnoses. It is best observed from above the patient.

— *Infection:* periorbital cellulitis (associated with marked eyelid swelling).
— Thyrotoxicosis.
— *Tumours:* capillary haemangioma, histiocytosis X, secondary deposits from a neuroblastoma (raccoon eyes) — the commonest childhood malignancy

to metastasize to the eyes, rhabdomyosarcoma (presents at around seven years of age), optic nerve glioma (there may be pre-existing neurofibromatosis in about 40–50% of cases), dermoid cysts appear as swellings on the upper orbit usually the temporal side, and rarely retinoblastoma.
— *Syndromes:* proptosis may be seen in various syndromes such as Crouzon syndrome. See chapter 14.

Bruising around the eye

May be a result of:

— Non-accidental injury (fundoscopy may reveal retinal haemorrhages)
— Bleeding disorder e.g. haemophilia
— Leukaemia (subconjunctival haemorrhages may be seen in addition)
— Neuroblastoma (raccoon eyes with or without proptosis)
— Basal skull fracture.

Subconjunctival haemorrhage

May be caused by:

— Trauma
— Non-accidental injury
— Bleeding disorders (including acute leukaemia)
— Whooping cough
— Spontaneous.

Optic atrophy

Seen as a very easily visible sharply demarcated pale disc.

— Post traumatic
— Raised intracranial pressure
— Optic nerve compression
— Vitamin B12 deficiency
— Retinal artery thrombosis leading to ischaemia
— Syndromes: Leber optic atrophy.

Papilloedema

The disc is difficult to focus on. The optic disc is swollen secondary to raised intracranial pressure.

Initially the disc is redder than normal because of hyperaemia, followed by blurring of the margins (nasal first). This is followed by dilatation and engorgement of the veins, and the smaller vessels sometimes dip over the edge of the optic disc. The optic cup (usually occupying the central third of the disc) is lost. This is followed by the development of small flame-shaped haemorrhages. In extreme cases the veins become even more dilated and the disc itself is elevated by pressure behind it and hard exudates may then develop.

Vision is initially unaffected but later the blind spot enlarges and this is followed by the development of optic atrophy.

Causes include raised intracranial pressure secondary to space-occupying lesions (tumour, abscess, intracranial bleed), meningitis, hydrocephalus, malignant hypertension, benign intracranial hypertension and infiltration of the disc, for example secondary to lymphoma and central retinal vein thrombosis.

Retinitis pigmentosa

The slide is easily recognisable with black pigmented particles (in 'bone spicule' formation) found throughout the fundus. The early symptoms consist of the development of night blindness (from rod cell damage) and there is then a progressive optic atrophy (the disc often appears waxy white/yellow in colour) and there is subsequently a loss of vision. Causes include:

— Post infection: congenital rubella, measles
— Cystinosis
— Refsum disease
— Abetalipoproteinaemia
— Inherited disorders for example Laurence–Moon–Biedl syndrome.

Corneal clouding

— Mucopolysaccharidoses: cloudiness usually develops by two years e.g. Hurler syndrome (not seen in Hunter)
— Trauma to the cornea
— Glaucoma
— Congenital TORCH syndrome
— Chronic keratitis.

Colobomata

A coloboma is an embryological developmental defect where the embryonic fissure of the optic cup does not completely fuse. The commonly shown slides are of the optic disc showing a shallow cup in the centre (not dissimilar to that seen in glaucoma). Alternatively sclera may be visible through a normal-looking surrounding retina. Alternatively a slide may show an iris which shows a notch usually in an inferonasal position. Colobomas of the eyelid are also occasionally seen. Associations include:

— Trisomy 13
— CHARGE syndrome
— Rieger syndrome (associated with glaucoma and dysmorphic facies)
— Isolated AD inherited familial condition
— Eyelid colobomas are associated with Goldenhar syndrome.

Uveitis

This describes an inflammation in the uveal tract (sometimes called iridocyclitis or iritis). This can occur in the iris, ciliary body or choroid. Anterior uveitis refers to inflammation as far back as the ciliary body and behind this it is referred to as posterior uveitis. The symptoms are of pain in the eye, photophobia, blurred vision and redness with increased lacrimation. Signs include erythema, pupillary miosis, perilimbal flush next to the limbus, keratic precipitates on the corneal endothelium, flare and cells (last three seen only on slit-lamp examination: these symptoms and signs refer mainly to anterior and intermediate uveitis). Posterior uveitis demonstrates vitreous inflammatory cells and possible shearing of retinal vessels. Chronic uveitis may in the long term result in glaucoma, cataract and retinal damage. Causes include:

— Juvenile rheumatoid arthritis — ANA associated (see chapter 11)
— Crohn disease and ulcerative colitis
— Behçet disease (seen in 75% of cases)
— Sarcoidosis
— Ankylosing spondylitis
— Reiter syndrome
— Toxoplasmosis (commonest cause of posterior uveitis)
— CMV infection
— Toxocariasis*
— TB
— Syphilis.

Treatment includes the use of local and systemic steroids.

*Toxocariasis (visceral larva migrans) is usually seen between the ages of 2–5 years. It is caused by the ingestion of eggs of nematode larvae (toxocara canis and catis) which hatch in the intestine and then invade and migrate through the body (producing an immunological response). It can present with a fever, cough, wheeze and sometimes with hepatomegaly. A chorioretinitis (which develops in older children and adults) may develop producing a granulomatous lesion on the retina near the macula (differential diagnosis of retinoblastoma). There is an eosinophilia, raised IgE levels and serological tests are available. Typically there are raised anti-A and anti-B isohaemagglutinin levels (in non-blood group A and B individuals). In the majority of cases recovery is spontaneous. Prophylaxis involves regular deworming of cats and dogs. Severe cases may require steroids and thiabendazole.

Aniridia

Be familiar with what this slide looks like. A light is shone into the eye and the red reflex is seen to cover the whole corneal diameter.

— Sporadic aniridia is associated with the onset of Wilm tumour in about one-fifth of cases
— Familial forms also exist.

Cataracts

These will give a white pupillary reflex (leukocoria). Cataract implies an opacification of the lens. There are many types and causes:

— *Post infection:* congenital infection (rubella leading to nuclear cataract, toxoplasmosis, CMV)

— *Metabolic causes:* Diabetes, galactosaemia (oil droplet cataract), Wilson disease (sunflower cataract) Fabry disease, hypocalcaemia and hypoparathyroidism

— *Secondary to ocular disease:* chronic uveitis, retinal detachment

— *Post traumatic:* Following an injury penetrating the anterior chamber

— *Syndromes:* Down syndrome (spoke-like cataract), trisomy 13, 18, Lowe syndrome, dystrophia myotonica and Conradi syndrome

— *Drugs:* Steroids (chronic use).

Blue sclerae

Seen in the following conditions:

— Normal children
— Osteogenesis imperfecta
— Osteopetrosis.

Additional slides

— You may be shown a slide of a baby or infant with large eyes, often asymmetrically so, and the cause will be *glaucoma*. Congenital glaucoma is called buphthalmos. The eyeball itself is large as a result of increased intraocular pressure. The cornea becomes thickened and cloudy (secondary to oedema), and with time the pupil becomes fixed and dilated. Other conditions in paediatrics associated with glaucoma are Rubinstein–Taybi syndrome, Lowe syndrome, Sturge–Weber syndrome, neurofibromatosis and following chronic uveitis.

— A common slide is of the bulbar telangiectasia seen on the conjunctivae of children with *ataxia telangiectasia*. Clues in the question may be the onset of clumsiness and ataxia or recurrent sinopulmonary infections.

— Know the slides of lens dislocation (ectopia lentis) in *Marfan syndrome* and homocystinuria. Remember that in Marfan the lens is dislocated upwards and outwards whereas in homocystinuria the lens is dislocated downwards and inwards.

— Be familiar with the cherry red spot of Tay–Sachs or Niemann–Pick (see chapter 10).

— Be familiar with the classic dendritic corneal ulcer resulting from *herpes simplex keratitis* (seen with fluorescein staining).

— Be familiar with congenital infection fundoscopic appearances:

   1. Toxoplasmosis retinitis produces a central white/yellow patchy area surrounded by peripheral pigmentation.

2. CMV retinitis causes haemorrhages and exudates causing the typical 'cottage cheese and tomato ketchup' picture.
3. Toxocariasis causes a granulomatous lesion on the back of the retina often with peripheral pigmentation.

— Retinoblastoma is another cause of a white pupillary reflex (leukocoria). There are two main types:

1. *Sporadic* (85% of cases). Unilateral and presents later than the inherited form, usually after 18 months–2 years.
2. *Inherited* (15% of cases). Autosomal dominant inheritance. Usually bilateral and presents at an earlier age than the sporadic type.

It may present as strabismus, leucokoria, glaucoma or a hyphaema. Once leucokoria is noted it is vital that a detailed ophthalmological examination is performed. Retinoblastoma is seen as an elevated mass arising from the retina, often yellow white in colour.

Other causes of leucokoria include cataract, corneal clouding, vitreous haemorrhage, toxocariasis and retinal detachment.

NB It is important that you know how to interpret visual field defects and relate them to defects in the visual pathway. This is discussed in chapter 5.

HEARING

Deafness

The causes of deafness can be categorised as follows:

Conductive hearing loss
Chronic serous otitis media (glue ear) is the commonest cause of conductive hearing loss in childhood. It may occur following acute otitis media or secondary to other abnormalities (such as cleft lip or palate or Down syndrome). Other causes include wax build up in the outer ear or a foreign body.

Sensorineural deafness
— *Prenatal* Congenital infection (TORCH syndrome), maternal drug ingestion (for instance aminoglycoside antibiotics), structural brain abnormalities, genetic (AD, AR) or as part of a syndrome, for example Waardenburg syndrome, Pendred syndrome, Treacher–Collins and mucopolysaccharidoses.

— *Perinatal* Prematurity, low birth weight, birth asphyxia and kernicterus (secondary to hyperbilirubinaemia).

— *Postnatal* Infection: mumps, meningitis, encephalitis, ototoxic drugs, head injury and lead poisoning.

Causes of chronic discharge from the ear

— Chronic middle ear infection
— Chronic otitis externa
— Cholesteotoma

— Histiocytosis X
— Rhabdomyosarcoma.

The commonest questions relating to hearing appear in the data interpretation section of the examination.

Tympanograms

In a tympanogram examination the external auditory meatus is sealed off with a probe to make an airtight seal. A range of pressures are then introduced into the outer ear and the compliance of the tympanic membrane is assessed at these varying pressures by measuring the reflection of sound off the ear drum. The pressures vary through positive and negative pressures. The compliance curve of the tympanic membrane is then transferred on to a graph. The technique is useful for looking at problems associated with the middle ear. The eardrum is at its most compliant when the pressures on either side of it are equalised (usually achieved by intermittent patency of the eustachian tube caused for example by swallowing). You should be familiar with the different tympanogram patterns (see Fig. 13.1)

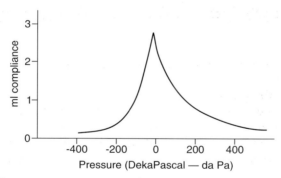

Fig. 13.1a This curve represents a normal tympanogram.

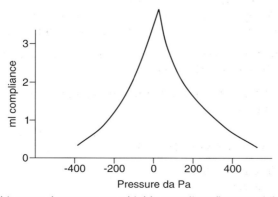

Fig. 13.1b This curve demonstrates a highly compliant (hypermobile) eardrum.

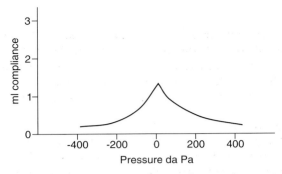

Fig. 13.1c This curve demonstrates a poorly compliant eardrum.

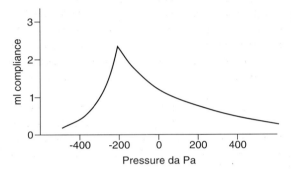

Fig. 13.1d This curve shows maximal compliance at a negative pressure and is typical of a blockage of the eustachian tube. This results in failure of the normal equilibration of the middle ear that occurs with swallowing. The air in the middle ear is resorbed resulting in negative pressure.

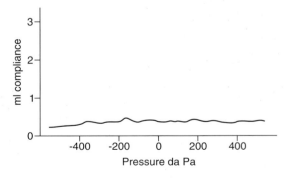

Fig. 13.1e This flat tympanogram results either from a perforated ear drum or from a completely fluid filled middle ear as might occur in glue ear resulting in a stiff non-compliant ear drum.

In most people (about 95%) a notch may be found on the tympanogram if a very loud sound is introduced into the ear and this simply represents the reflex contraction of the stapedius muscle.

Audiograms

Here pure tones at varying frequencies are introduced into the ear or on to the head at different intensities to determine the hearing threshold for the patient at each frequency delivered. This is carried out for air (into ear) and bone conduction (on to head) in turn. Audiogram questions are common and their interpretation is discussed here: each graph will represent one ear only.

Interpreting audiograms

Each graph will represent one ear only. The Y-axis is always the hearing loss (in dB). The X-axis is the frequency of the tones (in Hz). The points on the graphs represent the intensity threshold, at a particular frequency at which the child heard the sound. Thus the lower the point on the graph the worse the hearing. There will be a key alongside the graph indicating if the point refers to air or bone conduction. Grading hearing loss: Mild: 25–35 dB. Moderate: 40–60 dB. Severe: 60–90 dB. Profound: > 90 dB. It is important for you to know that sensorineural hearing loss causes a loss of hearing at higher frequencies and conductive hearing loss produces a hearing loss at the lower range of frequencies. Also conductive hearing loss does not cause hearing loss usually in excess of 50–60 dB.

Remember that when interpreting these audiograms if there is sensorineural deafness there will be a parallel drop in conductive hearing loss as well. This is because, despite the fact the conductive hearing loss is normal the sound will not be transmitted beyond the middle ear centrally to the auditory cortex.

Examples:
1.

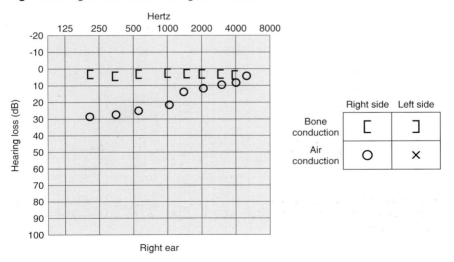

Fig. 13.2a Right conductive hearing loss — mild.

Here the hearing loss is seen in air conduction with no effect on bone conduction. The air conduction hearing loss is worse with the lower frequencies (as mentioned before a typically characteristic feature of conduction hearing loss).

2.

Fig. 13.2b Left moderate high frequency sensorineural deafness.

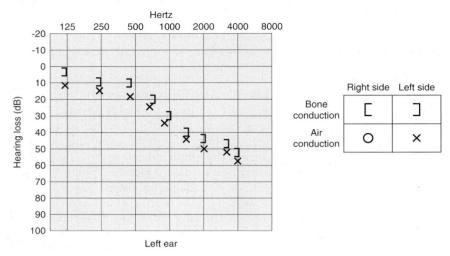

Here the hearing deficit is seen in both air conduction and bone conduction. As mentioned before if there is a sensorineural hearing loss then there will be a simultaneous conductive hearing loss on the audiogram. The hearing loss is greatest at higher frequencies which again corresponds to a sensorineural loss of hearing. This type of high frequency type of hearing loss is seen in kernicterus, birth asphyxia, Alport syndrome, Waardenburg syndrome, congenital rubella, drug toxicity (for example cisplatin and gentamicin) and post meningitis.

3. What does this show?

Fig. 13.2c Profound right sensorineural deafness.

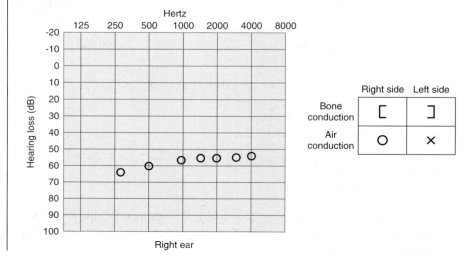

Here only the line corresponding to air conduction is shown on the audiogram. Despite this fact since the hearing loss is so great we can infer that the hearing loss is sensorineural to produce such a significant loss in hearing (as mentioned above).

Tuning fork tests

Sometimes included in data interpretation questions. They are used in clinical practice to help differentiate between conductive and sensorineural deafness.

1. *Weber's test* involves the base of the vibrating tuning fork being placed on the vertex of the skull and the patient asked to inform the examiner on which side he hears the sound loudest. If there is localisation of sound to one side this implies that there is either (a) conductive hearing loss on this side or (b) sensorineural deafness on the contralateral side.

2. *Rinne's test* involves placing the vibrating tuning fork next to the pinna (testing air conduction) and then placing the base on to the mastoid process (testing bone conduction) and asking the patient to indicate if the sound is louder via air or bone conduction. If both ears are functioning normally then air conduction is louder than bone conduction (Rinne's +ve). In the case of a conductive hearing loss bone conduction will be greater than air conduction (Rinne's −ve). In sensorineural deafness both the intensities of sound via bone and air conduction will be reduced but air conduction will still be louder. It is important to bear in mind that a falsely negative Rinne's test may possibly occur if there is a severe sensorineural deafness on one side such that the sound is picked up by the contralateral ear by bone conduction (resulting in bone conduction being greater than air conduction).

Examples:

— A child who has been referred to the outpatient department has the following tuning fork tests:
Weber's test: localisation to the right ear.
Rinne's test: L ear +ve, R ear −ve.
Answer: Conductive hearing loss of the right ear.

— A boy is examined because of parental concern about hearing loss:
Weber's test: localisation to the left ear.
Rinne's test: L ear +ve, R ear −ve.
Answer: Sensorineural deafness R ear.

— A child has been brought to the outpatient department because of hearing problems at home and school.
Weber's test: localisation to R ear.
Rinne's test: R ear +ve, L ear −ve.
Answer: Left severe sensorineural deafness. Here there is a falsely negative Rinne's on the left because of sound being picked up by the contralateral ear by bone conduction.

Paediatric syndromes

14

There are endless paediatric syndromes. Some of these you will have already encountered in clinical practice; some you will never encounter. Having said this you may well see them come up in the paediatric Part 2 examination. There are of course many textbooks devoted to the subject. What I aim to do in this chapter is to include the main syndromes that you are ever likely to come across in the examination and describe their pertinent features, which you will be expected to know. More detailed genetic explanations underlying some of the syndromes are found in the genetics chapter.

CHROMOSOMAL ABNORMALITIES

Down syndrome (Trisomy 21)

Incidence 1:800 live births (increasing risk with increased maternal age). See chapter 1.
● Short stature ● Intellectual retardation (most IQ < 50) and developmental delay ● Brachycephaly ● Third fontanelle ● Delayed fontanelle closure ● Central hypotonia (in 80% and disappears with time) ● Eyes: upward slanting palpebral fissures, brushfield spots, epicanthic folds, cataracts ● Upturned nose ● Small ears ● Hearing defects (increased incidence of middle ear infections) ● Downturned mouth ● Protruding tongue (secondary to hypotonia) ● Congenital hypothyroidism (1:300) and autoimmune type presenting later on in childhood ● Atlanto-axial articular laxity (10%) predisposing to C1–C2 dislocation (tell parents to report any neck pain, limb weakness or paraesthesiae and get a screening X-ray in those who might be involved in contact sports) ● Congenital heart disease (40%) especially AVSD which may need early intervention to prevent early pulmonary hypertensive changes ● Bowel — tracheo-oesophageal atresia, duodenal atresia (10%) (double bubble X-ray appearance), annular pancreas which can also result in obstruction, Hirschsprung disease (3%) ● Hands — short and broad hands and fingers and single palmar crease, clinodactyly ● Feet — short and broad feet and toes, increased space between the first and second toe (sandle toes) with underlying groove ● Skin — cutis marmorata, loosely adherent skin ● Increased risk of acute leukaemia (linked to chromosome 21) ● Increased risk of Alzheimer

disease (linked to chromosome 21) • Recurrent respiratory infections because of poor white cell function.
Prognosis: 15–20% die in first five years mainly as a result of the congenital heart disease but may live into their 60s or later.

Patau syndrome (trisomy 13)

Incidence 1:5000.

• IUGR • Cutis aplasia (scalp defect) most common over vertex of skull near midline seen as ulcers/crusts, secondary infection can occur but most heal in a few weeks • Microcephaly • Eyes — cataracts, colobomata, micro-ophthalmia and corneal opacities • Holoprosencephaly — failure of the midline division of the CNS structures giving e.g. one ventricle and in extremis cyclops • Low-set ears • Cleft lip/palate (60–80%) • Congenital heart disease (80%) mostly ASD, VSD, PDA. • Hands — post-axial polydactyly, hypoplastic nails, clinodactyly • Renal defects (60%) • External genitalia defects.
Prognosis: As for Edward syndrome.

Edward syndrome (trisomy 18)

Incidence 1:3000.
• Microcephaly • Prominent occiput • Micrognathia • Narrow forehead • Cleft lip/palate • Low-set ears • Congenital heart disease (ASD, VSD and PDA) • Short sternum • Hands — often clenched, overlapping fingers with index over the middle, and little over the ring finger, clinodactyly and hypoplastic nails • Rockerbottom feet caused by a vertical talus • Renal abnormalities • Apnoea very common and may be a cause of death.
Prognosis of trisomies 13 and 18: 60% dead in first two days and 90% in first year.

Turner syndrome (45XO)

Incidence 1:2500.

In utero Turner syndrome may be picked up as a result of generalised oedema or cystic collections such as a cystic hygroma that may be severe enough to cause obstruction to swallowing, resulting in polyhydramnios. In severe cases of oedema there may in addition be pleural and pericardial effusions.

At birth Turner might be considered if there is carpal or pedal oedema with hypoplastic nails (a common slide question).
• Short stature (height may be normal for the first four years and then fall away as the ovaries involute) • Intellect is low average but 10% have mental retardation. There may be problems with visuospatial relationships • Hearing problems with secretory otitis media is fairly common • Low hairline • Webbed neck • Widely spaced hypoplastic nipples • Increased carrying angle at the arms (cubitus valgus) • Congenital heart disease (20% — mainly coarctation of the aorta or bicuspid aortic valve. Remember that coarctation of the aorta is three times more common in males than females in the general

population, therefore if you have a girl with coarctation it is worthwhile getting her karyotype done ● Increased risk of raised blood pressure ● Shield shaped chest ● 20% renal abnormalities mainly horseshoe kidney ● Sexual immaturity because of streak ovaries ● Pigmented naevi ● Café au lait macules. Remember that because these girls only have one chromosome they will suffer the same incidence of X-linked conditions as boys ● Growth and sexual maturity can be stimulated hormonally. If Y chromosomes are present in the form of mosaicism then remove the gonads since there is a 50% risk of neoplasia.

Klinefelter syndrome (47XXY)

Incidence 1:1000 males.
● This syndrome is difficult to pick up before puberty since before adolescence, signs are minimal ● Tall with long limbs ● Normal intelligence, only 1:50 mentally retarded ● Problems in their use of language and perception of spoken language ● Thin and feminine shape to the body ● Gynaecomastia in approximately 40% ● Small firm testis, small penis and sometimes cryptorchidism ● Infertile.

Fragile X syndrome

There is an inherited fragility of the X chromosome (which can be detected on a folate deficient culture medium). It is the commonest cause of mental retardation in the world (30% of mental retardation in boys and 10% of mild retardation in girl heterozygotes) and the second most common chromosomal defect after Down syndrome. ● Head — macrocephaly, large ears, large jaw, prominent forehead, high-arched palate ● Hyperextensibility of joints (there is evidence of a connective tissue dysplasia), flat feet ● Mitral valve prolapse (related to connective tissue defect) ● Macrorchidism ● Most of these features are not detectable before the onset of puberty and therefore when one is investigating the cause of mental retardation one usually sends off a chromosomal analysis looking for fragile sites on the X-chromosome.

NON-CHROMOSOMAL SYNDROMES

Angelman syndrome

15q11–13 deletion (maternal) in 50% of cases.
● Microcephaly with brachycephaly ● Mental retardation ● Tend to have fair hair and blue eyes ● 'Happy puppet' with easily provoked paroxysms of laughter ● Variety of seizures, especially prone to salaam attacks ● Abnormal EEG with slow-wave cycles of 4–6/s ● Coarse facies, large tongue and prominent jaw ● Hypotonic with a stiff-legged broad based gait (puppet-like).

Cri du chat syndrome

Chromosome 5p deletion.
● Severe mental retardation ● Microcephaly ● Cat-like cry in first few months — pathognmonic (disappears later on in life).

Prader–Willi syndrome

15q 11–13 deletion (paternal) in 50–75% of cases.
● IUGR ● Short-stature ● Hypotonia ● Facies — almond-shaped eyes, long silky hair, small mouth with downturned corners ● Mental retardation ● Hypogonadal — small penis, cryptorchidism ● Feeding problems from birth but then at 2–3 years the child develops a pathological appetite including food craving and temper tantrums leading to obesity ● Later in life the child may develop diabetes mellitus that may be responsive to diet and oral hypoglycaemic agents ● Managing these children involves a combination of strict dieting and changing the lifestyle of the child ● Pickwickian syndrome ● Growth hormone might help with the short stature.

Laurence–Moon–Biedl syndrome

Autosomal recessive inheritance.
● Obesity ● Mental retardation ● Retinitis pigmentosa ● Knock-knees ● Polydactyly ● Hypogonadism ● Pickwickian syndrome.

William syndrome

Sporadic. This syndrome is common in the slide questions and in the clinical examination.
● Mild microcephaly ● Mental retardation ● 'Elfin-like' facies — short palpebral fissures, upturned nose, 'cupid bow' upper lip ● Lively 'cocktail party manner' ● They may have failure to thrive ● Supravalvular aortic stenosis and less commonly peripheral pulmonary artery stenosis ● Approximately 50% have hypercalcaemia which may be picked up radiologically in the orbits or metaphysis ● The hypercalcaemia may also produce a pressor effect and result in hypertension which in turn may result in renal damage ● Treatment involves giving the children a low calcium and vitamin D diet ● Steroids are sometimes used.

Noonan syndrome

Autosomal dominant with variable transmission. Normal karyotype M:F 1:1. Therefore if male and looks like Turner think of Noonan.
● These children look phenotypically like Turner syndrome children ● Short stature ● Triangular facies ● Eyes — hypertelorism, antimongoloid slant palpebral fissures and epicanthic folds ● Thin upper lip ● Pulmonary stenosis.

Fetal alcohol syndrome

There is a varying severity that appears to be related to the amount of alcohol consumption by the mother during pregnancy.
● IUGR ● Mental retardation ● Microcephaly ● Eyes — microphthalmia, short palpebral fissures and hypertelorism ● Maxillary hypoplasia (best seen from

the side), retrognathia, smooth philtrum and thin upper lip ● Cardiac defects (seen in 40%) — ASD, VSD are most common ● Joint contractures ● Renal defects ● Irritable babies and hyperactivity in childhood.

Russell–Silver syndrome/dwarfism

Sporadic.
● IUGR ● Short stature (with growth rate following the lower centiles but not crossing centiles) ● Normal intelligence ● Face — small triangular-shaped face, small and narrow jaw, thin lips and carp-shaped mouth ● Body assymetry with hemihypertrophy which may not be present at birth and becomes increasingly apparent with age ● Café-au-lait patches ● Hypospadias common ● Clinodactyly.

Waardenburg syndrome

Autosomal dominant.
● Square face and thin nose ● Dystopia canthorum (the medial canthi of the eyes are more lateral than expected – not hypertelorism) ● Heterochromia iridis – if complete can have different coloured eyes ● In approximately 80% of cases there may be sensorineural deafness ● Pigmentary changes in the skin and hair are common — white forelock in approximately 30% of cases which may be associated with patchy depigmentation of the skin.

Beckwith–Wiedemann syndrome

11p15 duplication found in some cases.
● Macrosomia — high birth weight ● Most have macroglossia ● Transverse linear groove in the ear lobe (60%) ● Hemihypertrophy ● Hyperinsulinism may give rise to neonatal hypoglycaemia ● A large proportion of these babies will have exomphalos ● These infants are at high risk of neoplasia: in particular Wilm tumour, renal cortical adenoma and hepatoblastoma, especially if hemihypertrophy is present ● Post-natal surveillance of tumours by serial abdominal ultrasounds is important.

Alagille syndrome (arteriohepatic dysplasia)

● Hypoplasia of intralobular bile ducts leading to neonatal hepatic cholestasis ● Facies: triangular thin face with prominent forehead and small chin ● Congenital heart disease: peripheral pulmonary stenosis ● Vertebral arch abnormalities: butterfly vertebrae ● Ocular abnormalities: persistent posterior embryotoxon ● Renal involvement ● Pruritis and xanthomas.

Schwachman–Diamond syndrome

● AR inheritance ● Pancreatic insufficiency leading to malabsorption (the second most common cause of pancreatic insufficiency after CF) ● Failure to thrive ● Leucopenia especially affecting neutrophils ● Severe gingivitis with possible mandibular alveolar bone destruction • Hepatomegaly and mild hepatic dysfunction • Renal tubular dysfunction.

Ehlers–Danlos syndrome

Autosomal dominant inheritance mainly but sometimes recessive. Defective type 3 collagen noted in some cases.
• Hyperextensibility of the skin, which after being stretched returns to its usual position • Poor wound healing • Hyperextensibility of the joints and increased risk of dislocation • Increased risk of dissection of the aorta and aortic regurgitation • Blue sclera may be a feature • There is an association with congenital diaphragmatic hernia and hiatus hernia • Increased risk of intracranial haemorrhage • Advise avoidance of trauma.

Marfan syndrome

Autosomal dominant inheritance, some sporadic.
• Tall with long limbs and the span of the outstretched arms is greater than the height of the individual, lower segment (pubis to heel) is greater than upper segment (pubis to vertex) • Ectopia lentis (lens dislocation) in 75% with lenses dislocated up and outwards, myopia is common • High arched palate • Increased joint laxity • Increased risk of hernias especially inguinal and femoral • Kyphoscoliosis and pectus excavatum • Medial necrosis in the aorta leading to a diffuse dilatation of the proximal aorta which may give rise to aortic regurgitation and dissection of the aorta. Risk of mitral regurgitation is also increased • Increased risk of pneumothorax (remember acute chest pain in a patient with Marfan may be caused by dissection of the aorta or pneumothorax).

Homocystinuria

Autosomal recessive inheritance. This syndrome is phenotypically very similar to Marfan syndrome with notable differences as follows.
• Vascular and arterial thromboses are common in homocystinuria and do not occur in Marfan syndrome. These thromboses account for the increased risk of cerebrovascular accidents, myocardial infarctions and mental retardation (the latter present in approximately 50%) • Lens dislocation is said to occur down and inwards in homocystinuria • In homocystinuria aortic and mitral regurgitation occur but there is no increased risk of aortic dissection • The two can be differentiated by means of their urine. In homocystinuria there is homocystine in the urine.

Caffey disease

This is an infantile cortical hyperostosis that mainly affects flat bones especially the skull, mandible, clavicles and tubular bones especially ulna and radius • The underlying pathology includes intraperiosteal inflammation with new bone formation and there is swelling over the bone in the soft tissue ● It may sometimes be confused with an injury secondary to child abuse.

Jeune asphyxiating thoracic dystrophy

Autosomal recessive inheritance.
● There is a very small narrow chest with a small AP diameter ● Because of the immobility of the chest wall the respirations are mainly diaphragmatic in nature ● The rest of the body is phenotypically normal ● The baby presents early with respiratory distress and the condition is commonly fatal in the neonatal period. Survival beyond this period is however possible in the milder forms.

Arthrogryposis multiplex

This condition is related to poor intrauterine mobility. This may be a result of oligohydramnios sometimes related to Potter syndrome with renal agenesis.
● There is a conglomeration of limb contractures (with fibrous ankylosis of joints) with the hips and wrists contracted in flexion (hip dislocation is common), knees are commonly flexed, elbows extended and digits flexed (club foot may occur) ● There is also muscular wasting. This may obviously be associated with reduced intrauterine movements ● Potter syndrome has associated pulmonary hypoplasia and characteristic facies with small low-set ears, micrognathia, beaked nose and widely set eyes.

Soto syndrome (cerebral gigantism)

● Macrosomia at birth ● Excessive growth during the first few years of life but normal adult height ● Large head, hands and feet ● Intellectual retardation is nearly always present with clumsiness (mild ventricular enlargement may be seen on CT scan).

Moebius syndrome

This is a congenital paralysis (usually bilateral) of the VIth and VIIth cranial nerves (as a result of agenesis of their corresponding brainstem nuclei). Associated with musculoskeletal defects.

Megalencephaly

There is a large head from birth due to increased brain size, with no hydrocephalus and normal CSF pressure (may be familial).

Marcus–Gunn syndrome

There is a unilateral ptosis, but on opening the mouth the ptosis is eliminated and the affected eyelid may rise to a higher than normal position.

Russell diencephalic syndrome

● Caused by a selective slow growing tumour of the anterior hypothalamus ● This condition usually presents from six months of age with severe failure to thrive and cachexia in a child with a normal food and calorie intake ● The child usually has an alert and wide-eyed startled appearance (as a result of upper eyelid retraction — Collier's sign) ● Hypoglycaemia, optic atrophy and nystagmus are common features ● Prognosis is poor.

CAP syndrome

Congenital **c**amptodactyly — fixed flexion deformity of the digits — **A**rthritis and **P**ericarditis (may cause confusion with JCA).

Pierre–Robin syndrome

Sporadic.
● High arched U-shaped palate ● Cleft palate ● Micrognathia ● Secondary posterior displacement of the tongue owing to the small mandible causing respiratory obstruction ● Feed with orthodontic teats and dental plates.

Stickler syndrome

Autosomal dominant inheritance.
 Pierre–Robin syndrome associated with severe myopia (which may result in retinal detachment in some), cataracts and deafness. Ophthalmological screening could be argued to be necessary in all cases of cleft palate to exclude Stickler syndrome.

Treacher–Collins syndrome

Autosomal dominant inheritance. A first branchial arch defect.
● Face — micrognathia, antimongoloid palpebral fissures, coloboma (most commonly of the lower eye lids), low-set ears, deafness, deformed external ears with preauricular sinuses, and sometimes absent external auditory canal ● CVS — most commonly VSD ● Musculoskeletal — fusion of radius and ulna ● Mental retardation in some.

Klippel–Feil syndrome

Sporadic. Females twice as common as males.
● Musculoskeletal — fusion of two or more cervical vertebrae into a single bony mass (occasionally extending down to the thoracic vertebrae) resulting in a short neck, low hairline, kyphoscoliosis, Sprengel's deformity ● CNS defects include cranial nerve palsies and a third may be deaf ● Syringomyelia and syringobulbia.

Meckel–Gruber syndrome

Autosomal recessive inheritance.

● Occipital encephalocoele ● Post-axial polydactyly ● Polycystic kidneys.

Encephalocoeles are seen as saccular protrusions from the skull usually in the midline and are occipital or nasal in position. They contain brain and meninges and protrude through a skull defect. The overlying skin is usually bald. If they are large neurological deficits can be seen. Investigation involves CT scan. Surgical removal is required and usually results in minimal neurological deficit. They may be confused with haemangiomas (especially those above the nose) or cephalhaematomas.

Goldenhar association (oculo–auricular–vertebral dysplasia)

Caused by abnormal development of first and second branchial arches.
● Face — asymmetry of the face ● Eye — coloboma, epibulbar dermoids ● Ears: low-set ears, abnormal outer ear, deafness ● Vertebra — fused vertebrae, short neck ● Renal and CVS abnormalities ● Mental retardation in some.

Poland syndrome

Sporadic.
● Complete or partial aplasia of the sternal head of pectoralis major which causes a flattening of the hemithorax of the same side ● Loss of breast and subcutaneous tissue ● Inversion of the nipple ● Associated with ipsilateral hand deformities, commonly syndactyly (in one-third of cases).

Lowe syndrome (oculo–cerebro–renal syndrome)

X-linked inheritance.
● Ocular involvement includes glaucoma and bilateral cataracts ● Cerebral involvement includes severe mental retardation and hypotonia ● Renal involvement includes Fanconi syndrome.

Rett syndrome

Affects females only.
● Normal at birth with normal development until the age of about six months ● Regression in milestones with irritability, speech disorder and a decline in the rate of head growth (these features thought to be caused by grey matter degeneration) ● Initial hypotonia later with spastic paraparesis and rigidity ● Scoliosis common ● Loss of purposeful hand movements ● Ataxia including gait ataxia ● Breathing stereotypes (hyperventilation) and hand stereotypes (hand wringing and clapping) ● Epilepsy in majority ● Characteristic EEG ● May cause initial diagnostic confusion with ataxic CP, leucodystrophies, Batten syndrome, autism and mitochondrial disorders.

Batten syndrome

Autosomal inheritance.

● Storage disorder resulting in progressive mental retardation and cerebral palsy ● Blindness with optic atrophy ● Seizures typically myoclonic fits ● Death by teenage years ● Diagnosis by electroretinogram (characteristic), EEG (shows high amplitude spikes produced by photic stimulation) or rectal biopsy.

Aicardi syndrome

Females only.
● CNS involvement includes severe mental and developmental retardation, infantile spasms, cortical and corpus callosum defects ● Eye defects include retinal lacunae (white punched-out lesions in the retina), choroidoretinitis and colobomata ● Costovertebral abnormalities.

Zellweger syndrome (cerebro–hepato–renal syndrome)

A peroxisomal disorder.
● CNS — congenital hypotonia, seizures, mental retardation ● Facies — dolicocephaly, narrow high forehead, large fontanelles ● Pigmentary retinopathy, corneal opacities and cataracts ● Hepatomegaly, hepatic fibrosis leading to cirrhosis ● Renal impairment and polycystic kidneys.

CHARGE syndrome

At least four out of six of following, always including colobomata or choanal atresia: **C**olobomas, **h**eart defects (commonly Fallot, VSD, aortic arch abnormalities), choanal **a**tresia, g**r**owth and mental **r**etardation, **g**enitourinary abnormalities (commonly hypoplasia), **e**ar abnormalities (including deafness).

Colobomata

Seen in CHARGE syndrome, Patau syndrome and Aicardi syndrome. May be idiopathic.

Riley–Day syndrome (familial dysautonomia)

Autosomal recessive inheritance commoner in Ashkenazi Jews.
● Failure to thrive ● Peripheral neuropathy with insensitivity to pain and temperature leading to unnoticed trauma, for example burns or fractures ● Lack of tendon reflexes ● Lack of tears leading to corneal abrasions ● Mental retardation and inco-ordination ● Poor temperature control (may result in hyperpyrexia and dehydration) ● Smooth tongue as a result of lack of fungiform papillae on the tongue ● Excessive sweating and drooling ● Paroxysmal hypertension, sweating and skin blotching ● Recurrent aspiration resulting in chest infections ● Test with subcutaneous histamine test where there is characteristically no wheal or pain ● Increased HMA and decreased VMA, lack of

miosis with 5% metacholine ● Death during childhood from chest infections or dehydration.

DIDMOAD syndrome

Diabetes insipidus, **d**iabetes **m**ellitus, **o**ptic **a**trophy, **d**eafness.

Bloom syndrome

● Small ● Micropcephaly ● Skin photosensitivity ● DNA fragility.

Rubinstein–Taybi syndrome

● Mental and growth retardation ● Hands have very broad thumbs with the distal phalynx displaced radially (talpism) ● Microcephaly with maxillary and mandibular hypoplasia with anteverted nose and antimongoloid slant to palpebral fissures.

Cornelia de Lange syndrome

● IUGR ● Subsequent mental and growth retardation ● Characteristic facies with confluent bushy eyebrows (synophrys), long curly eye lashes, low hair line, low-set ears, micrognathia, thin lips, anteverted nose and downturned mouth ● Limb defects include phocomelia and micromelia (small hands and feet) with the characteristic 'lobster hand' ● Excessive hair may be found on the limbs and trunk ● Cardiovascular defects most commonly ASD, VSD.

Leopard syndrome

Lentignes, **E**CG abnormalities, **o**cular hypertelorism, **p**ulmonary stenosis, **a**bnormalities of the genitalia, **r**etarded growth and **d**eafness.

Syndactyly

Fusion of fingers together.
Associated with Apert syndrome, Carpenter syndrome, Poland syndrome and trisomies 13 and 18.

Polydactyly

Extra digit.
Preaxial: on the radial side.
Postaxial: on the ulnar side.

Clinodactyly

Incurving of the fifth finger. Seen in normal people, Down syndrome and Russell–Silver syndrome.

Holt–Oram syndrome

Autosomal dominant inheritance.
- Limb defects: thumb/radius/ulna hypoplasia ● Cardiovascular defects (ASD:VSD 2:1).

Peutz–Jeghers syndrome

Autosomal dominant inheritance.
- Perioral pigmentation ● Intestinal polyposis.

Hereditary telangiectasia

Autosomal dominant inheritance.
- Multiple telangiectasia that can occur anywhere but especially skin, GI tract, brain, internal organs and increase in size and number with age ● Bleeding from telangiectasia causing complications at the site of bleed, for example intracerebral bleed ● Arteriovenous fistula (listen for bruits) which may produce cyanosis if R to L shunt occurs or heart failure if large.

Smith–Lemli–Opitz syndrome

- Microcephaly ● Initial hypotonia leading to hypertonia ● Seizures ● Cryptorchidism and hypospadias in males and hypoplastic labia in females ● Typical facies: broad upturned nasal tip, ptosis, micrognathia, low-set ears ● Clenched hand and syndactyly of the second and third toes are common ● CVS, renal and GI abnormalities can occur.

Septo-optic dysplasia

- Hypopituitarism ● Optic nerve hypoplasia and absence of the septum pallucidum.

VATER association

Sporadic.
  Vertebral (hemivertebrae and sacral defects — seen on X-ray), anal atresia, tracheo-esophageal fistula, oesophageal atresia, radial limb (radial aplasia, syndactyly, polydactyly, thumb deformities)/renal (renal hypoploasia, ectopic kidney — seen on renal ultrasound). It has been expanded to VACTERL with cardiac (often VSD) and limb defects. Usually of normal intelligence. Their growth is normal if co-existing defects are dealt with appropriately. These defects often occur all together.

Dwarfism

Remember that dwarfism is classified in many different types depending on the part of the body that appears shorter. In the case of the spine being shorter, then the prefix spondylo- is added. The metaphysis, epiphysis or diaphysis may also be involved (which may also be added to the name such as spondyloepiphyseal dysplasia). In disproportionate short stature there is a discrepancy between the limbs and the trunk.

Limb shortening may be classified into three types namely: rhizomelic if the proximal limb is involved for example the humerus or femur. Mesomelic if the middle segments are involved such as the radius, ulna and tibia. Acromelic describes the involvement of distal limb bones such as the carpal and metacarpal bones.

Achondroplasia

Autosomal dominant inheritance. Eighty per cent as a result of spontaneous mutation. Abnormal endochondral bone formation.
- This is a form of rhizomelic dwarfism. ● Head — large head when compared to the rest of the body with prominent frontal, parietal and occipital bones. Small foramen magnum: the resulting basilar compression may result in hydrocephalus ● Nose — saddle nose with a wide nasal bridge ● Concave posterior border of each vertebra, with the interpeduncular distance of the vertebrae decreasing as one descends from the top to the bottom of the spine ● Lumbar lordosis ● Vertebral disc herniation is common ● Spinal stenosis results in root compression which may cause neurological symptoms in the lower limbs resulting in a waddling gait and pelvic tilt ● Very short humerus (rhizomelic) ● Trident fingers — when the digits are in extension the distal ends of the fingers cannot touch each other.

Thanatophoric dwarfism

This is very rare but often comes up as a slide question. Make sure you see a picture of one before the exam.
- It is a lethal condition and babies are either stillborn or die shortly after birth
- The condition may resemble achondroplasia and the babies have extremely small chests ● X-rays are often shown in the exam and show the classical 'fishbone' vertebrae or 'telephone handle' femurs.

Osteogenesis imperfecta

This is a family of conditions and there is an abnormality in the formation of type 1 collagen. There are four main subtypes.

Type 1 (60–80% AD)
- Short stature ● Wormian bones on skull X-ray (often occipital) ● Bony fragility (diaphyseal > metaphyseal) which causes recurrent fractures and deformity. Frequency of fractures decreases after puberty ● Scoliosis ● Blue sclera ● Conductive hearing deafness in approximately half ● May have hypoplastic translucent teeth ● Aortic valve regurgitation associated.

Type 2 (AD/AR)
- Very severe ● Born with multiple fractures ● Sclerae are dark blue-grey ● Face is triangular with a beaked nose ● Stillborn or die shortly after birth.

Type 3 (AD/AR)

● Severe osteoporosis with resulting fractures. This causes progressive shortening and deformities of the long bones. ● Normal sclerae ● Abnormal teeth ● Easy bruising.

Type 4 (AD)

● Bony fragility varies from relatively mild to moderate ● Sclerae normal.

Ellis van Creveld syndrome

● Skeletal – short stature, post-axial polydactyly, acromelic dwarfism, short fingers (brachyactyly) with difficulty making a fist ● CVS — ASD most commonly ● Ectodermal dysplasia — fine diffusely sparse hair, hypoplastic small nails, teeth abnormalities (hypoplastic or peg teeth), congenital teeth may be present.

Conradi syndrome

Autosomal recessive inheritance.
● Looks similar to achondroplasia with short limbs ● In addition cataracts occur in 30% ● There is an abnormality of the cartilage with calcium stippling of the epiphyses ● Mental retardation occurs ● There is also an increased risk of cardiovascular disease (PDA, VSD).

Spondyloepiphyseal dysplasia

● Short stature ● Short trunk ● Kyphoscoliosis ● Mild rhizomelic limb shortening ● Flat face ● Myopia ● Epiphyseal fragmentation which may be seen on X-ray.

Cartilage–hair syndrome

● Resembles achondroplasia but with notable differences ● Hair is very sparse, short and brittle ● There is a normal head and no trident hands ● There is an increased risk of infections.

Cleidocranial dysostosis

Autosomal dominant inheritance.
● Mild dwarfing ● Delay in ossification of the fontanelles and sutures resulting in bossing of the frontal bone ● Small nasal bridge and shallow orbits give the impression of exophthalmos (pseudo-exophthalmos) ● Narrow thoracic cavity and absent lateral ends of the clavicles (some individuals with the condition can bring the shoulders to the front of the chest) ● Late eruption of teeth which are commonly deformed ● Narrow pelvis which in females can cause obstructed labour later in life ● There is no mental retardation and they live to an average age.

Congenital infections

- *Rubella*: IUGR, hepatosplenomegaly, jaundice, thrombocytopenia, chorioretinitis, cataracts, cardiac lesions (PDA) encephalitis, deafness, bony involvement ('celery stick' metaphysis) and purpura ('blueberry muffin' appearance).
- *CMV*: IUGR, hepatosplenomegaly, jaundice, chorioretinitis, microcephaly, encephalitis, cerebral calcification, deafness, purpura and pneumonitis. Diagnose with raised IgM to CMV and urinary CMV excretion.
- *Toxoplasmosis*: IUGR, hepatosplenomegaly, jaundice, chorioretinitis, encephalitis, cerebral calcification and deafness.

Low-set ears

Seen in a number of conditions, the commonest being Turner syndrome, Potter syndrome and Edward syndrome.

Cleft lip and palate

Seen in Pierre–Robin syndrome, trisomies 13 and 18, fetal phenytoin syndrome, Di George syndrome and Goldenhar syndrome.

Micrognathia

Seen in Pierre–Robin syndrome, Treacher–Collins syndrome, Russell–Silver syndrome and Potter syndrome.

Hypertrichosis

Seen in the mucopolysaccharidoses, Cornelia de Lange syndrome, leprechaunism and in children treated with cyclosporin.

The long case

15

The long case is the part of the examination in which you should feel perhaps more at ease compared with, for example, the short cases. Firstly it is the only time in the clinical examination in which you have some time to yourself and the parents and child. Secondly the scenario of clerking a patient is something that you do every working day and is therefore very familiar to you. You should bear in mind, however, that since you have more time with the patient than you would normally, a more detailed history should be taken, with special emphasis in particular places (see later). Always leave enough time to examine the child properly at the end, as well as time for organising your thoughts, history, formulating your differential diagnosis, relevant investigations and treatment.

After your allotted time with the patient and parents you are taken to the examiners. You will never be able to predict what the format of the next part of the long case (that is, the examiner interrogation) will consist of since it will range from a simple request to 'go ahead and present the history' to 'they tell me this child is on vigabatrin, just remind me of its mechanism of action'.

The well balanced long case viva should be a combination of finding out what you have gleaned from the patient and if you have picked up on the pertinent points, as well as asking some deeper probing questions that may arise from your description of the child's illness. Always appear interested in the case you are presenting, since the more inviting and interesting your tone of voice the more you will be able to say what you want to uninterrupted. The examiners are also looking for doctors who have a genuine interest in children's medicine and all other aspects involved in caring for sick children. Therefore try and sound fascinated by the case.

Always try and answer the question being asked. Try to avoid diving into your history at every possible opportunity, however tempting it may seem. However this does not mean that you cannot direct questions to your history. Very often (but not always) you will be taken back to the child to examine a system or demonstrate a physical sign. As in the short cases you should appear confident (but not too confident), courteous, caring, competent and show that you are good with children. You should address the child by his first name (especially since you have had some time to get to know him) and examine the system or demonstrate the sign being asked.

TAKING THE HISTORY

The following is a suggested format for taking the history. Indicate to the examiners who the history was taken from, that is, parent or child.

Name

Include here the name that people call the child: for example, the child's name may be William but he likes to be called Billy. This shows that you have a sensitivity towards the child.

Age

In the case of an infant born prematurely don't forget to give a corrected age.

Presenting complaint

If there is a long history of a particular disease it is wise to include the diagnosis here.

History of the presenting complaint

Here you should note how the disease first presented and progressed. Include here all the symptoms, investigations, treatments and admissions to hospital.

For any pain describe the onset, duration, frequency (of attacks), character, intensity/severity, precipitating factors, relieving factors, aggravating factors, diurnal or seasonal variation. This scheme can be applied to almost any presenting symptom.

Useful questions in children to indicate severity of symptoms are (a) whether the child is awakened by their symptoms at night (b) how many days of school the child has lost as a result of the illness (c) if the child has an appetite — since in sick children appetite is quickly affected; and finally (d) hospitalisations as a result of the illness (including duration of hospitalisation).

You can now perform a review of symptoms to elicit any related symptoms or features of the disease not mentioned. This can also be performed at the end of the history.

Past medical history

Any previous significant medical history should be included here. You should include any hospitalisations, treatments for the disease and any residual effects from the disease.

Neonatal history

Problems during the pregnancy (including any maternal illnesses or drug ingestion), gestation at birth, method of delivery, birth weight, postnatal problems or admission to NICU including details of management (e.g. ventilation including the number of days).

Developmental history

Choose some milestones that the child should have reached from gross motor, fine motor, vision, hearing and speech and personal and social skills.

Immunisations

Ask if the child is up to date with vaccinations. If necessary ask to see the child's record book.

Nutrition

Here you should include whether the baby was breast- or bottlefed, special milk formulas used (and why), any supplements, age at introduction of solids and cereals with gluten. Take a reasonably detailed dietary history of what the child currently eats. If a baby, then include volume and frequency of feeds.

Drugs

List all the medications that the child is taking. Include the doses and frequency.

Allergies

Ask about any known allergies to drugs or food. Then ask specifically about atopy including asthma, eczema or hay fever.

Family history

— You should draw an accurate family tree.
— You should ask about the country of origin and race of the parents.
— Ask about the possibility of consanguinity between the parents.
— Ask about any medical conditions that run in the family and specifically if there is someone else in the family with the presenting complaint of the child.

Social history

This should be detailed since questions relating to this are frequent in the long case.

— Include details about the ages, marital status and professions of the parents. Find out who else lives at home. Are there any pets? Does anyone in the household smoke?

— Find out about housing. This includes type of housing, flat or house (if flat what floor and whether or not there is a lift), rented, bought or council flat/house. Ask about type of heating and toilet facilities. Ask about any modifications that have been made to the house to accommodate the child's illness (for example, ramp to the house or rail in bathroom).

— Ask about any additional assistance the family might be getting in the form of financial support or people coming to the house. This will include home helps or nurses coming, for example, to change dressings or give injections.

— Get a detailed picture of the child's school life especially what type of school and reports from the teachers of any particular problems. Any accommodations made for the child at school because of the illness. Is the child happy at school, does he have friends? Is the child statemented? Has the child missed days from school because of his illness?

— What has the effect of the illness been on the child?

— What effect has the illness had on the siblings, parents and the family unit as a whole. Coping strategies?

Finally it is important to note what the parents' main concerns are at the present moment.

You should then perform a complete examination paying particular attention to the system affected by the illness. You will usually be supplied with height and weight of the child, so that you should plot these on the growth charts supplied. You will also usually be supplied with a urine specimen that you should dipstick. You will be expected to have taken the blood pressure yourself.

You should then bring your thoughts together. Make a problem list with as many different problems that you can find whether they relate to the disease itself or to the family or housing, for instance. It is useful making this list since it can act as a springboard for further discussion and it shows that you are a doctor who is sensitive to the various problems experienced by the child and his or her family.

Bibliography and recommended further reading list

Attard-Monalto S, Vaskar S 1994 Paediatric cases for postgraduate examinations. Butterworth-Heinmann Ltd. Oxford
Behrman RE, Kliegman RM 1994 Essentials of pediatrics. 2nd edn. W.B. Saunders Company, Philadelphia
Booth IW, Wozniak ER 1988 Paediatrics — pocket picture guides. Gower Medical Publishing, London
Cade A, Shetty A, Tinklin TS 1995 An aid to the paediatric MRCP viva. Churchill Livingstone, Edinburgh
Connor JM, Ferguson-Smith MA 1989 Essential medical genetics. 2nd edn. Blackwell Scientific Publications, Oxford
Davies AEM, Billson AL 1994 Key topics in paediatrics. Bios Scientific Publishers Ltd., Oxford
Dynski-Klein M 1994 A colour atlas of paediatrics. Wolfe Medical Publishing, London
Field DJ, Stroobant J, Fenton A, Maconochie I, O'Callaghan C 1995 Grey cases for paediatric examinations. Churchill Livingstone, Edinburgh
Habel A 1993 Aids to paediatrics. 3rd edn. Churchill Livingstone, Edinburgh
Habel A 1993 Synopsis of paediatrics. Butterworth-Heinmann Ltd., Oxford
Hampton J 1989 The ECG in practice. Churchill Livingstone, Edinburgh
Holmes JA, Kinsey S, Ludlum CA, Webb DK, Whittaker JA 1994 Self-assessment in clinical haematology. Wolfe Publishing, London
Hughes S 1989 A new short textbook of orthopaedics and traumatology. Edward Arnold, London
Hull D, Johnston DI 1999 Essential paediatrics. 4th edn. Churchill Livingstone, Edinburgh
Joss V, Rose S 1993 Case presentations in paediatrics. 2nd edn. Butterworth-Heinmann Ltd, Oxford
Kanski J 1992 Ophthalmology colour guide. Churchill Livingstone, Edinburgh
Langman J, Sadler TW 1995 Medical embryology. 7th edn. Williams & Wilkins, Baltimore
Levene MI, Tudehope D 1993 Essentials of neonatal medicine 2nd edn. Blackwell Scientific Publications, Oxford

Lote CJ 1982 Principles of renal physiology. Croom Helm, London & Canberra

Marshall WJ 1992 Clinical chemistry. 2nd edn. Gower Medical Publishing, London

Moore KL 1988 Essentials of human embryology. Decker, B.C., Ontario

Milner D 1994 Pediatrics — self-assessment picture tests in medicine. Mosby-Wolfe, London

O'Callaghan C, Stephenson T 1992 Data interpretation for paediatric examinations. Churchill Livingstone, Edinburgh

Polin RA, Ditmar MF 1989 Paediatric secrets. Hanley & Belfus Inc., Philadelphia

Reeves G, Todd I 1991 Lecture notes on immunology. 2nd edn. Blackwell Scientific Publications, Oxford

Reid JL, Rubin PC, Whiting B 1997 Lecture notes on clinical pharmacology. 5th edn. Blackwell Scientific Publications, Oxford

Reynolds DJ, Freeman HGM 1986 Aids to clinical chemistry. Churchill Livingstone, Edinburgh

Roberton NRC 1993 A manual of neonatal intensive care. 3rd edn. Edward Arnold, London

Rubenstein D, Wayne D 1997 Lecture notes on clinical medicine. 5th edn. Blackwell Scientific Publications, Oxford

Rudolph AM, Kamei RK 1994 Rudolph's fundamentals of pediatrics. Appleton & Lange, Connecticut

Stephenson T, Wallace H 1995 Clinical paediatrics for postgraduate examinations. 2nd edn. Churchill Livingstone, Edinburgh

Verbov J 1994 Diagnostic picture tests in paediatric dermatology. Wolfe Publishing, London

West JB 1999 Respiratory physiology: the essentials. 6th edn. Williams & Wilkins, Baltimore

Winrow AP, Gatzoulis M, Supramaniam G 1994 100 Paediatric picture tests. Churchill Livingstone, Edinburgh

Zitelli BJ, Davis HW 1994 Atlas of pediatric physical diagnosis. 2nd edn. Wolfe Publishing, London

Index

Note: page numbers in *italics* refer to figures and tables

A1AT deficiency, 143, 161, 166
Aarsog syndrome, 183
ABC resuscitation, 28
Abdomen
 clinical examination, 162–7
 palpation, 31
 scars, 167–8
 tumours, 159
Abdominal pain
 anaemia, 226–7
 and hyponatraemia, 139
 Mediterranean fever, 158, 159
 neurological features, 152
 recurrent, 151–2, 154
Abducens nerve, 124–5
Abetalipoproteinaemia, 116, 140, 152–3, 307
ABO incompatibility, 144, 146, 206, 208, *209*
Abscess, 113, 240
 cerebral, 95, 96, 103, 106
 lung, *59*
 pelvic appendix, 157
 retropharyngeal, 52
Acanthocytes, 203
Acanthocytosis, 152
Accessory nerve, 127
Acetazolamide, 74, 120, 265
Achondroplasia, 94, 183, 329
Aciclovir, 300–1
Acid lipase deficiency, 259
Acoustic neuroma, 96, 118
Acrodermatitis, 295
ACTH, 99, 173, 174, 175, 176
Acute intermittent porphyria, 77, 151, 152, 264
Acute renal failure, 69, 71–2
Addison disease, 75, 120, 151, 175, 194
 candidiasis, 240
 hyperkalaemia, 249
 metabolic acidosis, 265
 pigmentation, 303
Adenoma sebaceum, 289–90
Adenovirus, 57
ADH, 68, 190–2, 247–8
Adrenal carcinoma, 76

Adrenal hyperplasia, 76, 88, 174–5
Adrenal insufficiency, 174–5
Adrenal leucodystrophy, 114
Adrenal physiology, 172–3
Adult haemoglobin (HbA), 200, 209, 210
Aicardi syndrome, 326
AIDS, 58, 62
 investigation, 245
 management, *246*
 paediatric, 244–5, *246*
Alagille syndrome, 26, 144, 321
Albers–Schönberg disease, 102
Albinism, 298, 302
Alcohol, 26, 78, 100, 107, 180, 264
 abuse, 116, 266
 chronic ingestion, 201
 maternal consumption, 320
 poisoning, *268*
Alder–Reilly bodies, 256
Aldosterone, 68, 74, 76, 172–3
 deficiency, 75, 139
 resistance, 75
 see also Addison disease
Aldosterone-secreting adenoma, 76
Alkaptonuria, 77
Allergy, 155
Alopecia areata, 302
Alpha thalassaemia, 210–11
Alpha-fetoprotein, maternal serum, 10
Alport syndrome, 85, 86, 314
Alveolar/capillary membrane, 42
Alveolitis, extrinsic allergic, 56
Amiloride, 75, 76
Amino acidopathy *see* maple syrup urine disease
Aminoglycosides, 87, 310
Amiodarone, 56, 107, 138
Amniotic bands, 1
Amphoterocin, 74, 87, 239
Anaemia, 26, 30, 33, 43, 141
 abdominal pain, 154, 226–7
 aplastic, 201, 226–7
 arthritis, 227–8, 282
 classification, 200–1

Anaemia (*contd*)
cystic fibrosis, 45
folate deficiency, 203, *212–13*
haemolytic, 145, 154, 200, 201, 202
  autoimmune, 206
iron deficiency, 141, 201, 203, 204, *211–12*, *213*, 214
megaloblastic, 141, 201, 202, 204
microcytic hypochromic, 51–2
pernicious, 240
sideroblastic, 201, 202
vitamin B12 deficiency, 203, *212–13*
Anal membrane, 136–7
Androgens, 184, 187
Angelman syndrome, 11, 298, 319
Angio-oedema, 52
see also hereditary angio-oedema
Angiomyolipoma, 86
Angiotensin, 68, 173
Aniridia, 308
Anisocytosis, 201
Ankle jerk, absent, 107
Ankylosing spondylitis, 308
Anorectal agenesis, 137
Anorectal atresia, 151
Anorexia nervosa, 192
Anti-Ro antibodies, 20
Anticonvulsant drugs, 107
Antihistamines, 268
alpha-1 Antitrypsin deficiency *see* A1AT deficiency
Anus, bruising, 155
Aortic arch interruption, 14
Aortic atresia, 35
Aortic dissection, 52
Aortic regurgitation, 30
Aortic stenosis, 14, 24, 26, 31
  murmurs, 33
  see also coarctation of the aorta
Apert syndrome, 281
Aphthous ulcers, 156, 163
Aplasia, 200, 201, 218
Apnoea, obstructive, 40
Appley's law, 151
Aqueduct stenosis, 94
Aqueduct of Sylvius, 93, 94
Arachnoid granulations, 93, 94
Arachnoid villi, hypoplasia, 94
Arms, neurological examination, 127–8
Arnold–Chiari malformation, 94
Arterial occlusive disease, 113
Arterial trunk, common, 15
Arteriovenous malformation, 27
Arthritis, 271–2
  anaemia, 227–8, 282
  Henoch–Schönlein purpura, 82
  juvenile chronic, 271, 272–5, 294, 308
  pain, 275, 278
  reactive, 271
Arthrogryposis multiplex, 323
Arthropathy, psoriatic, 289
Ascariasis, 56
Ascites, 164

Aspergilloma, 57
Aspergillosis, 56–7, 241
Aspergillus fumigatus, 56, 57
Aspirin, 285
  see also salicylates
Association of malformations, 1–2
Asthma, 27, 37, 40–1, 42, 51
  allergic bronchopulmonary aspergillosis, 56–7
  clinical signs, 62–3
  CXR, 49
  differential diagnoses, 62
  growth retardation, 183
  PEFR, 62–3
  SIADH, 190
  TLCO, 43
Astrocytoma, 103, 116, 117
At risk register, 286
Ataxia, 116–17
  sensory, 132
Ataxia telangiectasia, 115, 116, 123, 179, 239–40, 309
Atopic eczema, 288–9
Atrial fibrillation, 22
Atrial flutter, *21*, 22
Atrial hypertrophy/enlargement, 18
Atrial natriuretic peptide, 68
Atrial septal defect, 16, *21*, 22, 23
  murmurs, 33–4
Atrioventricular canal defect, 14, 15
Atrioventricular septal defect, 22
Atrioventricular shunt, infected, 71
Audiograms, 313–15
Auscultation, 31, 64–5, 164
Auto antibodies, 245
Autosomal dominant (AD) inheritance, 3, 4, 5
Autosomal recessive (AR) conditions, 3, 4, 5, 6
Azathioprine, 206
AZT, 107, *246*

B cell
  abnormalities, 245
  function, 243
Babinski sign, 129
Bacterial endocarditis, 30, 71
Bacterial overgrowth, 140
Balloon atrial septostomy, 23
Barr bodies, 4
Bartter syndrome, 75–6, 139
Basophilia, 222
Basophilic stippling, 203
Batten disease, 115, 116, 325–6
BCG vaccination, 62
Becker muscular dystrophy, 110
Beckwith–Wiedemann syndrome, 88, 153, 159, 163, 180, 181
  obesity, 193
Behçet disease, 156, 294, 302, 308
Bell's palsy, 126
Benign essential tremor, 107

Benzodiazepines, *268*
Benzyl benzoate, 295
Berger disease, 86
Bernard–Soulier syndrome, *226*
Berry aneurysms, 85, 86
Beta thalassaemia, 3, 144, 163, 166
　anaemia, 201, 202, 203–4, 212
　haemoglobin electrophoresis, 210
　major, 102, 203–4, 217, 219
Bezoars, 157
Bicarbonate, 72, 73
Biliary atresia, 144, 167
Bilirubin
　abnormalities, 143–4, 145, 147–8
　metabolism, 142–3
Biochemistry errors, 228
Bird fancier's lung, 56
Birth asphyxia, 106, 180, 225, 310, 314
Blalock–Taussig (BT) shunt, 23, 24, 34
Blindness, 101
Blistering skin lesions, 296
Blood film abnormalities, 201–3
Blood gases, 41
　interpretation, 37–40
Blood group incompatibilities, 144, 146
Blood loss, 141
Blood swallowing, 154
Blood transfusion, 202, 203, 219
Bloom syndrome, 240, 327
Blue sclerae, 309
Bohr effect, 57
Bone
　age, 184
　anatomy, 275–7
　fibrous dysplasia, 117
　tumours, 280–1
Bone marrow, 200, 203, 205, 223
　transplantation, 219
Bordetella pertussis, 51
Borrelia burgdorferi, 271, 283
Bowel obstruction, intermittent, 51
Brachycephaly, 282
Bradycardia, 121
Breast feeding, 211
　contraindications, 138–9
Breast milk, 137–8
　jaundice, 145
Breath sounds, 65
Bronchiectasis, 37, 48, 57, 58
Bronchomalacia, 55
Bronchopulmonary dysplasia, 48
Brucellosis, 166
Brudinski sign, 105
Bruton disease, 237, *238*
Bulbar palsy, 57, 58
Bundle branch block, 20, *21*, 22
Buphthalmos, 309
Burns, 52, 202, 249, 302
Busulphan, 56
Byler disease, 144
Bypass surgery, 34

Caecum, arrested descent, 136
Café au lait patches, 117, 123, 303
Caffey disease, 282–3, 322–3
Calcification
　imaging, 105
　intracranial, 102, 103
　kidneys, 79
　neuroblastoma, 88
Calcipotriol, 289
Calcium
　physiology, 193–4
　see also hypercalcaemia; hypocalcaemia
Campylobacter, 83, 154
Candida infections/candidiasis, 239, 240, 241, 244, 287
Cannonball metastases, 88
CAP syndrome, 324
Captopril, 87
Carbamazepine, 112, 190
Carbimazole, 138, 171, 223
Carbon dioxide, 38, 39, 40
　respiratory failure, 41
Carbon monoxide, 42–3
　poisoning, 230
Carboxyhaemoglobin, 58, 230
Carcinoid syndrome, 195
Cardiac catheter, 15–17
Cardiac failure, 25, 26, 57, 58, 247
Cardiac operations, 23–4
Cardiac transplantation, 24
　rejection, 27
Cardiology, paediatric, 24–5
　see also heart
Cardiomyopathy, 14, 26, 83, 117
Cardiovascular cases, 30–5
Cardiovascular lesions, chronology, 14
Cardiovascular physiology, fetal, 13
Carditis, 28
Carnitine deficiency, 180
Carnitine palmitoyl transferase deficiency, 260
Carpenter syndrome, 281
Cartilage–hair syndrome, 330
Cataract, 308–9
Cavernous haemangioma, 291
Cell-mediated immunity disorders, 237–40
Central respiratory depression, 40
Cephalhaematoma, 302
Cephalosporin, 87
Cerebellar ataxia, acute of childhood, 116
Cerebellar lesions, 116
Cerebellar system examination, 130–1
Cerebral atrophy, 105
Cerebral malignancy, 96
Cerebral palsy, 116, 126
Cerebral thrombosis, 27
Cerebral tumour, 126
Cerebrospinal fluid (CSF)
　data interpretation, 94–7
　flow obstruction, 94
　microbiology, 96–7
　pathophysiology, 93–4
Cervical cord trauma, 106

Cervical lymph node, 64
Cervical spondylosis, 107
Charcot–Marie–Tooth disease, 118, 282
CHARGE syndrome, 1, 307, 326
Chediak–Higashi syndrome, 225, 241, 302
Chemotherapy, 142, 223, 232, 233
Cherry red spots, 256, 309
Chest
    bell-shaped, 57
    palpation, 64
    percussion, 64, 65
Chest X-ray (CXR), 46–9, 51, 56, 57, 243
Chickenpox, 113, 300–1
    see also varicella
Chignon, 302
Chinese herbal tea, 289
Chlamydia trachomatis, 60
Chloramphenicol, 138
Chlorpromazine, 223
Chlorpropamide, 190
Choanal atresia, 51
Cholecalciferol, 193–4
Choledocal cyst, 144
Cholestasis, 140, 144, 145, 266
Cholesteatoma, 310
Chondromalacia, 278
Chorea, 115–16
Choroid plexus calcification, 103
Chromosomal abnormalities
    neonatal, 106
    syndromes, 317–19
Chromosomes
    analysis, 6, 7–8
    nomenclature, 8–9
Chronic granulomatous disease, 241–2
Chronic renal failure, 72, 77, 87, 166, 194
Churg–Strauss syndrome, 56
Chylomicronaemia, familial, 265–6
Chylothorax, 43–4, 49
Cilia function, 58
Cisplatin, 107, 314
Cleft lip and palate, 1, 331
Cleidocranial dysostosis, 102, 277, 330
Clinistix, 78
Clinitest, 78, 259
Clinodactyly, 327
Cloacal membrane, 136
Clonus, 129–30
Clostridium difficile, 156–7
Clotting disorders, 214–17
Clotting factors, 158
Club foot, 121
Co-ordination testing, 128, 130
Coal tar preparations, 289
Coarctation of the aorta, 14, 16, 24, 34
Coeliac disease, 140, 141, 142, 156, 158, 228
Colchicine, 138
Cold antibodies, 207
Collagen vascular diseases, 271–2, 292
Colobomata, 307, 326
Colostomy, 168
Colostrum, 138
Coma, 25, 160–1

Common variable immunodeficiency, 237, 238
Complement defects, 242–3
Complement levels, 71
Condylomata acuminata, 297
Congenital abnormalities, 138, 178
    classification, 1–2
Congenital adrenal hyperplasia, 75, 81, 173–4, 185
    ambiguous genitalia, 187, 188, 189
Congenital heart disease, 13–15, 18, 22
    maternal diabetes, 178
    presentation, 25–6, 40
    respiratory distress, 50
    SVT, 28
Congenital infection, 1
Congenital nephrotic syndrome, 89
Congestive cardiac failure, 56, 143, 166, 183
Conn syndrome, 76, 77, 265
Conradi syndrome, 309, 330
Contact dermatitis, 296
Convergence reflex, 125
Cor pulmonale, 26, 57, 65
Cord compression, 113
Corneal clouding, 307
Corneal reflex, 125, 133
Cornelia de Lange syndrome, 296, 327, 331
Coronary artery
    aneurysms, 285
    anomalous left, 27
Corticosteroids, 120
Cortisol, 172, 173, 184
Corynebacterium, 118
Corynebacterium diphtheriae, 54
Cotrimoxazole, 239, 242, 246
Cough, nocturnal, 63
Cow's milk, 138, 211
    protein intolerance, 51, 141, 142, 154
Coxsackie virus, 295
Cranial nerve examination, 124–7, 133
Cranial ultrasonography, neonatal, 103–4
Craniopharyngioma, 103, 191
Craniosynostosis, 102, 281
Creatine phosphokinase (CPK), 3, 11, 119, 120
Creatinine, 69–70, 71
Cri du chat syndrome, 9, 319
Crigler–Najjar syndrome, 143, 145, 147–8
Crohn disease, 140, 141, 149, 155–6, 226, 308
Croup, 52, *60*
Crouzon syndrome, 281, 306
Cryoglobulinaemia, 71
Cryptococcus neoformans, 244
Cryptorchidism, 187
Cryptosporidium, 239, 244
CT scan
    renal, 80
    skull, 104
Cushing disease, 63, 120, 265, 303
Cushing reflex, 121

Cushing syndrome, 175–6, 183, 185
  glucose tolerance, 179
  hypertension, 81
  obesity, 193
Cutis marmorata, 296
Cyanosis, 14, 17–18, 28, 30
  central, 64
  methaemoglobin, 229
  respiratory distress, 51
Cyclophosphamide, 190
Cyclosporin, 83, 84, 230, 331
Cystic adenomatous malformations, 47
Cystic fibrosis, 3, 6, 11, 37, 44–6, 139
  allergic bronchopulmonary aspergillosis, 56–7
  bronchiectasis, 57
  clinical manifestations, 44–5, 63, 166
  CXR, 48
  diagnosis, 44, 166
  glucose tolerance, 179
  with haematemesis, 157–8
  hepatitis, 143
  malabsorption, 140
  with melaena, 157–8
  mutations, 44
  pneumonia, 58
Cystic fibrosis transmembrane regulator (CFTR), 11
Cystic hygroma, 55
Cysticercosis, 103
Cystinosis, 74, 253, 254–5, 307
Cystinuria, 77, 78, 253
Cytomegalovirus (CMV), 94, 103, 115, 143, 166
  cataracts, 309
  congenital, 331
  immune disorders, 238, 239
  retinitis, 310
  uveitis, 308
Cytotoxic drugs, 138

Dactylitis, sickle, 280
Dandy–Walker cyst, 94
Dapsone, 138
DDAVP, 190, 192
Deafness, 310
  sensorineural, 85, 86, 310, 313–14
Deformation, 1
Dehydration, 139
  renal vein thrombosis, 90
Dehydroepiandrosterone (DHEA), 172
Dementia, 107, 117
Dental hygiene, 30
Depigmentation, 302
Dermatitis
  artefacta, 302
  herpetiformis, 299
  infantile seborrhoeic, 287–8
  napkin, 287
Dermatology, clinical, 303
Dermatomyositis, 120, 283–4, 302, 305
Dermatophyte infections, 293

Dermoid cysts, 306
Development
  neurological examination, 132–3
  stages, 2
Developmental delay, 118, 256, 258
Developmental milestones, 122
  failure to reach, 114–15
Dexamethasone, 96
Dextrocardia, 21, 22, 31, 51, 148
Diabetes insipidus, 87, 183, 191
Diabetes mellitus, 83, 87, 176–9, 240
  cataracts, 309
  clinical examination, 197
  hyperlipidaemia, 266
  insulin-dependent, 151
  maternal, 49, 151, 178, 180, 193
  skin lesions, 296
Diabetic ketoacidosis, 179
Diamond–Blackfan syndrome, 218
Diamond–Schwachman syndrome, 140, 223, 321–2
Diaphragmatic hernia, 48
  congenital, 49
Diarrhoea, 139–40, 141, 160, 247, 249
  toddler's, 156
Diastomatomyelia, 120
DIDMOAD syndrome, 327
Diethylene triamine pentacetic acid *see* DTPA
DiGeorge syndrome, 240, 331
Digoxin therapy, 23
Dimercaptosuccinic acid *see* DMSA
Diphtheria, 54
Diplopia, 125
Discitis, 113
Disruption, 1
Disseminated intravascular coagulation, 216, 217, 225
Distal convoluted tubule (DCT), 68
Distal renal tubular acidosis, 73–4
Dithranol, 289
Diuretics, 249, 265
DMSA scan, 80
Dolicocephaly, 281
Down syndrome, 78, 106, 163, 170, 189, 317–18
  anaemia, 202
  cataract, 309
  cord compression, 113
  cutis marmorata, 296
  deafness, 310
  glucose tolerance, 179
  growth, 183
  inheritance, 9–10
  scabies, 295
  Wormian bones, 102, 277
  see also trisomy 21
Drawing images, 122, 123
Drop foot, 132
Drugs, 266
  abuse, 114
  chorea, 115
  nephrotoxic, 87

Drugs (contd)
  neutropenic, 223, 224
  ototoxic, 310, 314
  poisoning, 266, 267, 268–9
DTPA scan, 80–1
Dubin–Johnson syndrome, 144, 148
Duchenne muscular dystrophy, 3, 11, 37, 110, 118
  glucose tolerance, 179
  pes cavus, 282
Ductus arteriosus, patent, 15, 16, 17, 34
Ductus venosus, 13
Duodenal atresia, 149
Duodenum, 136
Dwarfism, 321, 328–9
  diabetic, 178
  thanatophoric, 329
Dysarthria, 131
Dysdiadochonesis, 128, 130
Dysmorphism, 183
Dystrophia myotonica, 309

Ears
  discharge, 310–11
  low-set, 331
Ebstein anomaly, 14, 22, 23, 25, 26
  SVT, 28
ECG, paediatric, 18–20, 21, 22–3
Ectopia lentis, 309
Eczema, 288–9
  herpeticum, 288
Edrophonium test, 107, 109
Edward syndrome, 7, 318, 331
  cutis marmorata, 296
  see also trisomy 18
EEG
  interpretation, 97–102
  optic pathway lesions, 101–2
  post-ictal, 101
Ehlers–Danlos syndrome, 322
Eisenmenger syndrome, 15, 17
Electrolyte imbalance, 23
Ellis van Creveld syndrome, 299, 330
Emphysema, 37, 43, 48
Empyema, 59
Encephalitis, 83, 94, 106, 113
  deafness, 310
  herpes simplex, 95–6, 99
  SIADH, 190
  varicella, 116
Encephalocoele, 119
Encephalopathy, 113–14, 115, 250–1, 252, 253
  EEG, 101
  hypertensive, 25, 85
Endocrine abnormalities, clinical examination, 196–7
Enzyme deficiencies, 141
Eosinophilia, 222
  pulmonary, 56
Eosinophilic granuloma, 290
Ependymoma, 117

Epidermolysis bullosa, 298–9
Epidermolytic hyperkeratosis, 298
Epidermophyton, 293
Epiglottitis, 53
Epilepsy
  benign Rolandic, 101, 112
  grand mal, 100
  Lennox–Gastaut, 101
  myoclonic, 100
  petit mal, 98
  photosensitive, 100
  temporal lobe, 112
Epiphysis, 275, 276, 277
Epstein–Barr virus, 166, 292
Erb palsy, 122
Erythema
  infectiosum, 302
  marginatum, 29, 294
  multiforme, 291–2
  nodosum, 292
Erythropoietic porphyrias, 264
Escherichia coli, 154, 241
  verotoxin, 83
Ethionamide, 61
Ewing sarcoma, 280
Exanthem subitum, 301
Exomphalos, 1
  see also omphalocoele
Extracellular fluid (ECF) osmolality, 248

Fabry disease, 309
Facial nerve, 125–6, 133
Factor VIII, 216
Fanconi syndrome, 74, 75, 85, 86, 87
  anaemia, 218–19, 228
  chromosomal fragility, 240
  cystinosis, 254–5
  lead poisoning, 152
  metabolic disease with hepatitis, 258
  radial aplasia, 277
  renal function, 253
Farber disease, 256
Farmer's lung, 56
Fasciculations, 107, 109
Fascioscapulohumeral dystrophy, 110
Fatty acid oxidation defects, 180, 251, 260
Femoral epiphyses, 276, 277, 279
Fetal alcohol syndrome, 320–1
Fetal haemoglobin (HbF), 200, 209–10
Fetal phenytoin syndrome, 331
Fibrosing alveolitis, 37, 56
Finger–nose test, 128, 130
Fits, 18, 25
  neonatal, 106–7
  see also seizures
Fixed airways obstruction, 42
Floppy infant, 106, 109
Focal abnormalities, EEG, 100
Fog's test, 129
Folate
  deficiency, 141, 203, 212–13
  supplementation, 219

Follicle stimulating hormone (FSH), 184, 185–6, 187
Fontan procedure, 24
Foramen of Magendie, 93, 94
Foramen of Monro, 93, 94
Foramen ovale, 13
Foraminae of Luschka, 93, 94
Forced expiratory volume (FEV1), 41
Forced vital capacity (FVC), 41
Foreign body, 154, 310
  inhaled, 54, 57, 58, 59
Formula milk, 138
Fractures, bone, 276, 286
  skull, 306
Fragile X syndrome, 12, 319
Friedreich ataxia, 3, 26, 107, 116, 117
  gait, 132
  glucose tolerance, 179
  pes cavus, 117, 118, 282
Fructosaemia, 143
Fructose intolerance, hereditary, 74, 253, 258

Gag reflex, 127, 133
Gait, 131
  drop foot, 132
  hemiplegic, 131
  limp, 277–8
  paraplegic, 131
  waddling, 132, 278
Galactosaemia, 74, 138, 143, 166, 180
  cataracts, 309
  metabolic disease
    affecting renal function, 253, 255
    with hepatitis, 258
Gallstones, pigment, 154
Gammaglobulin, 285
Gardner syndrome, 297
Gastritis, 141, 154
Gastro-oesophageal reflux, 56, 58, 154–5
Gastroenteritis, 154
Gastrointestinal bleeding, 154, 226, 230–1
Gastrointestinal perforation, 150
Gastroschisis, 136, 153
Gaucher disease, 114, 144, 256
Genetic anticipation, 12
Genetic pedigrees, 2–4, 5, 6
Genetic testing, 6
Genital lesions, mouth lesion association, 302
Genitalia, ambiguous, 187–9
Gentamicin, 314
Giardiasis, 140, 142, 158, 237, 239
Gilbert syndrome, 143, 145, 147
Glanzmann thrombasthenia, 226
Glaucoma, 307, 309
Glomerular filtration rate, 67, 69–71
Glomerulonephritis, 85, 86, 89
  mesangio-capillary, 71, 89
  post-streptococcal, 71, 82, 297
Glomerulosclerosis, 89
Glossopharyngeal nerve, 126–7

Glucose tolerance, impaired, 179
Glucose-6-phosphatase deficiency, 253
Glucose-6-phosphate dehydrogenase deficiency, 144, 207–8, 226, 242
Glue sniffing see solvent abuse
Gluten intolerance, 141
Glycogen storage disease, 26, 143, 166, 181, 266
  types 2, 4 and 5, 259–60
Glycolytic disorders, 260–1
Goitre, 171
  retrosternal, 55
Gold, 87, 89, 274
Goldenhar syndrome, 307, 325, 331
Gonococcal arthritis, 271
Goodpasture syndrome, 51
Gottron patches, 283
Gout, 78
Gower manoeuvre, 283
Gower sign, 110, 120, 131
Graft vs. host disease, 239
Granuloma annulare, 297
Graves disease, 171
Griseofulvin, 293
Growth
  abnormalities, 181–4
  rate, 182
  retardation with atopic eczema, 288
Growth hormone, 184
  deficiency, 183
Guillain–Barré syndrome, 40, 96, 110–12
  cord compression, 113
  facial nerve palsy, 126
Gum hypertrophy, 230
Gut embryopathology, 135–7

Haemangioblastoma, 116
Haemangioma, 154, 225, 291, 305
Haematinic deficiency, 200, 201, 223
Haematuria, 71, 77, 85, 86–7
  benign familial, 87
Haemochromatosis, 162
Haemoglobin, 58, 199–200
  electrophoresis, 209–11
Haemoglobinuria, 207
Haemolysis, 143, 205–8
  intravascular, 207
Haemolytic disorders, 147
Haemolytic uraemic syndrome, 83–4, 85, 205
Haemophilia, 231, 272, 306
  pain, 278
  radiology, 218
  treatment, 216
Haemophilia A, 215, 216
Haemophilia B, 3
Haemophilus influenzae, 53, 58, 59, 90, 96
  immune disorders, 237, 239, 242, 244
Haemoptysis, 56
Haemorrhagic disease of the newborn, 230–1

Haemosiderosis, 219
  pulmonary, 43, 51–2
Haemothorax, 43, 49
  white-out, 49
Halothane, 144
Hand, foot and mouth disease, 294–5
Hand–Schuller–Christian disease, 290
Hands, examination, 30, 63
Hartnup disease, 116
Hashimoto thyroiditis, 170, 171
Head injury, 106, 190, 191, 310
Headache, 121
Hearing, 310–15
  deficit, 126
  see also deafness
Heart
  apical beat, 64
  block, 19, 20, 21, 26
  murmurs, 31, 32–4
  see also cardiac entries
Heart sounds, 31, 34, 35
  displaced, 50
  second, 35
Heavy metals, 87, 89
  poisoning, 74
  see also gold; lead poisoning
Heel shin test, 130
Heel-to-toe test, 131
Heinz bodies, 202
Hemianopia
  bilateral, 101
  homonymous, 102
Hemiparesis, 27
Hemiplegia, 113, 131
Henoch–Schönlein purpura, 82, 86, 226, 271, 278
Hepatic dysfunction, 160–1
  see also liver disease
Hepatic portoenterostomy, 145–6
Hepatitis, 83, 166, 167
  chronic active, 74, 162
  idiopathic giant cell, 144
  infectious, 147
  maternal, 138
  metabolic diseases, 258–9
  neonatal, 143–4, 145
  non-neonatal, 144
Hepatitis B, neonatal immunisation, 148
Hepatoblastoma, 159, 185
Hepatomegaly, 161–2, 164, 166–7
Hepatorenal syndrome, 90
Hereditary angio-oedema, 242–3
Hereditary spherocytosis, 3, 154, 166, 202, 203, 205–6
Hereditary telangiectasia, 86, 297, 328
Hermaphroditism, true, 188, 189
Herpes simplex, 244, 288, 292
  encephalitis, 95–6, 99
  keratitis, 309
Herpetic whitlow, 295
Hindgut abnormalities, 136–7

Hip
  congenital dislocation, 276–7, 279–80
  irritable, 279
Hirschsprung disease, 137, 150, 159–60
Hirsutism, 296
Histiocytosis, 102
Histiocytosis X, 191, 277, 305, 311
  see also Langerhans cell histiocytosis
History taking, 334–6
HIV infection, 60, 115, 138, 157, 244, 245
Holt–Oram syndrome, 328
Homocystinuria, 252, 254, 309, 322
Hook-worm, 140, 141
Horner syndrome, 88, 305
Howell–Jolly bodies, 201–2, 203, 204
5HT, 195
Human herpes virus type 6, 301
Human papillomavirus (HPV) infection, 55, 297
Human parvovirus type B19, 302
Hunter syndrome, 256
Huntington chorea, 12, 106, 115
Hurler syndrome, 115, 256, 307
Hydatid disease, 166
Hydralazine, 284
Hydranencephaly, 104
Hydrocephalus, 93–4, 103, 107, 116
  puberty, 185
  tuberous sclerosis, 118
Hydronephrosis, 81, 86, 167
Hydroxychloroquine, 274
Hydroxycholecalciferol, 263
11β-Hydroxylase deficiency, 174
21-Hydroxylase deficiency, 173–4
Hyperalbuminaemia, 194
Hyperaldosteronism, 75, 76, 139, 249
Hyperbilirubinaemia, 140
  conjugated, 143–4, 145, 147
  unconjugated, 143, 145
Hypercalcaemia, 191, 194
Hypercalciuria, idiopathic, 87
Hypercapnia, 40–1
Hypercholesterolaemia, familial, 265
Hyperglycaemia, 177, 253
Hypergonadotrophic hypogonadism, 187
Hyperkalaemia, 249
Hyperlipidaemia, 265–6
Hypernatraemia, 248
Hyperoxaluria, 78, 79
Hyperoxic test, 17–18
Hyperparathyroidism, 78, 79, 103, 194
  idopathic primary, 78
Hypertension, renal disease, 76–7, 81–2
Hyperthyroidism, 170–1
Hypertrichosis, 296, 331
Hyperuricaemia, 78
Hyperventilation syndrome, 40
Hypoaldosteronism, 75
  see also Addison disease
Hypocalcaemia, 52, 194–5, 309
Hypogammaglobulinaemia, 142
Hypoglossal nerve, 127
Hypoglycaemia, 116, 152, 174, 179–81

Hypogonadotrophic hypogonadism, 187
Hypokalaemia, 23, 75, 76, 87, 191, 249, 265
Hypomagnesaemia, 194
Hyponatraemia, 139, 247–8
Hypoparathyroidism, 103, 194, 240, 309
Hypophosphataemia, 258
Hypopituitarism, 181, 183, 189, 302
Hypoplastic left heart syndrome, 24
Hyposplenism, 228
Hypothalamic disorders, 107
Hypothalamus, 233
Hypothermia, 23
Hypothyroidism, 116, 119, 143, 145, 163
  anaemia, 201
  congenital, 106, 170, 296
  growth retardation, 183
  hyperlipidaemia, 266
  juvenile, 170
  obesity, 193
  puberty, 185
  Wormian bones, 102, 277
Hypovolaemic shock, 27
Hypoxia, chronic, 26
Hypsarrythmia, 98–9

Ichthyosis, 298
Idiopathic thrombocytopenic purpura (ITP), 224–5
IgA nephropathy, 86
IgG, 236
  deficiency, 237, *238*
Ileostomy, 168
Imidazoles, 293
Immotile cilia syndrome *see* Kartagener syndrome
Immunity, antibody-mediated, 236–7
Immunocompromised patients, 58, *59*
Immunodeficiencies, 236–43
  antibody-mediated immunity, 236–7
  cell-mediated immunity, 237–40
  complement pathway disorders, 242–3
  investigation, 243
  phagocytic disorders, 240–2
  syndromes, 57
  see also AIDS; HIV infection; severe combined immunodeficiency (SCID)
Immunoglobulins, 236
Immunological disorders, investigation, 243
Immunology, 235
Impetigo, 292–3
Inborn errors of metabolism, 3, 138, 187
Incontinence, urinary/faecal, 107, 121
Incontinentia pigmenti, 4, 297–8
Indomethacin, 76, 138
Infantile spasms, 98, 99
Infections, *53*
  AIDS, 244
  antibody deficiencies, 237
  congenital, 331

Infections (*contd*)
  middle ear, 310
  neutropenia, 223
  pericarditis, 29
  see also bacterial endocarditis; parasitic infections; viral infections
Infectious mononucleosis, 204
Inflammatory bowel disease, 141, 154, 167, 272, 297
Influenza virus, *60*
Inheritance patterns, 4, *5*, 6
Insulin, 176, 180, 181
  stress test, 184
Interstitial lung disease, 41
Intestinal lymphangiectasia, 140
Intestinal obstruction, 144, 149, 157
Intestine
  atresia, 136
  duplication cysts, 136, 140
  embryology, 135–6
  incomplete rotation, 136
  malrotation, 135–6
  mucus production, 140
  stenosis, 136
Intra-uterine growth retardation (IUGR), 178, 180, 183
Intracranial bleed, 94, 103, 106
Intracranial calcification, 102, 103
Intracranial hypertension, 103
Intracranial pressure, raised, 86, 119–29, 121, 307
Intradural lipoma, 120
Intrauterine death, 10
Intravenous urography (IVU), 79
Intraventricular bleed, 94, 95, 103–4
Intussusception, 149–50, 154
Iron
  ingestion, *267*
  overload, 219
Islet cell adenoma, 180
Islet cell insulinoma, 180
Isoniazid, 61, 62, 107, 144, 284
Itraconazole, 293

Janeway lesions, 25
Jatene operation, 24
Jaundice, 206
  breast milk, 143
  first day of life, 144–5
  following prodromal illness, 146–7
  physiological of the newborn, 143
  recurrent, 147–8
  second day of life, 146
  three weeks of age, 145
Jejunal biopsy, abnormal, 141–2
Jervell–Lange–Nielson syndrome, 20
Jeune asphyxiating thoracic dystrophy, 57, 323
Job syndrome, 240
Joints
  anatomy, 275–7
  pain, 278

Kallman syndrome, 187, 189
Kartagener syndrome, 57, 58
Kasai procedure, 145–6, 167
Kassalbach–Merritt syndrome, 225, 291
Kawasaki disease, 285–6
Kayser–Fleischer rings, 161, 163, 166
Keratitis, 307, 309
Kernicterus, 115, 310, 314
Kernig sign, 105
Ketoacidosis, 151
  see also diabetic ketoacidosis
Kidney
  calcification, 79
  enlarged, 164, 165–6, 167
  functions, 67
  horseshoe, 79, 88
  see also polycystic kidney disease; polycystic kidneys; renal entries
Klebsiella, 58, 59, 96
Kleihauer test, 208
Klinefelter syndrome, 8, 9, 170, 187, 319
Klippel–Feil syndrome, 324
Klippel–Trenaunay syndrome, 290
Klumpke palsy, 122
Koebner phenomenon, 289
Kostman syndrome, 223
Kugelberg–Welander syndrome, 109–10
Kussmaul's sign, 29
Kvostek sign, 195
Kwashiorkor, 142
Kyphoscoliosis, 37
Kyphosis, 110

Labia majora bruising, 155
Labyrinthitis, 116
Lactic acidosis, 253, 264
Ladd's bands, 136
Landau–Kleffner syndrome, 111–12
Langerhans cell histiocytosis, 290
  see also histiocytosis X
Laryngeal papillomatosis, 55
Laryngeal web, 55
Laryngomalacia, 55
Laryngotracheobronchitis, acute, 52, 60
Laurence–Moon–Biedl syndrome, 193, 307, 320
Lazy leucocyte syndrome, 241
Lead poisoning, 78, 86, 105–6, 115, 152
  anaemia, 201, 203, 204, 226
  deafness, 310
  radiology, 217
  self-mutilation, 257
Leber hereditary optic neuropathy, 261, 306
Left axis deviation, 22
Legs
  neurological examination, 128–30
  paralysis, 107
  weakness, 121
  see also paraplegia
Leigh syndrome, 260
Leopard syndrome, 327
Leprechaunism, 331

Leprosy, 257, 302
Lesch–Nyhan syndrome, 78, 115, 257
Letterer–Siwe disease, 290
Leucocyte adhesion deficiency, 241
Leucoerythroblastic blood film, 203
Leukaemia, 95, 102, 166, 225, 228, 230
  bruising, 306
  classification, 231, 232
  investigations, 231–2
  presentation, 231
  prognosis, 232
  skull lesions, 277
  treatment, 232–3
Leukaemoid reactions, 202
Leukocoria, 310
Lichen planus, 302
Limb girdle-type dystrophy, 110
Limp, 277–8
Lindane, 295
Lisch nodules, 117
Lissencephaly, 105
Listeria monocytogenes, 96
Lithium, 26, 138, 191
Liver disease, 217
  chronic, 166
  rickets, 262
  see also hepatic dysfunction
Liver failure, hepatorenal syndrome, 90
Liver tumours, 166
Long case, 333–6
Long QT syndrome, 26
Loop of Henle, 68, 75
Lowe syndrome, 74, 253, 255, 309, 325
Lown–Ganong–Levine syndrome, 23
Lucey–Driscoll syndrome, 143, 145
Lumbar kyphosis, 107
Lumbar lordosis, 110
Lung
  biopsy, 34
  congenital lobar emphysema, 47–8
  fibrosis, 56
  perfusion, 23
  polycythaemia-induced stiffness, 49
  sepsis, 50
  shadows, 47
  shifting, 47
Lung disease
  obstructive, 37, 41, 42
  parenchymal, 43
  restrictive, 37, 41, 42
Lung function
  flow-volume loops, 41–2
  obstructive/restrictive pattern, 41
  tests, 41–4
Lupus
  drug-induced, 284
  nephritis, 71, 83
Luteinizing hormone (LH), 184, 185–6, 187
Lyme disease, 27, 271, 283
Lymphadenopathy, 227
Lymphocytosis, 51, 222
Lymphoma, 166

Lyonisation, 4, 207
Lysosomal storage diseases, 255–7

McCardle disease, 259–60
McCune-Albright syndrome, 185, 303
Macroglossia, 163
Macrogyria, 105
Macropenis, 189
MAG3 scan, 80
Malabsorption, 180, 182
    intraluminal, 140–1
    mucosal damage, 140
    syndromes, 139
Malaria, 166, 204
Malassezia furfur see *Pityrosporum orbiculare*
Malformation/malformation syndrome, 1
Mallory–Weiss tear/syndrome, 154
Malnutrition syndromes, 139
Maple syrup urine disease, 116, *250*
Marcus–Gunn syndrome, 323
Marfan syndrome, 252, *254*, 280, 309, 322
Marotaux–Lamy syndrome, 256
Mastoid surgery, 126
Mastoiditis, 126
Mauriac syndrome, 178, 193
May–Hegglin anomaly, 225
Measles, 57, 108, *300*, 307
Meckel–Gruber syndrome, 119, 324–5
Meckel's diverticulum, 135, 141, 154
Meconium aspiration syndrome, 48, *50*
Meconium ileus, *45*, 48, 63, 150–1
Mediastinal shift, 49
Mediastinum, 47
Mediterranean fever, 158–9
Medulloblastoma, 116, 117
Megalencephaly, 323
Melanin, 77
Melanocytic naevi, 291
MELAS syndrome, 6, 261
Meningioma, 117
Meningism, 105, 121
Meningitis, 94, 105, 106, 113
    CSF, *95*, 96
    deafness, 310, 314
    mumps, 96
    partially treated, 106
    SIADH, 190
    TB, 62, 96, 103
Meningococcal septicaemia, 302
Meningoencephalitis, 191
Menkes kinky hair disease/Menkes syndrome, 115, 258
Mental retardation, 118, 256, 258, 298
MERRF syndrome, 6, 260–1
Mesangiosclerosis, diffuse, 89
Metabolic acidosis, 39, 40, 84, 139–40
    with hypoglycaemia, 250
    hyponatraemic hypochloraemic, *45*
    with normal anion gap, 265
    with raised anion gap, 264–5
Metabolic alkalosis, 265
    hypochloraemic/hypokalaemic, 75–6, 139

Metabolic diseases/disorders, 249–51, *252*
    affecting muscle, 259–61
    hepatitis, 258–9
    renal function, 253–5
Metachromatic leukodystrophy, 106, 114, 116
Metaphysis, 275, 276
Methaemoglobin, 58
Methaemoglobinaemia, 18, 27, 229–30
Methotrexate, 56, 144, 275, 282, 284
Methyl malonic acidaemia, *251*
Metronidazole, 107, 157
Microcolon, 150–1
Micrognathia, 1, 331
Microgyria, 105
Micropenis, 189
Micropolyspora faenia, 56
Microsporum, 293
Micturating cystourethrogram (MCUG), 79
Mid-sternotomy scar, 34
Migraine, 113, 121
    basilar artery, 116
Milk
    nutrition, 137–8, 142
    see also breast milk; cow's milk
Milk–alkali syndrome, 78, 79, 194
Mitochondrial electron transport chain defects, 260–1
Mitochondrial inheritance, 6
Mitochondrial myopathies, 106
Mitral regurgitation, 33
Mobitz types 1 and 2, 20
Moebius syndrome, 323
Molluscum contagiosum, 295
Mongolian blue spot, 291
Monoarthritis, 271
Monocytosis, 222
Morphine, 190
Morquio syndrome, 256
Motor system examination, 127–30
Mouth lesions, genital lesion association, 302
Movement disorders, 115–16
Moya Moya disease, 113
MRI scan, skull, 104–5
Mucopolysaccharidoses, 114–15, 163, 166, 255–7, 310
    corneal clouding, 307
    hypertrichosis, 331
    scoliosis, 280
Multiple endocrine neoplasia (MEN), 195–6
Multiple sclerosis, 116
Mumps, 157, *300*, 310
    meningitis, 96
Munchausen by proxy, 180, 266, 286
Mustard operation, 24
Mutism, 111, 112
Myaesthenia gravis, 305
Myasthenia, congenital, 106
Myasthenia gravis, 109
Mycobacteria, atypical, 62
Mycobacterium avium-intracellulare, 62, 244
Mycoplasma, 59, 292

Myelofibrosis, 203
Myelomatosis, 203
Myelomeningocoele, 120
Myeloperoxidase deficiency, 242
Myeloproliferative disorders, 78
Myocarditis, 14, 22, 23, 83
Myopathy, 305
 congenital, 106
Myositis, 119
Myotonia congenita, 108–9
Myotonic dystrophy, 3, 12, 106, 108–9, 305

Na/K/H pump, 74
Naevi, 291
 pigmented, 291
 simplex, 302
Nail pitting, 302
Nappy rash, 287
Necrotising enterocolitis, 149, 154, 155
Neimann–Pick disease, 144
Neisseria meningitidis, 96
Nephritis
 interstitial, 74
 shunt, 86
Nephroblastoma, 81, 87–8, 159
Nephrocalcinosis, 74, 79
Nephrogram, 79
Nephropathy, obstructive, 74
Nephrotic syndrome, 89–90, 151, 247, 266
 renal vein thrombosis, 90
Nesidioblastosis, 88, 180
Neural tube defects, 10
Neuroblastoma, 88, 102, 117, 159, 166, 195, 225
 anaemia, 228
 bone metastases, 281
 periorbital bruising, 231, 306
 proptosis, 305
 skull lesions, 277
Neurofibromatosis, 81, 88, 117–18, 185, 195
 buphthalmos, 309
 café au lait papules, 117, 123, 303
 skin stigmata, 117, 123
Neurological examination, 122–3
 infant, 132–3
Neurological and renal combined signs, 85–6
Neurosyphilis, 96
Neutropenia, 222–4
Neutrophilia, 222
Niemann–Pick disease, 114, 256, 257, 309
Nikolsky sign, 292
Nitric oxide, 51
Nitroblue tetrazolium test, 242, 243
Nitrofurantoin, 56, 107
Nitrogen washout test *see* hyperoxic test
Non-accidental injury, 113, 231, 286
 eye, 306
 skin lesions, 296
Noonan syndrome, 22, 26, 189, 320
 growth retardation, 183
Norwood procedure, 24

NSAIDs, 56, 87, 141, 274, 283
Nutritional disorders, 182
Nutritional status, 137–9
Nystagmus, 126, 131
Nystatin, 293

Obesity, 40, 120, 192–3, 266
Obstructive sleep apnoea syndrome, 40
Oculomotor nerve, 124–5
Oesophageal atresia, 135
Oesophageal varices, 141
Oesophagitis, 154
Oesophagus, vascular rings, 54
Olfactory nerve, 124
Oligohydramnios, 1
Omphalocoele, 1, 135, 153–4
Opiates, *268*
Opsoclonus–polyclonus syndrome, 88
Optic atrophy, 117, 306
Optic disc, 306
Optic glioma, 117
Optic nerve, 124
 glioma, 306
Optic neuritis, 107
Optic pathway lesions, 101–2
Organic acidaemia, *251*
Organogenesis, 2
Ornithine transcarbamylase deficiency, *252*
Osgood–Schlatter disease, 276, 278
Osler nodes, 25
Osteochondritis, 278
Osteochondroma, 281
Osteogenesis imperfecta, 106, 286, 309, 329–30
Osteoid osteoma, 280–1
Osteopenia of prematurity, 263
Osteopetrosis, 74, 102, 203, 277, 309
Osteosarcoma, 272, 277, 280
Otitis externa, 310
Otitis media, 105, 120, 310
Ovarian cyst/tumour, 185
Oxygen, 38, 39, 40
 dissociation curve, 57–8
 respiratory failure, 41
 saturation, *15*, 40

P wave, 18, 20
Pancreatic insufficiency, *45*
Pancreatitis, 83, 140, 159, 194
Pancytopenia, 227
Papilloedema, 306–7
Paracetamol, 144, *267*
Parainfluenzae, *60*
Paralytic ileus, 150
Paraplegia
 acute, 112–13
 gait, 131
 hysterical, 113
Parasitic infections, 56, 140, 155, 166
Parathyroid hormone (PTH), 193, 194
Paris nomenclature, 8–9

350

Parotitis, 157
Paroxysmal cold haemoglobinuria, 207
Patau classification, 6
Patau syndrome, 318
　see also trisomy 13
Patent ductus arteriosus, 15, 16, 17, 34
Peak end expiratory pressure (PEEP), 38, 39
Peak expiratory flow measurements (PEFR), 41, 62–3, 65
Pelvic appendix abscess, 157
Pendred syndrome, 170, 310
Penicillamine, 87, 89, 274
Penicillin, 87, 283, 292
Peptic ulceration, 141, 154
Pericarditis, 29–30
　constrictive, 27
Periorbital bruising, 231
Peripheral neuropathy, 107
Periventricular leucomalacia, 104
Peroxisomal defects, 261
Persistent fetal circulation, 49
Perthe disease, 276, 278–9
Pertussis, 51, 57, 306
Pes cavus, 117, 118, 121, 282
Peutz–Jeghers syndrome, 163, 293, 297, 328
Phaeochromocytoma, 81, 117, 195
Phagocytic disorders, 240–2
Phenothiazines, 268
Phenylketonuria, 138, 257, 298, 302
Phenytoin, 26, 107, 230
Phosphate metabolism, rickets, 262–3
Pierre–Robin syndrome, 1, 324, 331
Pigmentation, 303
Pituitary gland, 184, 233
　tumours, 183
Pityriasis, 302
　rosea, 296
Pityrosporum orbiculare, 294
Plain abdominal X-rays, 79, 148–51
Plantar reflex, 129
Plasmodium, 204
Platelet defects, 225, *226*
Pleural effusion, 49
　aspirates, 43–4
Pneumococcus, 59, 90
Pneumoconiosis, 56
Pneumocystis carinii, 60, 238, 239, 244
Pneumomediastinum, 49
Pneumonia, 49, *50*, 58–9, *60*, 105
　SIADH, 190
Pneumonitis
　hypersensitivity, 55–6
　lymphocytic interstitial, 244–5
Pneumopericardium, 49
Pneumothorax, 49, *50*, 52, *59*
Poikilocytosis, 202
Poisoning, 266, *267*, 268–9
　accidental, 114
　ataxia, 116
　see also lead poisoning
Poland syndrome, 325
Poliomyelitis, 107, 110–11

Polyarteritis nodosa, 82
Polyarthritis, 28, 271
Polycystic kidney disease, 84–5, 86
Polycystic kidneys, 3
Polycystic ovarian disease, 193
Polycythaemia, 18, 27, 43, 49, 58
　hyperbilirubinaemia, 143
　maternal diabetes, 178
　neonatal, 228–9
　older children, 229
　renal vein thrombosis, 90
Polydactyly, 1, 327
Polydypsia, 179, 191–2
Polyuria, 87, 179, 191–2
Porencephaly, 104
Porphobilinogen, 78
Porphyrias, 116, 263–4
Port wine stain, 290
Portal hypertension, 167
Posterior column disease, 131
Potassium
　urinary excretion, 249
　see also hypokalaemia
Potter syndrome, 331
Pox virus, 295
PR interval, 23
Prader–Willi syndrome, 11, 106, 179, 320
　delayed puberty, 187
　growth abnormality, 183
　micropenis, 189
　obesity, 193
Precocious puberty, 183, 185–6, 189
Prednisolone, 99
Prematurity, 180, 183, 194, 202, 310
　rickets, 263
Prerenal failure, 69, *70*
Propionic acidaemia, *251*
Propranolol, 107, 171
Proptosis, 305–6
Propylthiouracil, 284
Prostacyclin, 51, 83
Prostaglandins, 68, 75
Protein C deficiency, 90, 113
Protein-losing enteropathy, 160
Proteinuria with absent red reflex, 255
Proteus, 78
Proximal convoluted tubule (PCT), 67–8
Proximal myopathy, 131
Proximal renal tubular acidosis, 73, 74–5, 85
Prune belly syndrome, 91
Pseudohermaphroditism, 187–8, 189
Pseudohyperkalaemia, 249
Pseudohyperparathyroidism, 194
Pseudohypoaldosteronism, 175
Pseudohyponatraemia, 248
Pseudomembranous colitis, 156–7
Pseudomonas, 59, 96, 302
Pseudoptosis, 305
Pseudopuberty, 185
Psoralens, 289
Psoriasis, 289, 302
Psoriatic arthropathy, 272

Psychosis
  acute, 106
  manic depressive, 112
Psychosocial deprivation, 183
Ptosis, 305
Puberty, 184–5
  delayed, 186–7
  see also precocious puberty
Pulmonary acidosis, 49
Pulmonary artery banding, 34
Pulmonary atresia, 14, 23, 24, 35
Pulmonary blood flow
  murmur, 34
  reduced, 43
Pulmonary embolus, 40, 43
Pulmonary eosinophilia, 56
Pulmonary fibrosis, 40
Pulmonary haemorrhage, 43, 50
Pulmonary hypertension, 25, 26, 43, 49, 51
  chronic, 57
  cystic fibrosis, 45
  persistent, 38
Pulmonary hypoplasia, 1, 48, 57
Pulmonary interstitial emphysema, 38
Pulmonary metastases, 88
Pulmonary oedema, 40, 53, 58
Pulmonary sequestration, 47
Pulmonary stenosis, 14, 22, 24, 26
Pulse, water hammer, 30
Pulsus paradoxus, 27
Purine, dietary, 78
Pus collection, 153
Pyelonephritis, 105
  chronic, 74, 75
Pyloric stenosis, hypertrophic, 139, 148–9
Pyrazinamide, 61
Pyridostigmine, 109
Pyridoxine deficiency, 253
Pyruvate kinase deficiency, 208

Q waves, 19
QRS complex, 18, 19, 22, 23
QRS progression, 19–20
QT interval, 20, 23
Quadrantic field loss, 102

Radial aplasia, 277
Radiology, paediatric, 24–5
Ramsay Hunt syndrome, 126
Rashkind procedure, 23, 144
Red cells
  aplasia, 218
  enzyme defects, 202
  life cycle, 200
  membrane defects, 144
5-alpha Reductase deficiency, 187
Reflex sympathetic dystrophy, 121–2
Reflexes
  infants, 132
  testing, 128, 129
Reflux oesophagitis, 141

Refsum disease, 116, 307
Reiter syndrome, 271, 308
Renal artery stenosis, 76, 118
Renal biochemistry, 71–2
  see also kidney
Renal collecting system duplication, 79
Renal disease
  presentation, 69
  rickets, 262
Renal failure, 69, 71–2, 183, 247, 249, 265
  hepatorenal syndrome, 90
  hyperlipidaemia, 266
  laboratory investigations, 70
  skin rash, 82–3
  see also chronic renal failure
Renal function, metabolic diseases, 253–5
Renal hypertension, 76–7, 81–2, 85
Renal and neurological combined signs, 85–6
Renal physiology, 67–8
Renal radiography, 79–81
Renal stones, 78, 86
Renal transplantation, 74, 75, 83
Renal tubular acidosis (RTA), 72–5, 78, 79, 183, 265
  type 1, 73–4
  type 2, 74–5
  type 4, 75
Renal tubules, 67–8
Renal tumours, 77
Renal vein thrombosis, 74, 90, 167
Renin, 68, 75, 76, 172–3
Respiratory acidosis, 38, 39, 40
Respiratory alkalosis, 38, 40
Respiratory disease, radiological findings, 46–9
Respiratory distress, 25–6, 49–52
Respiratory distress syndrome (RDS), 38, 48, 50
Respiratory failure, 40–1
Respiratory neuromuscular disease, 40
Respiratory syncytial virus (RSV), 26, 60
Respiratory system, examination, 63–5
Reticular dysgenesis, 223
Reticulocytosis, 200, 201, 203
Retina
  detachment, 309
  renal hypertension, 81–2
Retinal artery thrombosis, 306
Retinal haemorrhage, 25, 83
Retinal phakoma, 118
Retinitis
  CMV, 310
  pigmentosa, 152, 307
  toxoplasmosis, 309
Retinoblastoma, 3, 310
Rett syndrome, 115, 325
Reye syndrome, 114, 160–1, 166, 180
Rhabdomyolysis, 119
Rhabdomyosarcoma, 306, 311
Rhesus haemolytic disease, 208, 209
Rhesus incompatibility, 144, 146, 180, 208, 209

Rheumatic fever, 23, 27, 28–9, 294
   Jones' major manifestation, 115
   post-streptococcal, 297
Rickets, 261–3
   hypophosphataemic, 75
   phosphate metabolism, 262–3
   prematurity, 263
   X-linked hypophosphataemic, 4, 5
Rieger syndrome, 307
Rifampicin, 61, 144, 190
Right axis deviation, 22
Riley–Day syndrome, 257, 326–7
Rinne test, 126, 315
Ritter syndrome, 292
Robertsonian translocation, 9, 10
Romano–Ward syndrome, 20, 26
Romberg's test, 131
Roseola infantum, 301
Roth spots, 25
Rotor syndrome, 144, 148
Rouleaux formation, 202
Rubella, 300
Rubella, congenital, 1, 26, 143, 258, 331
   hearing defects, 314
   visual defects, 307, 309
Rubinstein–Taybi syndrome, 309, 327
Russell diencephalic syndrome, 324
Russell–Silver syndrome, 183, 303, 321, 331

Sacrococcygeal teratoma, 107
Sagittal sinus thrombosis, 94
St Vitus dance *see* Sydenham chorea
Salicylates, 78, 180, 264, 267
Salmon patches, 302
Salmonella, 83, 96, 154, 237, 241, 271
Sanfilippo syndrome, 256
Sarcoidosis, 56, 79, 194, 308
   TB differential diagnosis, 62
Sarcoptes scabei (scabies), 295
Scalded skin syndrome, 292
Scaphocephaly, 281
Scarlet fever, 297
Scars, thoracic, 34
Scheie syndrome, 256
Schilling test, 214
Schistocytes, 203
Schistosomiasis, 56, 166
Schizencephaly, 105
Schizophrenia, 112
Scimitar syndrome, 47
Scoliosis, 40, 41, 110, 117, 280
Scotoma, central, 102
Seizures, 85, 116, 119
   focal frontal, 112
   grand mal, 99, 100
   infantile spasms, 98, 99
   Landau–Kleffner syndrome, 111
   myoclonic epilepsy, 100
   petit mal, 98
   tuberous sclerosis, 118
   see also fits
Selective IgA deficiency, 237, 238

Self-mutilation, 119, 257
Senna, 138
Senning operation, 24
Sensation testing, 128, 130
Sensory system examination, 127–30
Sepsis, 143, 145, 166, 202, 225, 240
Septic arthritis, 271
Septo-optic dysplasia, 328
Sequence, 1
Serratia marcescens, 77, 241
Severe combined immunodeficiency
   (SCID), 142, 237–9
Sex chromosomes, 3, 6
Sexual abuse, 155, 286
Shigella, 83, 154
Shivering artefact of ECG, 23
Short stature, 182
Shunting, 15, 17, 18
   palliative, 23
Sick sinus syndrome, 28
Sickle cell crisis, 152, 154, 221, 222, 278, 280
Sickle cell disease, 3, 58, 74, 86, 113, 144, 162
   arthritis, 272
   blood films, 204
   clinical features, 219–22, 226, 228
   diabetes insipidus, 191
   haemoglobin electrophoresis, 209–10
   hyposplenism, 228
   radiology, 218
   splenomegaly, 166
   treatment, 221
Single ventricle, 35
Sinus arrhythmia, 18
Sinus tachycardia, 27–8
Sjögren syndrome, 74, 302
Skin
   examination, 303
   gut lesion association, 297
   rash and renal failure, 82–3, 86
   stigmata, 117, 123
Skull
   fracture, 306
   multiple lesions, 277
   X-rays, 102–3
Slipped upper femoral epiphysis (SUFE),
   276, 279
Slow waves, 98
Smith–Lemli–Opitz syndrome, 189, 305, 328
Smogyi effect, 177–8
Sodium *see* hypernatraemia;
   hyponatraemia
Sodium valproate, 100
Solvent abuse, 114, 116, 144, 268–9
Soto syndrome, 193, 323
Soya milk protein intolerance, 142
Space occupying lesions, 113, 190, 307
Spastic diplegia, 131
Spasticity, 121
   knife-clasp, 127, 129
Speech development, 111, 112
Spherocytes, 202, 206
Spherocytosis *see* hereditary spherocytosis
Spider naevi, 163

Spike waves, 98
Spina bifida, 107, 118, 133, 282
    occulta, 129, 164
Spinal block, 96
Spinal cord
    subacute combined degeneration, 107
    trauma, 112
Spinal dysraphism, occult, 120–1
Spinal muscular atrophy *see*
    Werdnig–Hoffman disease
Spinal shock, 112
Spirometry, 41, *42*
Spironolactone, 75, 76
Spleen, enlarged, 164, 165–7, 222
Splenectomy, 58, 202, 203
Spondyloepiphyseal dysplasia, 330
Sprengel deformity, 282
Staphylococcus, 58, 292
Staphylococcus aureus, 53, *59*, 96, 157
    AIDS, 244
    chronic granulomatous disease, 241
    eczema, 288
    infections in immunodeficiency, 237, 244
    septic arthritis, 271
Staphylococcus epidermidis, 96, 118
Stein–Leventhal syndrome, 193
Steroids, 274–5, 284, 289, 309
Stevens–Johnson syndrome, 292, 302
Stickler syndrome, 324
Still's murmur, 33, 34
Stork mark, 302
Strawberry naevi, 291
Streptococcal disease, renal, 71, 82
Streptococcus, 244, 271, 292, 297
    group B, 40, 96, 271, 289
Streptococcus pneumoniae, 58, *59*, 83, 96, 237, 239, 242
Streptococcus pyogenes, 157
Stridor, 52–8, 63, 291
    investigations, 53–5
String sign, 148
Strongyloides, 140
Sturge–Weber syndrome, 103, 123, 290, 309
Subacute sclerosing panencephalitis (SSPE), 99, 106, 108, 115
Subaponeurotic haemorrhage, 302
Subconjunctival haemorrhage, 306
Subdural haematoma, 96, 103, 113
Subglottic haemangioma, 55
Subglottic stenosis, *55*
Sulphasalazine, 274
Sulphonamides, 56, 138, 292
Supraventricular tachycardia (SVT), 14, 26
    paroxysmal, 27–8
Sweat test, 44, 45–6
Sydenham chorea, 28, 115
Synacthen tests, 175
Syndactyly, 327
Syndrome of inappropriate ADH secretion (SIADH), 56, 106, 151, 190–2, 247
Synovitis, transient, 279
Syphilis, 27, 96, 202, 308
Syringomyelia, 107

Systemic hypoperfusion, 14
Systemic lupus erythematosus (SLE), 27, 74, 86, 115, 271, 284–5
    maternal, 20, 285
    neonatal, 284–5
    nephritis, 82, 83
    nephrotic syndrome, 89
    urticaria, 294
Systolic murmurs, 32

T cell
    abnormalities, 245
    function, 243
T waves, 20, *21*, 22–3
Tachycardia, 22
    see also supraventricular tachycardia (SVT)
Tactile vocal fremitus (TVF), 64, 65
Talipes, 1
Tamponade, 27
Tanner staging, 185
TAR syndrome, 219, 225, 277
Target cells, 201, 203
Tay-Sachs disease, 114, 256, 309
Teenagers, poisoning, 114
Teeth, 299
Telangiectasia, 141, 163, 328
    see also ataxia telangiectasia; hereditary telangiectasia
Tendon reflexes, 128, 129
Tension pneumothorax, 27, 49
Teratogenesis, 2
Teratogens, 1, 26
Testicular feminisation syndrome, 187, 189
Testicular tumour, 185
Tetany, 195
Tethered spinal cord syndrome, 118, 120–1, 282
Tetracyclines, 56, 74, 138, 299
Tetracyline, 120
Tetralogy of Fallot, 14, 15, 16, 23, 24, 28
    omphalocoele, 153
    second heart sound, 35
Thalassaemia *see* alpha thalassaemia; beta thalassaemia
THAM, 39
Theophylline, 138
Thiazide diuretics, 78, 194, 266
Thiouracil, 138
Third nerve palsy, 305
Thoracotomy scar, 34
Threadworms, 155
Thrombocytopenia, 224–5
Thrombocytopenic purpura, 302
Thrombophilia, 90
Thyroid binding globulin, 90
Thyroid function investigations, 171–2
Thyroid hormones, 169, 171–2
Thyroid physiology, 169
Thyroid releasing hormone (TRH), 169, 172
Thyroid stimulating hormone (TSH), 169, 170, 172

Thyroid storm, 171
Thyrotoxicosis, 115, 172, 194, 305
Thyroxine, 184
Tight filum terminale syndrome, 120
Tinea, 293
  versicolor, 294
Tinnel sign, 195
Todd palsy, 113
TOGA procedures, 23, 24
Tolazoline, 51
Tonsillitis, 105
TORCH syndrome, 307, 310
Torticollis, 282
Total anomalous pulmonary venous drainage (TAPVD), 14, 16, 25
Toxic shock syndrome, 293
Toxocariasis, 308, 310
Toxoplasmosis, 94, 103, 143, 166, 202
  congenital, 331
  visual defects, 308, 309
Trachea, vascular rings, 54–5
Tracheitis, bacterial, 53
Tracheo-oesophageal fistula (TOF), 48
  H-type, 56
  repair, 55
Tracheomalacia, 53, 55
Transfer factor (TLCO), 42–3
Transient erythroblastopenia of infancy (TEC), 218
Transient tachypnoea of the newborn (TTN), 48, 49
Transposition of the great arteries, 14, 17, 24
Transverse myelitis, 113
Trauma, 113, 126, 185, 249, 306
  eye, 309
  pain, 278
Treacher–Collins syndrome, 310, 324, 331
Trendelenburg gait, 110, 257
Triamterine, 75
Trichophyton, 293
Tricuspid atresia, 22, 23, 24
Tricuspid regurgitation, 33
Tricyclic antidepressants, *268*
Trigeminal nerve, 125
Triple test, 10
Trisomy 13, 307, 309, 318, 331
Trisomy 18, 309, 318, 331
  see also Edward syndrome
Trisomy 21, *8*, 10, 317–18
  see also Down syndrome
Trochlear nerve, 124–5
Tropical sprue, 142, 228
Trypsin, serum immunoreactive, 44
Tuberculosis, 60–2, 153, 166, 271, 308
  anaemia, 202, 203
  diagnosis, 61–2
  hypercalcaemia, 194
  maternal, 138
  meningitis, 62, 96, 103
  pneumonia, 58, *59*
Tuberous sclerosis, 3, 86, 103, 118, 123
  adenoma sebaceum, 289
  café au lait patches, 303

Tubulointerstitial disease, 75
Tumour lysis syndrome, 78, 233, 249
Tuning fork tests, 315
Turner syndrome, 4, 7, 9, 10, 318–19
  ears, 331
  growth retardation, 183
  Hashimoto thyroiditis, 170
  impaired glucose tolerance, 179
Tympanograms, 311–12
Tyrosinaemia, 74, 143, 253, 258–9

Ulcerative colitis, 149, 156, 228
Ultrasound, renal, 80
Umbilical vessels, 13
Umbilicus, discharge, 153
Upper airway obstruction, 53
Urea, 70–1
Urea cycle defects, *252*
Urethral valves, posterior, 85
Urinary acidification, normal, 72–3
Urine
  colour, 77–8
  microscopy, 71
  pH, 75, 78
  tests, 77–8
Urobilinogen, 78
Urography, intravenous (IVU), 79
Urticaria, 294
UV light, 289
Uveitis, 307–8, 309

V/Q scan, 23
Vagus nerve, 126–7
Vancomycin, 157
Varicella, 300–1
  encephalitis, 116
  zoster, 244
  see also chickenpox
Vascular malformations, 113
Vascular rings, 54–5
Vasculitides, 56
Vasculitis, 154, 226, 283
Vasoactive intestinal peptide (VIP), 88
Vasovagal attacks, 26
VATER association, 328
VATER/VACTERL syndrome, 1, 277
Vein of Galen, aneurysm, 94
Venous hum, 34
Venous thrombosis, 113
Ventilation–perfusion mismatch, 40, 43
Ventilator, 38–40
Ventral suspension, 132
Ventricular dominance, 19
Ventricular fibrillation, 23
Ventricular hypertrophy, 19, 22, 26
Ventricular septal defect, 14, 15, 16, 26
  murmurs, 33
  tetralogy of Fallot, 28
Ventricular tachycardia, 22
Ventriculo-atrial shunt, 118
Ventriculo-peritoneal shunt, 86, 118

Verne–Morrison syndrome, 88
Verruca, 297
Vertigo, benign paroxysmal, 119
Vesicoureteric reflux, 83
Vestibulocochlear nerve, 126
Vigabatrin, 99
Vinblastine, 107
Vincristine, 107, 190
Viral exanthemem, 299, *300, 301, 302*
Viral infections, 57, 271
    ataxia, 116
    cord compression, 113
    teratogenic, 1
Vision, 305–10
Vitamin B12 deficiency, 107, 140, 141, 306
    anaemia, 203, *212–13*
    Schilling test, 214
Vitamin D, 193–4
    deficiency, 194
    metablism, *262*
    rickets, 261–2
Vitamin D-binding globulin, 90
Vitamin K
    absorption, 158
    deficiency, *217*, 230
Vitelline cysts, 136
Vitelline duct, 135–6
Vitiligo, 302
Vocal cord palsy, *55*
Volvulus, 136, 150, 154
Vomiting, 139, 160, 247, 249, 265
Von Gierke disease, 180
Von Willebrand disease, *215*, 216

Waardenburg syndrome, 310, 314, 321
Waiter's tip sign, 122
Walking, delay, 107
Warts, 297
Water deprivation test, 191–2

Waterhouse–Friederichsen syndrome, 175
Weber test, 126, 315
Wegener granulomatosis, 82
Werdnig–Hoffman disease, 3, 48, 57, 107, 108, 109
Wheezing, 52
White cell counts, 222
Whooping cough *see* pertussis
William syndrome, 26, 81, 320
Wilm tumour, 86, 87, 167, 308
Wilson disease, 74, 85, 106, 115, 116, 144
    abdominal pain, 152
    cataracts, 309
    presentation, 161, 163, 166
    proteinuria, 255
    renal function, 253
Wiskott–Aldrich syndrome, 225, 239
Wolff–Parkinson–White syndrome, 19, *21*, 22, 23
    SVT, 28
Wolman disease, 143
Wormian bones, 102, 277

X chromosome, 3, 6, *7–8*
X-linked dominant conditions, 4, *5*
X-linked recessive conditions, 3–4, *5*
X-rays
    orthopaedics and rheumatology, 275–7
    skull, 102–3
    see also chest X-ray (CXR); plain abdominal X-rays

Y chromosome, 3, 6, *7–8*

Zellweger syndrome, 144, 261, 326
ZIG (*Varicella* immunoglobulin), 300
Zinc supplementation, 295